Anatomical Basis
OF
Low Back Pain

Anatomical Basis

OF

Low Back Pain

L.G.F. GILES, M.Sc., D.C.(C), Ph.D.

Senior Research Fellow
Division of Science and Technology
Griffith University
Nathan, Brisbane, Queensland, Australia

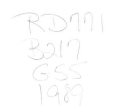

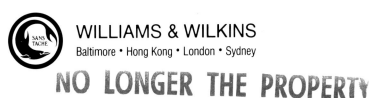

WILLIAMS & WILKINS
Baltimore • Hong Kong • London • Sydney

Editor: Timothy S. Satterfield
Associate Editor: Linda Napora
Copy Editor: Deborah Klenotic
Design: Norman W. Och
Illustration Planning: Ray Lowman
Production: Raymond E. Reter
Cover Design: Norman W. Och

Library of Congress Cataloging-in-Publication Data

Giles, L. G. F.
 Anatomical basis of low back pain.

 Includes bibliographies and index.
 1. Backache—Pathophysiology. 2. Lumbosacral
region—Anatomy. 3. Spine—Histopathology. I. Title.
[DNLM: 1. Backache. 2. Lumbosacral Region—
anatomy & histology. WE 755 G472a]
RD771.B217G55 1989   617′.56   88-20772
ISBN 0-683-03525-8

             89 90 91 92
   1 2 3 4 5 6 7 8 9 10

Preface

The principal aim of this text is to give some insight into the complex problem of low back pain, which confronts so many groups of health professionals. This text is written mainly for chiropractors, medical practitioners, osteopaths, and physiotherapists. Much of the pertinent literature on lumbosacral anatomy and on low back pain with or without leg pain is reviewed first. References are provided to enable the reader to consult original literature on the various topics discussed. The results of my investigations encompassing lumbosacral spine gross dissection, histology, and clinical studies are then presented. The final chapter summarizes the basic anatomical findings, their possible role in low back pain with or without leg pain, and the rational steps for differential diagnosis of this common condition which are necessary to indicate the appropriate treatment regimen. It is not my objective to go into detail regarding differential diagnosis, as there are numerous textbooks on this topic. Appendices are included which define some of the terms used in this textbook.

To a large extent, this text forms a personal record based on 13 years of clinical practice, followed by 10 years of postgraduate scientific investigation involving a detailed study of the gross and histologic anatomy of the spine—particularly of the posterior spinal elements of the lumbosacral spine.

There is a long-standing controversy regarding the etiology of many low back pain conditions. This is particularly true with respect to the possible relationship between biomechanical stresses and low back pain with or without sciatica, when no obvious pathology, such as intervertebral disc nucleus pulposus extrusion, can be demonstrated. This prompted me to investigate both the clinical and anatomical aspects of leg length inequality, with postural scoliosis, with particular reference to the posterior spinal elements, since I had the clinical impression that chronic low back pain sufferers with a significant leg length inequality (9 mm or more) benefited from shoe-raise therapy coupled with spinal manipulation.

Perhaps the histologic studies have not previously been undertaken because of the time-consuming and specialized techniques which I had to devise for my postgraduate studies at The University of Western Australia in order to obtain good-quality large histologic sections of bone with adjacent soft tissues from cadavers. The average time taken to process each large block of osseous tissue was 5 months. Also, the collection of numerous surgical specimens for nerve studies was time consuming, and existing histologic techniques had to be modified in order to obtain acceptable results with fresh surgical material.

I hope that this text will stimulate further interest in the costly and debilitating condition of low back pain with or without sciatica, particularly as it relates to the posterior spinal elements and the common condition of leg length inequality and postural scoliosis, which is largely ignored by many health practitioners.

There is some repitition among the chapters as a result of summarizing various anatomical and radiographic findings and correlating these findings with likely explanations for the multifactorial mechanisms involved in low back pain with or without sciatica and the rationale for treatment. The section on normal biomechanics of the lumbar spine is not intended to be a definitive discussion of this topic, since many authors have contributed to this topic in the literature over the years.

It is my concern that this work should lead to a better understanding of low back pain and, therefore, benefit some low back pain sufferers. I hope it will stimulate further clinical and anatomical investigations in the field of low back pain and be a guide for future investigations. For this reason, an Appendix is included detailing the histologic techniques which I developed for spinal histology, particularly the processing of large blocks of bone with their adjacent soft tissue structures.

Acknowledgments

I am grateful to Associate Professor J. R. Taylor for the time he spent in discussing numerous aspects of my research and co-authoring some papers, and to Emeritus Professor D. C. Sinclair for his helpful suggestions regarding parts of this text.

I gratefully acknowledge the suggestions made by Dr. W. F. C. Blumer regarding photography, Dr. M. Grounds regarding mounting medium for immunohistochemistry, Professor A. R. Harvey regarding immunohistochemistry processing, and Dr. A. S. Wilson regarding silver and gold chloride impregnation studies.

I am grateful to Dr. J. Polak, Department of Histochemistry, Hammersmith Hospital, Royal Postgraduate Medicine School, London, for providing me with substance P antibody.

I am indebted to the members of the faculty and technical staff in the University of Western Australia's departments of anatomy and human biology, pathology, and radiology, who willingly helped me with numerous aspects of this study.

I am particularly grateful for the technical assistance provided by H. Baggett, A. Cockson, K. Cole, M. Holmes, D. Kirk, P. Mees, and B. Wyatt. I am grateful to Sally McConnell, Fiona McLeod, and Laszlo Bubrik for carefully reproducing the many photographs and to Martin Thompson for most of the line drawings.

I am indebted to the individuals who offered to act as an asymptomatic control group in the clinical study and to the individuals who bequeathed their bodies to the University of Western Australia.

The statistical evaluation of data by Dr. M. Thornett is gratefully acknowledged, as is the valued assistance provided by Kevin Singer, DipPT., MSc., with regard to gross dissection of lumbosacral spinal nerves.

I am indebted to my wife and to my receptionist Mrs. B. Napier for their valuable and willing assistance in helping to record the data for the clinical study.

I express my gratitude for the financial support received from the Foundation for Chiropractic Education and Research (United States) and the Australian Spinal Research Foundation Limited, which partly funded the costs associated with the histologic studies.

I thank Professor D. B. Allbrook and his successors as head of the department of anatomy and human biology, Dr. L. Freedman, Reader, and Associate Professor N. W. Bruce, for enabling me to perform much of the histologic work in their department. I also thank Dr. T. Chakera and Dr. L. Matz of the Departments of Radiology and Pathology at the Royal Perth Hospital for making it possible for me to perform some of this work in their departments.

I gratefully acknowledge the receipt of numerous surgical specimens which were provided by Dr. R. J. Vaughan, FRACS, neurosurgeon, as well as specimens provided by orthopaedic surgeons Drs. N. Anastas, FRACS, B. Slinger, FRACS, and Professor S. Nade during routine surgical procedures.

I am grateful to Drs. H. F. Farfan, FRCS(C), and S. Haldeman, FRCP(C), who have not only contributed so much knowledge on the topic of spinal problems themselves, but have encouraged me, over many years, to continue to pursue spinal research. They have willingly and generously spent time discussing research with me, and they have given me much valued advice.

I appreciate the helpful assistance extended to me by Mr. T. S. Satterfield, Acquisitions Editor, and the other members of the Williams & Wilkins staff who have been involved in the production of this text.

I thank J. I. Giles for her encouragement and assistance, which made this research possible, and for her tireless efforts in typing this text; and M. E. Giles for her valuable assistance in proofreading this text.

I sincerely thank the publishers of the following journals who have given me permission to reproduce the contents of manuscripts which were initially published in their journals:

- Giles LGF, Taylor JR: Low back pain associated with leg length inequality. *Spine* 6:510-521, 1981; Giles LG, Taylor JR: Lumbar spine structural changes associated with leg length inequality. 7:159-162, 1982; Giles LG: Lumbosacral radiography. 9:842, 1984; Lippincott/Harper and Row.
- Giles LGF: Lumbosacral facetal "joint angles" associated with leg length inequality. *Rheumatology and Rehabilitation* 20:233-238, 1981; Bailliere Tindall.
- Giles, LGF, Taylor JR: Intra-articular synovial protrusions in the lower lumbar apophyseal joints. *Bulletin of the Hospital for Joint Diseases Orthopaedic Institute* 12:248-255, 1982.
- Giles LGF, Taylor JR: Histological preparation of large vertebral specimens. *Stain Technology* 58:45-49, 1983; Williams & Wilkins.
- Giles LGF, Taylor JR: The effect of postural scoliosis on lumbar apophyseal joints. *Scandinavian Journal of Rheumatology* 13:209-220, 1984; The Almqvist and Wiksell Periodical Company.
- Giles LGF: Lumbar apophyseal joint arthrography. *Journal of Manipulative and Physiological Therapeutics* 7:21-24, 1984; Giles LGF, Taylor JR: Osteoarthrosis in human cadaveric lumbosacral zygapophyseal joints. *J Manipulative Physiol Ther.* 8:239-243, 1985; Williams & Wilkins.
- Giles LGF, Taylor JR, Cockson A: Human zygapophyseal joint synovial folds. *Acta Anatomica* 126:110-114, 1986; S. Karger AG, Basel.
- Giles LGF: Lumbo-sacral and cervical zygapophyseal joint inclusions. *Manual Medicine* 2:89-92, 1986; Springer-Verlag.
- Giles LGF: Pressure related changes in human lumbo-sacral zygapophyseal joint articular cartilage. *The Journal of Rheumatology* 13:1093-1095, 1986.
- Giles LGF, Taylor JR: Innervation of lumbar zygapophyseal joint synovial folds. *Acta Orthopaedica Scandinavica* 58:43–46, 1987; Munksgaard International Publishers Ltd.
- Giles LGF, Taylor JR: Human zygapophyseal joint capsule and synovial fold innervation. *British Journal of Rheumatology* 26:93-98, 1987; Giles, LGF, Harvey AR: Immunohistochemical demonstration of nociceptors in the capsule and synovial folds of human zygapophyseal joint. 26:362-364; Bailliere Tindall.

- Giles LGF: Lumbo-sacral zygapophyseal joint tropism and its effect on hyaline cartilage. *Clinical Biomechanics* 2:2-6, 1987; John Wright.
- Giles LGF: Human lumbar zygapophyseal joint inferior recess synovial folds: a light microscopy examination. *The Anatomical Record* 220:117–124, 1988; Alan R. Liss, Inc.

CONTENTS

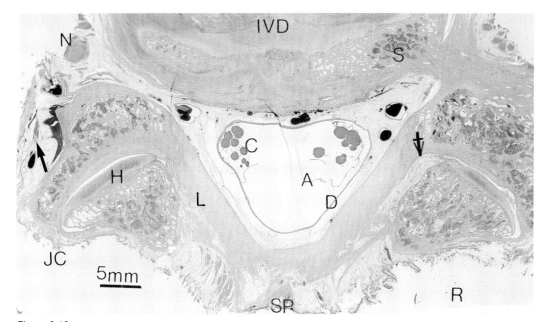

Figure 3.10

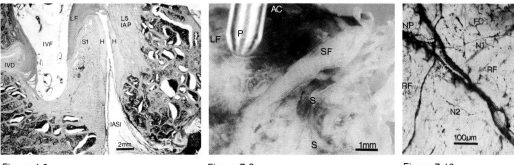

Figure 4.3

Figure 7.2

Figure 7.18

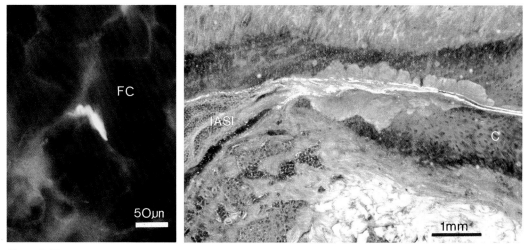

Figure 7.25

Figure 9.3

CHAPTER 1

General Introduction to Low Back Pain

Magnitude of the Problem of Low Back Pain

Low back pain is one of the most common and incapacitating disorders in modern society (1–5). About 80–88% of people experience incapacitating low back pain during their adult lives (6–12), but frequently its cause is not known (13–18). Jayson (19) concurs that our understanding of the problem is very limited. According to Dixon (2), in 9 out of 10 instances low back pain is transient, it is related to some posture or strain, and recovery can take place in a short time. However, chronic back pain and its associated disabilities represent a significant health problem (20) in which physical signs are often totally lacking (21).

Back pain is the second leading cause of industrial absenteeism, behind only the common cold (16, 22, 23), and is a problem of daunting proportions (24–26). Friberg and Hirsch (27) examined 1500 patients with a history of back pain and found that symptoms began in the late 20s, with the highest incidence between the ages of 30 and 50 years and equal incidence in men and women. In spite of the common nature of this costly complaint, which was responsible for an economic loss of some 300 million pounds a year to Britain (28), its causes remain largely obscure except in cases of acute low back pain with sciatica. The latter condition is, in many instances, almost certainly related to a prolapsed intervertebral disc (29).

According to Haldeman (30), two important factors compound the problem of back pain mechanisms: (*a*) Back pain may have a multifactorial etiology, and (*b*) there may be several types of back pain which closely mimic each other. Baldwin (31) states that part of the problem lies in the fact that the low back region is extremely complex, both anatomically and functionally. We await further elucidation of the pathophysiology of the back problem since the pathologic etiology of many varieties of back pain remains undiscovered (13–15, 17, 18, 32–40). However, most painful conditions of the lumbar spine affect the lower lumbar mobile segments (41).

Motion (Mobile) Segment and Its Parts

The mobile segment (42) is conveniently subdivided into anterior and posterior elements (43). It is claimed, on the basis of clinical and experimental observations, that degeneration of the intervertebral disc and associated osteoarthritis of the zygapophyseal joints can cause low back pain (42, 44, 45–54). Some authors (55) stress psychologic factors. However, it has been suggested that pain can also be experienced in the absence of degenerative joint disease, or other pathologic changes, as a result of traction on normal pain-sensitive structures, for example, the joint capsules (56, 57), or pinching and tractioning of the intra-articular synovial fold inclusions within the zygapophyseal joints (58–61).

The joint capsule forms superior and inferior recesses which are filled with small synovial "fat pads" (62). In contrast to the the upper lumbar spine inferior recesses, the lower lumbar inferior recesses, particularly at the lumbosacral joint, have large synovial fold inclusions (59, 61). These synovial fold inclusions have been shown to have small paravascular nerve fibers as well as nerve fibers which are unrelated to blood vessels coursing through them (63, 64). The lumbosacral inferior joint recess differs dramatically from the inferior recesses of other lumbar joints, partly because of the differences in the bony anatomy of the lumbosacral level compared with the remaining lumbar zygapophyseal joints. Thus, in this text, the large lower lumbar zygapophyseal joint inferior recesses and their synovial fold inclusions are described in detail, and the relatively small superior recesses, which are not normally amenable to surgical procedures, are only briefly described.

Diagnostic Problems

Diagnostic problems relate to (*a*) inadequacies in the precise knowledge of the lumbosacral spine and (*b*) the limitations of many diagnostic procedures.

For example, controversy exists regarding the source of the innervation of zygapophyseal joint capsules and the innervation of human synovial folds within the zygapophyseal joints. Bogduk (65), Reilly et al (66), Bradley (3), Moore (67), Lynch and Taylor (68), and Giles (64) show a dual innervation for each joint. Sunderland (69) states that each vertebral joint is innervated from at least two spinal nerves, while Wyke (70, 71), Paris et al (72), and Paris (73) claimed innervation of each joint from at least three spinal nerves.

Hadley (74) and B. D. Wyke (personal communication, 1983) were unable to find nerves in the synovium of human zygapophyseal joints. Wyke (75) refers to mechanoreceptors in animal fibrous capsules and fat pads, but in 1967 (75) and 1972 (76) and with Nade et al (77), he stated that no receptor endings of any description are present "in the synovial tissue" of zygapophyseal joints. However, Giles et al (63) and Giles (64) showed that small-diameter nerve fibers are present in human lower lumbar zygapophyseal joint synovial folds; these are both paravascular and remote from blood vessels.

In many cases of acute low back pain with sciatica, intervertebral disc prolapse was described by Mixter and Barr (29). Other investigators have confirmed this pathology (50, 78–85), but according to Wiesel et al (86) herniated lumbar intervertebral discs are often asymptomatic when a spinal canal is not narrow (87). However, many authorities believe that disc lesions have been overemphasized as the principal source of back pain. Alternative, or multifactorial, sources of back pain are also frequently involved, including pathology of the zygapophyseal joints and the related ligaments and muscles, which are supplied by the posterior primary rami (30, 88–93). Some authors have focused particular attention on the zygapophyseal joints (68, 94–101), but our understanding of their pathology and its relation to painful syndromes is limited (19). In patients presenting with local tenderness in the low back, muscle spasm, and low back pain referred to the back of the thigh, to the mid-calf, or to the ankle, it is often thought that the pain arises from the zygapophyseal joints (37, 102). The alleviation of the pain by injection of local anesthetic, with or without steroid suspension, into the joints, under fluoroscopic control, supports this diagnosis (103–108).

The importance of fluoroscopic control is stressed for positioning a hypodermic needle in ligaments (109) and in zygapophyseal joints (37, 68, 110).

The continuing interest shown in recent years in low back pain syndromes by epidemiologists, pathologists, rheumatologists, bioengineers, and other biomedical researchers reflects both the magnitude of the problem and the lack of definitive solutions (111).

Limitations of Investigative Methods

Routine plain-film radiologic demonstration of the zygapophyseal joints is not easy, because only one plane of the curved or "biplanar" (112) articular surface presents itself tangentially to the x-ray beam (113, 114). Joint radiographs can be informative but have limitations (115), and there is sometimes a discrepancy between the degree of pain and the severity of radiographic changes (116). Disabling zygapophyseal joint facet syndromes can be associated with normal or nearly normal plain-film radiographs (101). While computerized tomography scans give fuller information

(117), they are not applicable to all cases of low back pain (118) and do not generally reveal soft tissue pathology. Thus, radiologically "normal" but painful spines (119) may have "pathologic changes" which cannot be demonstrated radiologically (120). On the other hand, many individuals with radiologic abnormalities of spinal joints remain pain free, and the relation between these radiologic abnormalities and symptoms is not understood (121, 122). Many spinal structures probably play a role in pain production, and all innervated structures in the motion segment are possible sources of pain (30, 123).

The patient who complains of low back pain without sciatica presents unusual diagnostic difficulties, and in most cases it is impossible to make a precise anatomical and pathologic diagnosis (124).

Pain-Sensitive Structures of the Lumbosacral Spine and Pelvis

The main structures of the lumbosacral spine which are considered to be pain sensitive are shown in Figure 1.1

Table 1.1 briefly summarizes some possible causes of low back pain, with or without leg pain.

Figure 1.2 summarizes some well-established causes of low back pain which are due to the lumbar spine, and some of its ad-

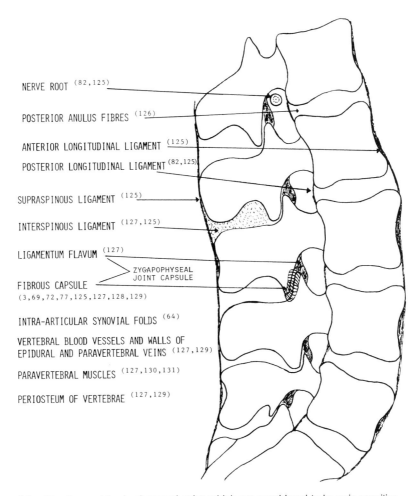

NERVE ROOT (82,125)

POSTERIOR ANULUS FIBRES (126)

ANTERIOR LONGITUDINAL LIGAMENT (125)

POSTERIOR LONGITUDINAL LIGAMENT (82,125)

SUPRASPINOUS LIGAMENT (125)

INTERSPINOUS LIGAMENT (127,125)

LIGAMENTUM FLAVUM (127)

ZYGAPOPHYSEAL JOINT CAPSULE

FIBROUS CAPSULE
(3,69,72,77,125,127,128,129)

INTRA-ARTICULAR SYNOVIAL FOLDS (64)

VERTEBRAL BLOOD VESSELS AND WALLS OF EPIDURAL AND PARAVERTEBRAL VEINS (127,129)

PARAVERTEBRAL MUSCLES (127,130,131)

PERIOSTEUM OF VERTEBRAE (127,129)

Figure 1.1. Structures of the lumbosacral spine which are considered to be pain sensitive.

Table 1.1.

Some Possible Causes of Low Back Pain, With or Without Leg Pain

Nerve root conditions
- Adhesions between dural sleeves and the joint capsule with nerve root fibrosis (132, 133)
- Intervertebral disc degeneration (134) and fragmentation (135) or nucleus pulposus extrusion (29)
- Lumbosacral arachnoiditis (136)

Zygapophyseal joint conditions
- Joint derangement due to ligamentous and capsular instability (91, 128, 137)
- Joint capsule tension, encroachment of the intervertebral foramen lumen; impingement of the articular process tip against the pedicle above and the lamina below (128)
- Joint degenerative changes, e.g., "meniscal" incarceration (42), osteoarthrosis (101)
- Joint effusion with capsular distension which may exert pressure on a nerve root (138) or cause capsular pain (132) or nerve root pain by direct diffusion (30)
- Joint capsule adhesions (139)
- Intra-articular synovial fold inclusions tractioning against the pain-sensitive joint capsule (128, 140)

Miscellaneous conditions
- Spinal stenosis (141)
- Intervertebral foramen venous stasis (142, 143)
- Myofascial genesis of pain (trigger areas) (130, 131)
- Hypertension in the bone marrow of the vertebral body or in the juxtachondral space of osteoarthritic intervertebral joints (49)

jacent soft tissue structures, as well as pelvic lesions.

It is not possible to list all the causes of pelvic pain in this text, but it is worth noting the contribution made by the sacroiliac joints and the sacroiliac ligaments (145).

The percentage of various conditions causing low back pain, with or without leg pain, is shown in Ghormley's (146) etiologic grouping of 2000 patients who sought help regarding their low back pain (Table 1.2).

Note that the biomechanical disturbances combined with osteoarthritis together form by far the largest group, that is, more than 50% of Ghormley's (146) cases. When it is remembered that abnormal joint biomechanics can cause degenerative joint changes in the articular triad, it appears that abnormal joint function is responsible for a large number of cases of low back pain.

Etiological groupings of conditions thought to cause low back pain, using radiographic criteria (7, 146–151), do not mention whether leg length inequality was taken into account when evaluating low back pain. However, epidemiologic surveys have linked the possibility of low back pain's being associated with leg length inequality (152–161). Some of these authors have attempted to correlate leg length inequality and low back pain by comparing the prevalence of leg length discrepancies in low back pain and control groups. However, it is still maintained by a large body of orthopedic opinion (162, 163) that a 1-cm leg length deficiency gives rise to an innocuous postural scoliosis with no structural changes, although it is not known whether a leg length inequality of 1–2 cm predisposes to back problems in later life (164). However, some evidence is now available on the long-term effects of leg length inequality of the order of 1–2 cm which produces minimal lumbar scoliosis of the order of 5–10° (59, 165). In spite of this, not many clinical trials have used carefully standardized erect posture radiography to evaluate lumbopelvic functional biomechanics in relation to low back pain.

Not taking leg length inequality into account when evaluating low back pain appears to ignore an important factor outside the spine which can affect all parts of the mobile segment by influencing its posture.

Low back pain is frequently due to irritation of pain-sensitive structures in the spinal canal, the intervertebral canals, the zygapophyseal joints, and the associated ligaments and muscles. Since the pain is commonly movement related, the pain-sensitive structures of the motion segment of Junghanns (42) must be irritated (see Fig. A1.3). The mechanism by which leg length equality may produce low back pain must involve (*a*) some lumbar spine pathology, whether structural or functional; (*b*) possible sacroiliac joint dysfunction, (*c*) possible pelvic–lumbar muscle dysfunction, or (*d*) a combination of these factors.

In spite of the current concepts of low back pain etiology, outlined above, a controversy persists as to which pathologic or radiologic abnormalities may be of signifi-

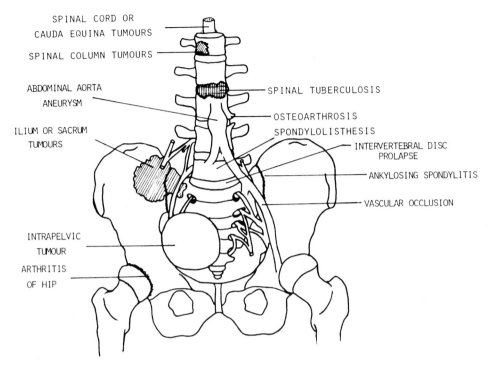

SPINAL CORD OR
CAUDA EQUINA TUMOURS

SPINAL COLUMN TUMOURS

ABDOMINAL AORTA
ANEURYSM

ILIUM OR SACRUM
TUMOURS

INTRAPELVIC
TUMOUR
ARTHRITIS
OF HIP

SPINAL TUBERCULOSIS

OSTEOARTHROSIS
SPONDYLOLISTHESIS

INTERVERTEBRAL DISC
PROLAPSE

ANKYLOSING SPONDYLITIS

VASCULAR OCCLUSION

Figure 1.2.   Some causes of low back pain, with or without leg pain, which must be considered in differential diagnosis. Modified from Adams JC: *Outline of Orthopaedics*, ed 9. Edinburgh, E.S. Livingstone, 1981, p 208.

cance in back pain (166). Also, for any one individual patient there can be a lack of close correlation between the degree of observed morbid change and the subjective severity of the complaint (167, 168).

One important aspect in the investigation of causes of low back pain is the biomechanical analysis of loads on the lumbar spine and their relation to pain, although no direct means exist which measure these loads in vivo (169). In spite of the numerous clinical and anatomical studies outlined, there are still many different opinions concerning the interpretation of causes, sources, and mechanisms of low back pain (94, 170).

The stresses sustained by the spine are multiple, including vertical compression, horizontal shear, angular torque, and a variety of combinations of these (111).

Farfan (48) and Hutton and Adams (171) found that the zygapophyseal joints accept a proportion of body weight. Using excised, embalmed cadaveric spines, with an inter-vertebral load cell at the L2–3 level, Hakim and King (172) estimated that the articular facets carry 20–40% of the total compressive spine load in the erect posture. Jayson (173) confirmed that compressive forces are considerable in the posterior elements of the vertebra and that they are increased by extension.

The biomechanical stresses of the lumbosacral junction in a person with a normal sacral base angle of approximately 41° and equal leg lengths are summarized in Figure 1.3.

Because the human erect posture involves a permanent lordosis, the lower lumbar joints are always subject to a shearing force even in the relaxed upright stance (178). This load-bearing shearing force will be influenced by spinal posture and the associated joint plane angle. Some authors have stressed that humans' erect posture predisposes them to low back pain (179, 180) and that changes in posture may influence the load borne by zygapophyseal joints.

Table 1.2.
Etiologic Grouping of 2000 Cases of Low Back Pain, Sciatic Pain, or Both[a]

	Number	%
Compensation neurosis	1	0.1
Partial sacralization	2	0.1
Gynecologic disease	5	0.2
Neoplasms of cord and adjacent soft tissues	6	0.3
Neoplasms of vertebrae	14	0.7
Scoliosis	11	0.6
Previous operation for disc (with or without fusion)	11	0.5
Syndromes (facet, interspinous, fibrositis)	14	0.7
Spondylolysis with or without spondylolisthesis	57	2.9
Miscellaneous (Pagets, coccygodynia, osteoporosis)	94	4.6
Trauma with or without fractures	108	5.5
Inflammatory (vertebral epiphysitis, rheumatoid spondylitis)	177	8.7
Suspected protruded intervertebral disc	445	22.3
Osteoarthritis	511	25.6
Indeterminate causes of static disturbances	544	27.2
Total	2000	100.0

[a]Modified from Ghormley RK: An etiologic study of back pain. *Radiology* 70:649-652, 1958.

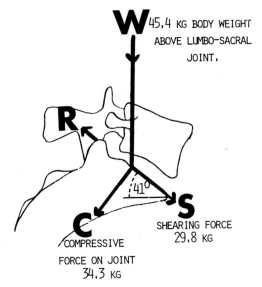

Figure 1.3. Biomechanical forces at the lumbosacral junction. Sacral superior articular facets have a counter reactive force (R) to the shearing force (S). (Modified from Davis PR: Human lower lumbar vertebrae: some mechanical and osteological considerations. *J Anat* 95:337-344, 1961; Kapandji IA: The physiology of the joints. In: *The Trunk and the Vertebral Column*. Edinburgh, Churchill Livingstone, 1974, Vol 3, p 78; Lafferty JF, Winter WG, Gambaro SA: Fatigue characteristics of posterior elements of vertebrae. *J Bone Joint Surg (Am)* 59:154-158, 1977; and LeVeau B: *Williams and Lissner: Biomechanics of Human Motion*, ed 2. Philadelphia, W.B. Saunders, 1977.)

The clinical importance of leg length inequality depends on the degree of inequality (163, 181) and relates to a number of associated conditions and problems, some of which may have the following consequences:

1. A possible correlation between the resultant pelvic obliquity and any degenerative changes in the lumbar spine, such as osteoarthritis, spondylosis, etc. (59, 182, 183);
2. A possible association with low back pain (152, 156, 160);
3. Excessive unilateral stress on the sacroililiac joint capsule; its ligaments, and its articular cartilage (184);
4. A correlation with hip joint degenerative changes (osteoarthritis) (155, 183, 185, 186);
5. A correlation with knee joint degenerative changes—osteoarthrosis, "long leg arthropathy" (187);
6. Psychologic difficulties associated with the aesthetic consequences of the postural deformity (163, 188, 189).

The most common cause of pelvic obliquity is inequality of length of the lower limbs (190), which may also be implicated in early degenerative changes in the zygapophyseal joints of the lumbar spine (183) since it may alter the mechanical stresses in these joints.

In the scoliotic spine, the articulating surfaces of the zygapophyseal joints are probably no longer fully congruous, and consequently increased friction may occur at some point of the gliding movement (137). According to Huskisson and Hart (191), abnormally shaped or positioned zygapophyseal joint surfaces appear to be a cause of osteoarthritis.

Unequal growth may result from pathologic involvement of long bone epiphyses by infection, trauma, radiation, Perthes disease, and paralysis of associated muscle groups. In addition, during growth or after completion of growth, leg length inequality may result from fracture.

However, the vast majority of patients with leg length inequality of 1 cm or more have no known etiology for this inequality (192), which arises during normal growth without any apparent pathology. This asymmetrical growth of the lower extremities is very common and, according to Taylor and Halliday (193), is associated with "out of phase" growth in length of the long bone(s) of the lower limbs. This tendency and the amount of inequality persisting at maturity may be determined by hereditary factors (194).

It is very rare to find individuals with exactly equal leg lengths. In a normal community, leg length inequality appears to develop frequently in individuals who appear skeletally normal.

In order to understand a low back pain sufferer's signs and symptoms, it is necessary to clearly understand the complex anatomy of the lower lumbosacral spine. Therefore, in this text the anatomy of the lower lumbosacral spine is reviewed, followed by a review of the pathologic changes associated with degenerative motion segment disorders.

References

1. Wedge JH: The natural history of spinal degeneration. In Kirkaldy-Willis WH (ed): *Managing Low Back Pain*, New York, Churchill Livingstone, 1983, pp 3-8.
2. Dixon ASt:Diagnosis of low back pain—sorting the complainers. In Jayson M (ed): *The Lumbar Spine and Back Pain*. London Sector Publishing, 1976, pp 77-92.
3. Bradley KC: The posterior primary rami of segmental nerves. In Dewhurst D, Glasgow EF, Tahan, P, Ward AR, Idczak RM (eds): *Aspects of Manipulative Therapy, Proceedings of a Multidisciplinary International Conference in Manipulative Therapy*, Melbourne, Ramsay Ware Stockland, 1980, pp 56-59.
4. Andersson GBJ: Epidemiology of low back pain. In Buerger AA, Greenman PE (ed): *Empirical Approaches to the Validation of Spinal Manipulation*. Springfield, IL, Charles C. Thomas, 1985, pp 53-70.
5. Sedlak K:Low-back pain. Perception and tolerance. *Spine* 10:440-444, 1985.
6. Nachemson AL:Low-back pain—its etiology and treatment. *Clin Med* 78:18-24, 1971.
7. Nachemson AL:The lumbar spine: an orthopaedic challenge. *Spine* 1:59-71, 1976.
8. Nachemson AL: Pathophysiology and treatment of back pain. A critical look at different types of treatment. In Buerger AA, Tobis JS (eds): *Approaches to the Validation of Manipulation Therapy*. Springfield, IL, Charles C. Thomas, 1977, pp 42-57.
9. Haldeman S: The spine as a neuro-musculoskeletal organ. In: *A Comprehensive Interdisciplinary Approach to the Management of Spinal Disorders*. Haldeman Interprofessional Conference on the Spine. Las Vegas, 1980.
10. Friedman WA: New techniques for treatment of disk disease. *Geriatrics* 39:41-53, 1984.
11. Kirkaldy-Willis WH, Cassidy J: Spinal manipulator in the treatment of low back pain. *Can Fam Physican* 31:535-540, 1985.
12. Jayson, MIV: The inflammatory component of mechanical back problems. *Br J Rheumatol* 25:210-213, 1986.
13. Park WM, McCall IW, O'Brien JP, Webb JK: Fissuring of the posterior annulus fibrosus in the lumbar spine. *Br J Radiol* 52:382-387, 1979.
14. Mehta M: Current views on non-invasive methods in pain relief. In Swerdlow M (ed): *The Therapy of Pain*. Lancaster, MTP Press, 1981, pp 171-187.
15. Feldman F: The symptomatic spine: relevant and irrelevant roentgen variants and variations. *Orthop Clin North Am* 14:119-145, 1983.
16. Lewinnik GE: Management of low back pain and sciatica. *Int Anesthesiol Clin* 21:61-78, 1983.
17. Mooney V: The syndromes of low back disease. *Orthop Clin North Am* 14:505-515, 1983.
18. Yong-Hing K, Kirkaldy-Willis WH: The pathophysiology of degenerative disease of the lumbar spine. *Orthop Clin North Am* 14:491-504, 1983.
19. Jayson MIV: Back pain, spondylosis and disc disorders. In Scott JT (ed): *Copeman's Textbook of Rheumatic Diseases*, ed 5. London, Churchill Livingstone, 1976, pp 960-985.
20. Kepes ER, Dunclaf D: Treatment of backache with spinal injections of local anaesthetics, spinal and systemic steroids. A review. *Pain* 22:33-47, 1985.
21. Mellin G: Chronic low back pain in men 54–63 years of age. *Spine* 11:421-426, 1986.
22. Kiernan PJ: Monitoring spinal movement relating to back pain. *Rheumatology and Rehabilitation* 20:143-147, 1981.
23. Bronfort G, Jochumsen OH: The functional radiographic examination of patients with low back pain. A study of different forms of variations. *J Manipulative Physiol Ther* 7:89-97, 1984.
24. Anderson JAD: Back pain and occupation. In Jayson MIV (ed): *The Lumbar Spine and Back Pain*, ed 2. Kent, Pitman Medical, 1980, pp 57-82.
25. Wood PHN, Badley EM: Back pain in the community. *Clin Rheum Dis* 6:3-16, 1980.
26. Spengler DM, Bigos SJ, Martin NA, Zeh J, Fisher L, Nachemson A: Back injuries in industry: A retrospective study. 1. Overview and cost analysis. *Spine* 11:241-245, 1986.
27. Friberg S, Hirsch C: On late results of operative treatment for intervertebral disc prolapses in the lumbar region. *Acta Chirurgic Scand* 93:161-168, 1946.
28. Robertson AM: Manipulation for back pain. *Lancet* 1:1190, 1979.
29. Mixter WJ, Barr JS: Rupture of the intervertebral disc with involvement of the spinal canal. *N Engl J Med* 211:210-215, 1934.
30. Haldeman S: Why one cause of back pain? In

Buerger AA, Tobis TS (eds): *Approaches to the Validation of Manipulation Therapy*. Springfield, IL, C.C. Thomas, 1977, pp 187-197.

31. Baldwin KW: A critique of the low back pain problem. In Buerger AA, Tobis JS (eds): *Approaches to the Validation of Manipulation Therapy*. Springfield, IL, Charles C. Thomas, 1977, pp 303-307.

32. Brown JR: The etiology of low back pain and vertebral traumatic pathology. In: *Manual Lifting and Related Fields. An Annotated Bibliography*. Ontario, Canada, Ontario Ministry of Labor, Labor Safety Council, 1976, p 30.

33. Glover JR: Prevention of back pain. In Jayson M (ed): *The Lumbar Spine and Back Pain*. London, Sector Publishing, 1976, pp 47-54.

34. Editorial: Apophyseal joints and back pain. *Lancet* 2:247, 1978.

35. Crown S: Psychosocial factors in low back pain. *Clin Rheum Dis* 6:77-92, 1980.

36. Nachemson AL: A critical look at conservative treatment of low back pain. In Jayson MIV (ed): *The Lumbar Spine and Back Pain*, ed 2. Kent, Pitman Medical, 1980, pp 453-466.

37. Kirkaldy-Willis WH: The pathology and pathogenesis of low back pain. In Kirkaldy-Willis WH (ed): *Managing Low Back Pain*. New York, Churchill Livingstone, 1983, pp 23-43.

38. Cassidy JD, Kirkaldy-Willis WH, McGregor M: Spinal manipulation for the treatment of chronic low-back and leg pain: An observational study. In Buerger AA, Greenman PE (ed): *Empirical Approaches to the Validation of Spinal Manipulation*. Springfield, IL, Charles C. Thomas, 1985, pp 119-150.

39. Pearcy M, Portek I, Shepherd J: The effect of low back pain on lumbar spinal movements measured by three-dimensional x-ray analysis. *Spine* 10:150-153, 1985.

40. Tajima N, Kawano K: Cryomicrotomy of the lumbar spine. *Spine* 11:376-379, 1986.

41. Ehni G: Historical writings on spondylotic caudal radiculopathy and its effect on the nervous system. In Weinstein PR, Ehni G, Wilson CB (eds): *Lumbar Spondylosis: Diagnosis, Management and Surgical Treatment*. Chicago, Year Book Medical Publishers, 1977, pp 1-12.

42. Schmorl G. Junghanns H: *The Human Spine in Health and Disease*. ed 2. New York, Grune and Stratton, 1971, pp 22, 37, 148, 197.

43. Andersson GBJ: The biomechanics of the posterior elements of the lumbar spine. *Spine* 8:326, 1983.

44. Hadley LA: Subluxation of the apophyseal articulations with bony impingement as a cause of back pain. *AJR* 33:209-213, 1935.

45. Sashin D: Relation of Pathologic changes of the intervertebral discs to pain in the lower part of the back. *Arch Surg* 32:932-944, 1936.

46. Harris RI, Macnab I: Structural changes in the lumbar intervertebral discs. Their relationship to low back pain and sciatica. *J Bone Joint Surg* 36B:304-322, 1954.

47. Lewin P: *The Back and Its Disc Syndromes*. Philadelphia, Lea and Febiger, 1955.

48. Farfan HF, *Mechanical Disorders of the Low Back*. Philadelphia, Lea and Febiger, 1973.

49. Arnoldi CC: Intraosseous Hypertension. *Clin Orthop* 115:30-34, 1976.

50. Crock HV: Isolated lumbar disk resorption as a cause of nerve root canal stenosis. *Clin Orthop* 115:109-115, 1976.

51. Culberson JL: Origins of low back pain—the intervertebral foramen. In Kent B (ed): *Proceedings, International Federation of Orthopedic Manipulative Thera-*

pists, 1977, pp 21-34.

52. Hastings DE: Back pain: a multifaceted syndrome. *Postgrad Med* 62:159-165, 1979.

53. Kirkaldy-Willis WH: Five common back disorders: how to diagnose and treat them. *Geriatrics* 22:32-41, 1978.

54. Kirkaldy-Willis WH, Farfan HF: Instability of the lumbar spine. *Clin Orthop* 165:110-123, 1982.

55. Hoehler FK, Tobis JS: Psychological factors in the treatment of back pain by spinal manipulation. *Br J Rheumatol* 22:206-212, 1983.

56. Mehta M, Sluijter ME: The treatment of chronic back pain. *Anesthesia* 34:768-775, 1979.

57. Budd K: The use of non-pharmaceutical methods in the treatment of arthritic pain. *Clin Rheum Dis* 7:437-454, 1981.

58. Kos J, Wolf J: Les Menisques Intervertebraux et leur Role Possible dans les Blocages Vertebraux. *Annals de Medicine Physique* 15:203-217, 1972.

59. Giles LGF, Taylor JR: Intra-articular synovial protrusions in the lower lumbar apophyseal joints. *Bull Hosp Jt Dis* 42:248-255, 1982.

60. Kirkaldy-Willis WH: The relationship of structural pathology to the nerve root. *Spine* 9:49-52, 1984.

61. Giles LGF: Lumbo-sacral and cervical zygapophyseal joint inclusions. *Manual Medicine* 2:89-92, 1986.

62. Lewin T, Moffett B, Viidik A: The morphology of the lumbar synovial intervertebral arches. *Acta Morphol Neerlando-Scandinavica* 4:299-319, 1961.

63. Giles LGF, Taylor JR, Cockson A: Human zygapophyseal joint synovial folds. *Acta Anat* 126:110-114, 1986.

64. Giles LGF: *The anatomy of human lower lumbar and lumbo-sacral zygapophyseal joint inferior recesses with particular reference to their synovial fold innervation*. Ph.D. thesis, Department of Anatomy and Human Biology, University of Western Australia, Nedlands, Western Australia, 1987.

65. Bogduk N: The anatomy of the lumbar intervertebral disc syndrome. *Med J Aust* 1:878-881, 1976.

66. Reilly J, Yong-Hing K, MacKay RW, Kirkaldy-Willis WH: Pathological anatomy of the lumbar spine. In Helfet AJ, Gruebel DM (eds): *Disorders of the Lumbar Spine*. Philadelphia, J.B. Lippincott, 1978, pp 26-50.

67. Moore KL: *Clinically Oriented Anatomy*. Baltimore, Williams & Wilkins, 1980.

68. Lynch MC, Taylor JF: Facet joint injection for low back pain. A clinical study. *J Bone Joint Surg* 68B:138-141, 1986.

69. Sunderland S: Anatomical perivertebral influences on the intervertebral foramen. In Goldstein M (ed): *The Research Status of Spinal Manipulative Therapy* (Monograph No. 15). Bethesda, MD, National Institute of Neurological and Communicative Disorders and Stroke, 1975, pp 129-140.

70. Wyke BD: The neurology of low back pain. In Jayson MIV (ed): *The Lumbar Spine and Back Pain*, ed 2. Kent, Pitman Medical, 1980, pp 265-339.

71. Wyke BD: The neurology of joints: a review of general principles. *Clin Rheum Dis* 7:223-239, 1981.

72. Paris SV, Nyberg R, Mooney V, et al: What's new for low back pain and just plain pain. *Medical World News* 21:2128-2143, 1980.

73. Paris SV: Anatomy as related to function and pain. *Orthop Clin North Am* 14:475-489, 1983.

74. Hadley LA: *Anatomico-Roentgenographic Studies of the Spine*. Springfield, IL, Charles C. Thomas, 1976.

75. Wyke BD: The neurology of joints. *Ann Engl R Coll Surg* 41:25, 1967.

76. Wyke BD: Articular neurology: a review. *Physiotherapy* 58:94-99, 1972.

77. Nade S, Bell S, Wyke BD: The innervation of the lum-

bar spinal joints and its significance. *J Bone Joint Surg Proc* 62B:255, 1980.

78. Love JG, Camp JD: Root pain resulting from intraspinal protrusion of intervertebral discs. *J Bone Joint Surg* 19B: 776-804, 1937.

79. Adson AW: Chronic recurring sciatica: diagnosis and treatment of protrusions of ruptured intervertebral discs. *Arch Phys Ther* 20:325-330, 1939.

80. Craig WMcK, Walsh MN: The diagnosis and treatment of low back and sciatic pain caused by protruded intervertebral disc and hypertrophied ligaments. *Minn Med* 22:511-517, 1939.

81. Spurling RG,Grantham EG: Neurologic pictures of herniations of the nucleus pulposus in the lower part of the lumbar region. *Arch Surg* 40:375, 1940.

82. Smyth MJ, Wright V: Sciatica and the intervertebral disc. *J Bone Joint Surg (Am)* 40:1401-1418, 1958.

83. Taylor TKF, Akeson WH: Intervertebrai disc prolapse: a review of morphologic and biochemical knowledge concerning the nature of prolapse. *Clin Orthop* 76:54-79, 1971.

84. Hazlett JW: Low back pain with femoral neuritis. *Clin Orthop* 108:19-26, 1975.

85. Rothman RH, Simeone FA: Lumbar disc disease. In Rothman RH, Simeone FA (eds): *The Spine*. Philadelphia, W.B. Saunders, 1975, p 442.

86. Wiesel SW, Tsourmas N, Feffer HL, and associates: A study of computer-assisted tomography: 1. The incidence of positive CAT scans in an asymptomatic group of patients. *Spine* 9:549:551, 1984.

87. Heliovaara M, Vanharanta H, Korpi J, Troup JDG: Herniated lumbar disc syndrome and vertebral canals. *Spine* 11:433-435, 1986.

88. Putti V: New conceptions in the pathogenesis of sciatic pain. *Lancet* 2:53, 1927.

89. Jackson RK: Lumbar disc lesions: facts and fallacies. *Hospital Update* 1:431-459.

90. Haldeman S: The pathophysiology of the spinal subluxation. In Goldstein M (ed): *Research Status of Spinal Manipulative Therapy* (Monograph No. 15). Bethesda, MD, National Institute of Neurological and Communicative Disorders and Stroke, 1975, pp 217-226.

91. Macnab I: *Backache*. Baltimore, Williams & Wilkins, 1977.

92. Yang KH, King Al: Mechanism of facet load transmission as a hypothesis for low back pain. *Spine* 9:559-565, 1984.

93. Chusid JG: *Correlative Neuroanatomy and Functional Neurology*, ed 19. Los Altos, CA, Lange Medical Publications, 1985, p 376.

94. Hirsch C, Ingelmark BE, Miller M: The anatomical basis for low back pain. *Acta Orthop Scand* 33:1-17, 1963.

95. McCall IW, Park WM, O'Brien JP: Induced pain referral from posterior lumbar elements in normal subjects. *Spine* 4:440-446, 1979.

96. Bogduk N: The anatomy and physiology of lumbar back disability. *Bulletin of the Post-Grad Committee in Medicine*, University of Sydney, Australia 36:2-17, 1980.

97. Rauschning W: Topographic and functional anatomy of the lumbar zygapophyseal joints (abstract). Presented at a meeting of the International Society for the Study of the Lumbar Spine, Dallas, 1986.

98. Shirazi-Adl A, Drouin G: A quantitative analysis of the load-bearing role of the lumbar facets in compression. The effects of posture and nucleus dissolution (abstract). Presented at a meeting of the International Society for the Study of the Lumbar Spine, Dallas, 1986.

99. Giles LGF, Taylor JR: Human zygapophyseal joint capsule and synovial fold innervation. *Br J Rheumatol* 26:93-98, 1987.

100. Giles LGF, Taylor JR: Innervation of human lumbar zygapophyseal joint synovial folds. *Acta Orthop Scand* 58:43-47, 1987.

101. Eisenstein SM, Parry CR: The lumbar facet arthrosis syndrome. Clinical presentation and articular surface changes. *J Bone Joint Surg* 69B:3-7, 1987.

102. Kirkaldy-Willis WH, Cassidy JD: Toward a more precise diagnosis of low back pain. In Genant HK (ed): *Spine Update 1984. Perspectives in Radiology, Orthopaedic Surgery, and Neurosurgery*. San Francisco, Radiology Research and Education Foundation, 1984, pp 5-16.

103. Mooney V, Robertson J: The facet syndrome. *Clin Orthop* 115:149-156, 1976.

104. Carrera GF: Lumbar facet arthrography and injection in low back pain. *Wisc Med J* 78:35-37.

105. Destouet JM, Gilula LA, Murphy WA, Monsess B: Lumbar facet joint injection: indication, technique, clinical correlation and preliminary results. *Radiology* 145:321-325, 1982.

106. Kirkaldy-Willis WH, Tchang S: Diagnosis. In Kirkaldy-Willis WH (ed): *Managing Low Back Pain*. New York, Churchill Livingstone, 1983, pp 109-127.

107. Aprill C: Lumbar facet joint arthrography and injection in the evaluation of painful disorders of the low back (abstract). Presented at a meeting of the International Society for the Study of the Lumbar Spine, Dallas, 1986.

108. Lewinnik GE, Warfield CA: Facet joint degeneration as a cause of low back pain. *Clin Orthop* 213:216-222, 1986.

109. Sinclair DC, Feindel WH, Weddell G, Falconer MA: The intervertebral ligaments as a source of segmental pain. *J Bone Joint Surg* 30B:515-521, 1948.

110. Burnell A: Injection techniques in low back pain. In Twomey LT (ed): *Low Back Pain* (proceedings of a conference on low back pain). Perth, Australia, Western Australian Institute of Technology, 1974, pp 111-116.

111. Harvey GR: The engineering aspects of the human trunk. In: *Engineering Aspects of the Spine*. London, Mechanical Engineering Publications, 1980, pp 97-102.

112. Taylor JR, Twomey L: Age changes in lumbar zygapophyseal joints: observations on structure and function. *Spine* 11:739-745, 1986.

113. Reichmann S: Radiography of the lumbar intervertebral joints. *Acta Radiol* 14:161-170, 1973.

114. Park WM: The place of radiology in the investigation of low back pain. *Clin Rheum Dis* 6:93-132, 1980.

115. Carroll GJ: Spectrophotometric measurement of proteoglycans in osteoarthritic synovial fluid. *Ann Rheum Dis* 46:375-379, 1987.

116. Stockwell RA: *A Pre-clinical view of osteoarthritis*. A Sir John Struthers Lecture. Teviot Place, Edinburgh, The Medical School, 1985.

117. Chafetz NI, Mani JR, Genant HK, Morris JM, Hoaglund FT: CT in low back pain syndrome. *Orthop Clin North Am* 16:395-416, 1985.

118. LaMasters DL, Dorwart RH: High-resolution, cross-sectional computed tomography of the normal spine. *Orthop Clin North Am* 16:359-379.

119. Benson DR: The spine and neck. In Gershwin ME, Robbins DL (eds): *Musculoskeletal Diseases of Children*. New York, Grune and Stratton, 1983, p 469.

120. Dixon AS: Diagnosis of low back pain—sorting the complainers. In Jayson M (ed): *The Lumbar Spine and Back Pain*. ed 2. Kent, Pitman Medical 1980, pp 135-156.

121. Isherwood I, Antoun NM:CT scanning in the assessment of lumbar spine problems. In Jayson MIV (ed): *The Lumbar Spine and Back Pain*, ed 2. Kent, Pitman Medical, 1980, pp 247-264.

122. Vanharanta H, Korpi J, Heliovaaram, Troup JDG: Radiographic measurements of lumbar spinal canal size and their relation to back mobility. *Spine* 10:461-466, 1985.
123. Nachemson AL: Advances in low-back pain. *Clin Orthop* 200:266-278, 1985.
124. Taylor JR: Pathology of the lumbar disc prolapse. In Twomey LT (ed): *Low Back Pain* (proceedings of a conference on low back pain). Perth, Australia, Western Australia Institute of Technology, 1974, pp 27-35.
125. Farfan HF: Mechanical factors in the genesis of low back pain. In Bonica JJ and associates (eds): *Advances in Pain Research and Therapy*. New York, Raven Press, 1979, Vol 3, pp 635-645.
126. White AA,III, Panjabi MM: *Clinical Biomechanics of the Spine*. Philadelphia, J.B. Lippincott, 1978.
127. Wyke BD: The neurological basis of thoracic spinal pain. *Rheumatol Phys Med* 10:356-367, 1970.
128. Hadley, LA: *Anatomico-Roentgenographic Studies of the Spine*. Springfield, IL, Charles C. Thomas, 1964.
129. Bogduk N: The innervation of the lumbar spine. *Spine* 8:286-293, 1983.
130. Travell J, Rinzler SH: Myofascial genesis of pain. *Postgrad Med* 11:425-434, 1952.
131. Bonica JJ: Management of myofascial pain syndromes in general practice. *JAMA* 164:732-738, 1957.
132. Jackson R: *The Cervical Syndrome*. ed 3. Springfield, IL, Charles C. Thomas, 1966.
133. Sunderland S: *Nerves and Nerve Injuries*. Edinburgh, E.S. Livingstone, 1968.
134. Nachemson A: Intradiscal measurements of pH in patients with lumbar rhizopathies. *Acta Orthop Scand* 40:23-42, 1969.
135. Schiotz EH, Cyriax J: *Manipulation Past and Present*. London,William Heinemann Medical Books, 1975.
136. Spiller WG, Musser JH, Martin E: Arachnoidal cysts. *University of Pennsylvania Medical Bulletin* 16:27-30, 1903.
137. Cailliet R: Low Back Pain Syndrome, ed 2. Philadelphia, F.A. Davis, 1968.
138. Mennell JMcM: *Back Pain. Diagnosis and Treatment using Manipulative Techniques*. ed 1. Boston, Little, Brown, 1960.
139. Farfan HF: The scientific basis of manipulative procedures. *Clin Rheum Dis* 6:159-178, 1980.
140. Giles LGF: Leg length inequality with postural scoliosis: its effect on lumbar apophyseal joints. M.Sc thesis, University of Western Australia, Perth, Western Australia, 1982.
141. Sachs ES, Fraenkel J: Progressive ankylotic rigidity of the spine. *J Nerv Ment Dis* 27:1, 1900.
142. Giles LGF: Spinal fixation and viscera. *Journal of Clinical Chiropractic Archives* 3:144-165, 1973.
143. Sunderland S. The anatomy of the intervertebral foramen and the mechanisms of compression and stretch of nerve roots. In Haldeman S (ed): *Modern Developments in the Principles and Practice of Chiropractic*. New York, Appleton-Century-Crofts, 45-64, 1980.
144. Adams JC: *Outline of Orthopaedics* ed 9. Edinburgh, E.S. Livingstone, 1981, p 208.
145. Barbor R: A treatment for chronic low back pain. *Excerpta Medica International Congress Series* 107:661-664, 1964.
146. Ghormley RK: An etiologic study of back pain. *Radiology* 70:649-652, 1958.
147. Conn HR: The acute painful back among industrial employees alleging compensable injury. *JAMA* 79: 1210-1212, 1929.
148. White AWM: Low back pain in men receiving workmen's compensation. *Can Med Assoc J* 95:50-56, 1966.
149. Stevens J: Pain and its clinical management. *Med Clin North Am* 52:55-71, 1968.
150. Anderson JAD: Back pain in industry. In Jayson M (ed): *The Lumbar Spine and Back Pain*, London, Sector Publishing, 1976, pp 29-46.
151. Witt I, Vestergaard A, Rosenklink A: A comparative analysis of x-ray findings of the lumbar spine in patients with and without lumbar pain. *Spine* 9:298-300, 1984.
152. Rush WA, Steiner HA: A study of lower extremity length inequality. *AJR* 56:616-623, 1946.
153. Stoddard A: *Manual of Osteopathic Technique*. London, Hutchinson Medical Publications, 1959, p 212.
154. Nichols PJR: Short-leg syndrome. *Br Med J* 1:1863-1865, 1960.
155. Gofton JP, Trueman GE: Unilateral idiopathic osteoarthritis of the hip. *Can Med Assoc J* 87:1129-1132, 1967.
156. Sicuranza BJ, Richards J, Tisdall LH: The short leg syndrome in obstetrics and gynecology. *Am J Obstet Gynecol* 107:217-219, 1970.
157. Bourdillon JF: *Spinal Manipulation*. London, William Heinemann Medical Books, 1970.
158. Yates A: The lumbar spine and back pain. In Jayson M (ed): *Treatment of Back Pain*. London, Sector Publishing, 1976, pp 341-353.
159. Hazelman B, Bulgen D: Low back pain. International Medicine 1 (Part 2):486-491, 1981.
160. Giles LGF, Taylor JR: Low back pain associated with leg length inequality. *Spine* 6:510-521, 1981.
161. Subotnick SI: Limb length discrepancies of the lower extremities (the short leg syndrome). *J Orthop Sports Phys Ther* 3:11-16, 1981.
162. Fisk JW, Baigent ML: Clinical and radiological assessment of leg length. *NZ Med J* 81:477-480, 1975.
163. Amstutz HC, Sakai DN: Equalization of leg length (editorial comment). *Clin Orthop* 136-2-5, 1978.
164. Sikorski JM: *Understanding Orthopaedics*. Sydney, Butterworths, 1986, p 68.
165. Giles LGF, Taylor JR: The effect of postural scoliosis on lumbar apophyseal joints. *Scand J Rheumatol* 13:209-220, 1984.
166. Currey HLF: An introduction to clinical rheumatology: degenerative joint disease II. In Mason M, Currey HLF (eds): *Spondylosis and Disc Lesions*, ed 2. Kent, Pitman Medical, 1975, pp 222-234.
167. Dixon AStJ: Progress and problems in back pain research. *Rheumatology and Rehabilitation* 12:165-175, 1973.
168. Meachim G: Cartilage breakdown. In Owen R, Goodfellow J, Bullough P (ed): *Scientific Foundation of Orthopaedics and Traumatology*. London, William Heinemann Medical Books, 1980, pp 290-296.
169. Marras WS, King Al, Joynt RL: Measurements of loads on the lumbar spine under isometric and isokinetic conditions. *Spine* 9:176-187, 1984.
170. OBrien JP: The multidisciplinary approach to back pain disorders. *Clin Rheum Dis* 6:133-142, 1980.
171. Hutton WC, Adams NA: The forces acting on the neural arch and their relevance to low back pain. In: *Engineering Aspects of the Spine*. London, Mechanical Engineering Publications, 1980, pp 49-55.
172. Hakim NS, King AI: Static and dynamic articular facet loads. In: *Proceedings, 20th Stapp Car Crash Conference*. 1976, pp 609-637.
173. Jayson MIV: Compression stresses in the posterior elements and pathological consequence. *Spine* 8:338-339, 1983.
174. Davis PR: Human lower lumbar vertebrae: some mechanical and osteological considerations. *J Anat*

95:337-344, 1961.

175. Kapandji IA: The physiology of the joints. In: *The Trunk and the Vetebral Column*. Edinburgh, Churchill Livingstone, 1974, Vol 3, p 78.

176. Lafferty JF, Winter WG, Gambaro SA: Fatigue characteristics of posterior elements of vertebrae. *J Bone Joint Surg (Am)* 59:154-158, 1977.

177. LeVeau B: *Williams and Lissner: Biomechanics of Human Motion*. ed 2. Philadelphia, W.B. Saunders, 1977.

178. Farfan HF: The biomechanical advantage of lordosis and hip extension for upright man as compared with other anthropoids. *Spine* 3:336-345, 1978.

179. Friberg S: Anatomical studies on lumbar disc degeneration. *Acta Orthop Scand* 17:224-230, 1948.

180. Rasch PJ, Burke RK: *Kinesiology and Applied Anatomy*. ed 3. Philadelphia, Lea and Febiger, 1967, p 375.

181. Nichols PJR: *Rehabilitation Medicine. The Management of Physical Disabilities*. ed 2. London, Butterworths, 1980, pp 110-116.

182. Giles LGF: Leg length inequalities associated with low back pain. *Journal of the Canadian Chiropractic Association* 20:25-32, 1976.

183. Morscher E: Etiology and pathophysiology of leg length discrepancies. In Hungerford DS (ed): *Leg Length Discrepancy. The Injured Knee* (Progress in Orthopedic Surgery, Vol 1) New York, Springer-Verlag, 1977, pp 9-19.

184. Dihlmann W: *Diagnostic Radiology of the Sacroiliac Joints*. Chicago, Year Book Medical Publishers, 1980, pp 92-93.

185. Gofton JP: Studies in osteoarthritis of the hip: Part IV Biomechanics and clinical considerations. *CMAJ* 104:1007-1011, 1971.

186. Pauwels F: *Biomechanics of the Normal and Diseased Hip* (translation of German 1973 edition) Berlin, Springer-Verlag, 1976.

187. Dixon AST, Campbell-Smith S: Long leg arthropathy. *Ann Rheum Dis* 28:359-365, 1969.

188. Hughes JL, Hogue RE: Basic rehabilitation principles of persons with leg length discrepancy: an overview. In Hungerford DS (ed): *Leg Length Discrepancy. The Injured Knee*. (Progress in Orthopedic Surgery, Vol 1) New York, Springer-Verlag, 1977, pp 3-8.

189. Wagner H: Surgical lengthening or shortening of femur and tibia. Techniques and indications. In Hungerford DS (ed): *Leg Length Discrepancy. The Injured Knee* (Progress in Orthopaedic Surgery, Vol 1). New York, Springer-Verlag, 1977, p 71.

190. Cailliet R: *Scoliosis Diagnosis and Management*. Philadelphia F.A. Davis, 1975, p 44.

191. Huskisson EC, Hart FD: *Joint Disease: All the Arthropathies*. ed 3. Bristol, John Wright and Sons, 1978.

192. Ladermann JP: About inequalities of the lower extremities. *Annals of the Swiss Chiropractors Association* 6:37-57, 1976.

193. Taylor JR, Halliday M: Limb length asymmetry and growth. *J Anat* 126:634-635, 1978.

194. Halliday M: Limb length asymmetry and scoliosis. Bachelor of science honors thesis, Department of Anatomy and Human Biology, University of Western Australia, Perth, Australia, 1976.

CHAPTER 2

Anatomy of the Lumbosacral Spine with Particular Reference to the Zygapophyseal Joints

The human vertebral column is a remarkable structure consisting of many parts, which should be considered as an integrated unit (1, 2). It combines strength and flexibility by alternately interposing rigid bony vertebrae with deformable cartilaginous discs (3). The intervertebral disc lives because of movement (4).

In the average adult male, the lumbar spine is 18 cm in length. Normally there are five lumbar vertebrae, each of which comprises two principal parts: (*a*) the posterior vertebral arch with its processes, and (*b*) the anterior vertebral body, which is composed of spongy bone covered by a thin layer of compact bone (5).

Motion Segment

Lewin et al (6) and Hirsch et al (7) pointed out that the basic anatomical and functional unit of the vertebral column is the articular triad, consisting of the fibrocartilaginous intervertebral joint and the two synovial zygapophyseal joints. The intervertebral joints in the spine are primarily responsible for (*a*) the flexibility of the spine, allowing a variety of movements such as flexion, extension, lateral bending, and axial rotation; and (*b*) load transmission and shock absorption, as a result of the mechanical properties of the disc (8, 9).

Joints between the Vertebral Bodies

The intervertebral discs are the largest avascular structures in the human body (10). They are load-bearing structures with a central gel-like nucleus enclosed by the lamellae of the anulus fibrosus (11). The intervertebral discs consist of three distinct and separate subunits: an outer lamellar anulus fibrosus (blending with the ring apophysis, via Sharpey's fibers, and the hyaline cartilage end-plates) which envelops a "semifluid" nucleus pulposus (12-14); this unique amphiarthrosis with its associated ligaments forms the strongest part of the mobile segment (15).

The anulus fibrous is inhomogeneous, while the nucleus pulposus is homogeneous and has a relatively high proportion of mucopolysaccharides causing it to behave as an incompressible fluid which is confined to a constant volume in a hydrostatic state of stress (5).

The fibers of the anulus fibrosus exhibit a biaxial orientation, which allows a variation in distance between vertebrae to accommodate the various modes of movement (16). The anulus fibrosus is able to contain high pressures and at the same time be compressed, rotated, or bent, because of its unique arrangement of collagen fibers (17).

The disc is unique as a compressive unit, because it shows stiffening with increasing force; also it becomes "stiffer" the faster it is loaded (18). Furthermore, the disc exhibits "creep"; that is, under constant compressive force it tends to compress with time (19). These observations were made on cadavers.

The hyaline cartilage end-plate is similar architecturally to the articular cartilage of synovial joints, and in discs of elderly patients in which the disc height is maintained, the end-plates are indistinguishable from younger discs (20).

The anterior and posterior longitudinal ligaments form ties between adjacent discs, and in addition, the anterior longitudinal ligament helps bind adjacent vertebral bodies together (15).

In early life the nucleus pulposus contains 80–90% water and the anulus fibrosus contains 78% water (21). There is a reduction in the water content of both the nucleus pulposus and the anulus fibrosus to approximately 70% with aging (22) and degeneration (23).

Because the intervertebral discs in the adult do not possess any blood vessels, they receive their nutrient substances merely by diffusion across the vertebral end-plate, and metabolic waste products are eliminated in a similar fashion (24, 25). The intradiscal space, cartilaginous plates, anulus fibrosus, paravertebral tissues, and spongiosa of the adjacent vertebrae constitute an osmotic system, and fluid shifts due to pressure, thereby promoting the exchange of substances in the disc (24).

Using fresh cadaveric lumbar motion segments, Nachemson et al (26) found that age does not seem to consistently affect the mechanical behavior of adult cadaveric lumbar motion segments in any pronounced way. However, female motion segments were somewhat more flexible than those of males in response to bending movements and compression loads.

Using cadaveric lumbar intervertebral joints subjected to physiologic loads to simulate flexion, Adams et al (27) found that flexion of a lumbar intervertebral joint is resisted primarily by the capsular ligaments of the zygapophyseal joints and by the intervertebral disc, with the ligamentum flavum and the interspinous and supraspinous ligaments making lesser contributions.

A more detailed review of the intervertebral disc and its associated structures is not required here since this text is primarily concerned with the anatomy and innervation of the "posterior element" structures.

Joints between the Vertebral Arches

Zygapophyseal Joints

The lumbar zygapophyseal joints lie posterolateral to the lumbar spinal canal and posterior to the intervertebral foramina or "canals" (28). The lumbar articular pro-

cesses and zygapophyseal joints, originally oriented in the coronal plane, assume their final form and orientation during childhood (29). These joints are approximately sagittally oriented in the upper lumbar spine, "rotating" toward the coronal plane at the lumbosacral junction (30, 31) (Fig. 2.1).

The lumbar zygapophyseal joints are "biplanar," with the major posterior parts of the joint approximated to the sagittal plane (32).

There is a wide range of variability of the lumbosacral joint planes in the horizontal plane, and asymmetry in the joint planes comparing left and right sides is common (33) (Fig. 2.2).

A relationship exists between the orientation of the zygapophyseal joints and the orientation of their related laminae; for example, at L5–S1 the zygapophyseal joints

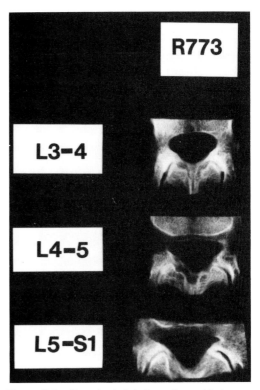

Figure 2.1. Superior-to-inferior radiographic images of the L3–S1 zygapophyseal joints of a 36-year-old female. Note that the horizontal plane of the L3–4 zygapophyseal joint is more sagittal than that of the L5–S1 zygapophyseal joint.

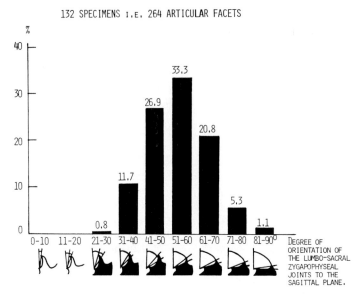

Figure 2.2   The variability of lumbosacral joint planes. (Modified from Cihak R: Variations of lumbosacral joints and their morphogenesis. *Acta Universitatis Carolinae Medica* 16:145-165, 1970.)

and the laminae are more coronally oriented (34).

The superior articular processes project upward, curving dorsally and laterally from the junction of the pedicle and upper margin of the lamina, and have a smooth concave cartilaginous articular surface averaging 10 × 18 mm in adults (35). On the posterior aspect of the base of the superior articular process, extending posteriorly, is a protuberance of variable size called the mamillary process (36), and at the base of the transverse process, posteriorly, is a small accessory process (37, 38). Between the mamillary and accessory processes a fibrous band, called the mamillo–accessory ligament (39, 40), usually bridges over a groove of variable depth forming a tunnel about 6 mm long (41). This ligament is occasionally ossified, rather than being fibrous (39), and can then be seen on radiographs (42). This tunnel transmits the medial branch of the posterior primary ramus, as it descends from the intervertebral canal immediately above (43), as well as small blood vessels to the posterior paraspinal muscles (37).

The zygapophyseal joint is a synovial joint which is formed by the convex laterally

facing inferior articular process of the upper vertebra and the concave medially facing superior articular process of the lower vertebra (5, 32, 44). It is a true diarthrodial joint, complete with a joint capsule and synovial lining (45). The *posterolateral fibrous capsule* of the zygapophyseal joint resembles that of other synovial joints, but the *medial capsule* is formed by the ligamentum flavum (7, 46). The joint "cavity" is normally potential rather than real because it contains only a very small volume of synovial fluid (47). Parts of the lumbar zygapophyseal joint synovial folds project into the joint cavity, particularly from the inferior recess (48–52). The normal appearance of L4–5 and L5–S1 zygapophyseal joint inferior recesses during arthrography showed that the inferior recess is much larger at L5–S1 than at L4–5, and the contrast medium appeared below the level of the lumbosacral joint capsule (48).

Each inferior articular recess lies caudal and anteromedial to the tip of the inferior articular process, where its location is identified by a conspicuous bony fossa on the dorsal surface of the adjacent lamina of the lower vertebra (6). The lateral boundary of this fossa is formed by a ridge of bone which runs from the lamina to the base of the superior articular process; the inferior recess of the lumbosacral joint is marked by a similar but larger fossa on the dorsal aspect of the sacrum (6).

Function of the Zygapophyseal Joints

The function of the lumbar zygapophyseal joints is to guide and restrain movement between vertebrae and to protect the discs from shear forces, excessive flexion, and axial rotation (32, 53, 54).

According to Hakim and King (55), who used an intervertebral load cell (a transducer [56] inserted into the inferior portion of a cadaveric lumbar vertebral body to deduce facet loads), normal lumbar facets may carry up to 40% of the incumbent body weight. Using a similar method, Yang and King (57) found that normal facets carry up to 25% of the incumbent body weight. Using cadaveric lumbar spines on a hydraulic servo-controlled testing machine, which gave outputs of applied force against deformation, Hutton and Adams (58) found that an average of 16% of the axial load is carried by the facets. It is difficult to account for the large discrepancy between these estimates obtained by different investigators. In cadaveric osteoarthritic joints, facet loading may increase to as high as 47% of the total axial load (57). According to Gregersen and Lucas (59), the lumbar facets are orientated so as to restrict axial rotation of the lumbar vertebral column to less than 9°, and the facets and the disc both play major roles in resisting axial torsion movements (60, 61). The restraints to movement at each joint are of two types: passive restraint (due to the articular facet orientation and resistance in joint capsules, the adjacent ligaments, and the intervertebral disc) and active restraint (provided by muscular contraction) (62). The principal plane of movement in the lumbosacral spine is flexion–extension (35).

Articular Cartilage of Zygapophyseal Joints

Hyaline articular cartilage is a highly specialized form of connective tissue which lines all sliding joint surfaces (63–66). Its chemical content and cell density vary in different parts of the same joint and at different depths within the tissue (67). Its histologic zones are shown in Figure 2.3.

Using scanning electron microscopy to examine the surface of hyaline articular cartilage from weight-bearing areas of adult rat femoral condyles, Bloebaum and Wilson (69) showed that the surface is smooth in the normal state.

Hyaline articular cartilage has a special shock-absorbing property which may be explained by the interaction among collagen, proteoglycans, and the extracellular fluid as a response to loading (70). Normal adult cartilage is composed of approximately 75% water and 25% solids (71–74). It is said to be an aneural and avascular tissue (75–79) except at its periphery (67). According to Kellgren and Samuel (80), articular cartilage gives rise to no sensation when it is stimulated. It is nourished by the synovial fluid, and in young cartilage, before the calcified zone is fully developed, the deeper parts of cartilage also receive nutrition from capillary loops in the underlying bone (78). Cartilage thickness varies in different parts of the same joint (81, 82), but it is generally thicker at the periphery of concave surfaces and at the center of convex surfaces (66). The combined thickness of the two articular cartilages across the center of the zygapophyseal joints in the lumbar spine is approximately 2–2.4 mm (49, 83).

According to Woessner et al (84) and von der Mark and Conrad (85), hyaline articular cartilage may be viewed in simplistic terms as a dense extracellular matrix populated by a sparse, diffuse population of chondrocytes; there is no direct cell-to-cell interaction (86). The major components of the matrix are long fibers of collagen which form an oriented meshwork and proteoglycans which fill the interstices of this meshwork. Benninghoff (87) described the arcade arrangement of collagen fibers in articular cartilage with fibers orientated perpendicular to the subchondral bone plate and arching round to become tangential to the articular cartilage surface.

Normal adult human articular cartilage contains only type II collagen (88), the functions of which are to protect the chondrocytes, provide attachment for proteoglycans, resist tensile stresses produced

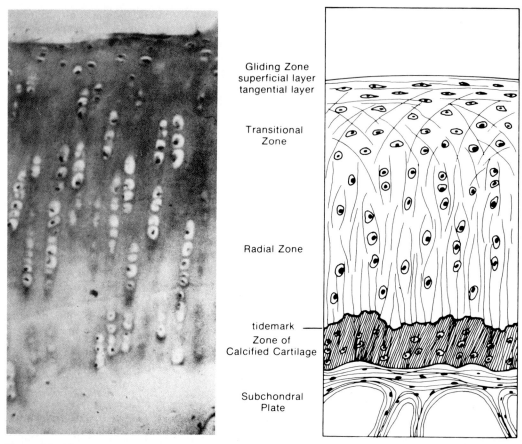

Gliding Zone
superficial layer
tangential layer

Transitional
Zone

Radial Zone

tidemark
Zone of
Calcified Cartilage

Subchondral
Plate

Figure 2.3 Histologic zones of adult articular cartilage. The predominant collagen bundle orientation changes from being horizontal in the gliding zone to vertical in the radial zone. (Reproduced with permission from Edwards CC, Chrisman OD: Articular cartilage. In Albright JA, Brand RA (eds): *The Scientific Basis of Orthopedics.* New York, Appleton-Century-Crofts, 1979, p 316.)

by compression, and anchor the cartilage to the subchondral bone (73, 89–92).

The calcified cartilage zone is the narrow band between the tide line and the compact lamellar subchondral bone which unites the articular cartilage to the subchondral bone and which contains some living cells (93). Articular cartilage is covered neither by perichondrium nor by synovial membrane (78). Cartilage, as a whole, serves to transmit loads and allows repetitive joint motion without breakdown (68, 79). Its elastic properties are essential to normal joint function (94, 95); its ability to deform under load achieves greater congruency between the opposing sides of the joint, thereby spreading the load over a greater surface area (68, 79). With active motion, there is compres-

sion of the articular cartilage in one area and decay of previous compression in another, resulting in a pumping action with movement of synovial fluid through the cartilage matrix, which aids in the nutrition of the chondrocytes as well as in the maintenance of proper joint lubrication (96). The compressive load-bearing properties of articular cartilage arise principally from the physiologic interplay between the collagen fibers and the hydrated proteoglycan complexes (97).

Zygapophyseal Joint Capsule

Lumbar zygapophyseal joint capsules differ from those of other synovial joints in having a quite unique capsular structure anteromedially—the ligamentum flavum—while posterolaterally having a typical fibrous capsule (7, 98, 99). The fibrous capsule is relatively loose above and below where it forms superior and inferior recesses which are filled with small synovial "fat pads" (6), and it is relatively thinner above and around the superior recess (54). The "capacity" of each joint capsule is 0.5–1 cm³ in the lower lumbar spine (31). The capsule is attached close to the dorsal and ventral margins of the joint (7). Fibrous strands from the interspinous ligament are said to reinforce the lower part of the dorsal capsule (54, 100). According to Farfan's (37) measurements, the average length of the capsular ligaments is 12.7 mm; however, it is difficult to distinguish them from the ligamentum flavum anteriorly and, in some areas, from the tendon of the multifidus posteriorly (53, 101).

The posterior capsule is predominantly fibrous; its cells are mainly fibrocytes or fibroblasts, with minimal ground substance, and its fibers are mainly white collagenous fibers, arranged in bundles of parallel fibers with a diameter of 0.3–0.5 μm (102). These fibers are seen by electron microscopy to consist of fine cross-banded fibrils of about 100 μm in diameter, with an axial periodicity of about 690 Ångstroms (102).

The fibrous capsule has a relatively poor blood supply; therefore, once it is damaged, it is slow to heal (102).

Multifidus Muscle

The mutifidus muscle covers the posterior joint capsule and the joint recesses (6, 7, 103, 104). A tendon of the multifidus muscle is clearly applied to the fibrous capsule as it crosses the joint to attach to the mamillary process and to the posterior aspect of the joint capsule (32, 53, 101, 102). Deep to the multifidus muscle there may be some adipose tissue which extends into the inferior recess of the joints (7).

The multifidus muscle consists of a number of fleshy and tendinous fasciculi which fill the groove beside the spines of the vertebrae from the sacrum to the axis; they are best developed in the lumbosacral region (105). Fasciculi are attached inferiorly to the back of the fourth sacral level, the posterior

sacroiliac ligament, and lumbar mamillary processes; they pass obliquely upwards and medially to an upper attachment to the whole length of the spinous process of a vertebra two or three segments above; the fasciculi vary in length, with the deepest fasciculi connecting contiguous vertebrae (105, 106).

Ligamentum Flavum

The ligamenta flava are a series of interlaminar ligaments located within the spinal canal (107, 108), covering most of the dorsal bony wall of the spinal canal (109, 110). Perpendicular fibers of yellow elastic tissue extend horizontally from the articular capsules laterally, to the midline where the laminae fuse to form the spinous process (105). Here, the ligamenta flava meet the membranous interspinous ligament posteriorly (99, 105, 111–113). Small midline intervals are present in the ligamenta flava for the passage of vessels (105). However, according to Brown (114), Ramsey (115), Kapandji (116), Ellis and Feldman (117), and Lee and Atkinson (118), the posterior margins of the ligamenta flava completely fuse in the midline. The fiber direction is said to be essentially longitudinal in the medial interlaminar portion and slightly oblique in the capsular portion (115, 119). The anteromedial border of each ligament passes around the joint, skirts the posterior edge of the intervertebral foramen (114) and forms its roof (115). The medial part of each ligament is thicker and unites the laminae, while the lateral thinner portion surrounds the joints and blends with their fibrous capsules (120).

In ventroflexion of the lumbar spine the ligamenta flava are stretched, while in lordosis the fibers of the ligamenta flava become slack and the cross-sectional thickness of the ligaments increases (121). These ligaments act to some degree as check ligaments in preventing hyperflexion, their elasticity serving to reestablish and maintain normal posture after flexion and rest (35). However, according to Twomey (110), the posterior ligaments play only a minor role in limiting ventroflexion and their main function is to maintain the posterolateral wall of the spinal canal smooth in all postures of the spine.

The ligamentum flavum not only has the structure and function of a ligament, but also acts as a fibrous capsule on the ventral surface of the lumbar zygapophyseal joint and as an elastic band keeping the spinal nerves free from compression when passing through the intervertebral canal during movements in the lumbar spine (7). The main function of the ligamentum flavum is probably to provide a smooth covering for the posterior part of the spinal canal in all positions of the spinal column (109).

Numerous measurement studies of the ligamentum flavum thickness variously report them as 2–10 mm thick (12, 49, 99, 111, 115, 122–127). The variation would depend, in part, on where the measurements were made (49). According to Horwitz (111), they are thickest at the L4–5 and L5–S1 levels, and their height varies from 1.0 to 2.0 cm (123).

Microscopically, the ligamenta flava consist of elastic connective tissue fibers (80%) with collagen fibers (20%) interspersed among the elastic fibers (115, 128). The elastic fibers measure about 1 μm in diameter and consist of fine, parallel fibers, without striations, when viewed by transmission electron microscopy (102). The adult ligamentum flavum is quite cell poor, and the basic cell appears to be the spindle-shaped fibrocyte (115).

The ligamentum flavum is described as having only a few irregularly dispersed blood vessels which are said to be capillaries and other small, thin-walled blood vessels (115). No lymphatics have been observed in the body of the ligamentum flavum (115, 122).

Structure and Function of Synovial Folds of Zygapophyseal Joints

Synovial Membrane

The synovial membrane which lines synovial folds is one of the characteristic features of synovial joints (63). It is a complex lining tissue (129, 130) which is necessary to maintain the normal function of the synovial joint; it is the conduit for the exchange of nutrients and waste between blood and the joint tissues, and its cells synthesize and secrete the proteins and pro-

teoglycans necessary for normal joint lubrication (131). The synovial membrane has three principal functions: (*a*) secretion of synovial fluid hyaluronate, (*b*) phagocytosis due to the phagocytic capacity of the "A" cells involved in the clearing of waste materials, and (*c*) regulation of the movement of solutes, electrolytes, and proteins (132). Normal synovium is sustained by low levels of glycolysis and oxidative metabolism (133).

The synovial membrane lines not only the inner surface of the fibrous articular capsule but also those intracapsular parts of the bone which are not covered by articular cartilage, and it extends around fat pads which fill joint recesses (102, 134, 135) (Fig. 2.4). There is no distinct basal membrane between the synovial lining membrane and the subsynovial tissue (131, 135, 136).

According to Barnett et al (102), the synovial membrane of synovial joints overlaps the nonarticular margins of the cartilage, becomes gradually thinner, then terminates without a clear line of demarcation. This overlapping part of the synovial membrane contains the "circulus articuli vasculosus," i.e., a fringe of looped vascular anastomoses. It is considerably more vascular than the fibrous periarticular structures supporting

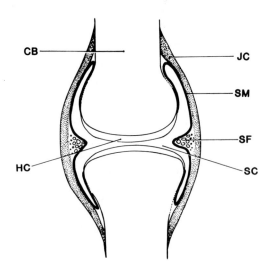

Figure 2.4. Synovial joint. CB = cancellous bone; HC = hyaline articular cartilage; JC = fibrous joint capsule; SC = synovial (joint) "cavity"; SF = synovial fold with synovial lining membrane and subsynovial tissue; SM = synovial lining membrane.

the joint, such as the capsule, ligaments, and tendons (137).

The *synovial membrane* usually consists of two parts (*a*) a lining layer bounding the joint space referred to as the *synovial lining* or the synovial intima (predominantly cellular with an abundant blood supply), and (*b*) a supportive or backing layer which should be called the subintima but is usually referred to as the *subsynovial layer* or subsynovial tissue (formed of loose fibrous connective tissue rich in blood vessels, lymphatics, and adipose tissue in varying proportions (75, 132, 138).

Synovial Lining (Intimal) Layer

The surface of the synovial membrane is smooth, moist, and glistening, with small villi and fringelike folds (75, 132, 139) (Fig. 2.5).

The cells of the synovial lining layer, which are secreting fibroblasts, form an intricate meshwork between the joint cavity and the underlying capillary bed (64, 140, 141). The synovial cells do not form a continuous compact layer like true epithelium (75); rather, they form a layer which varies

in depth, or they may be absent, leaving minute gaps in the synovial lining layer (142) (Fig. 2.6).

As seen by electron microscopy, the synovial lining is formed by 1–3 layers of cells of two types, i.e., A and B cells (144, 145). The A cells have a phagocytic function and the B cells probably represent different functional stages of the same cell type (145). This layer varies considerably in structure in different regions of the joint (138) (Fig. 2.7), and no stable intercellular attachments, such as tight junctions, are present (142).

Where the synovium lines extra-articular bone and the fibrous capsule, the subsynovial layer may be absent and the synovial lining layer blends into the intraarticular periosteum and the fibrous capsule (75).

Subsynovial (Subintimal) Layer

The structure of the subsynovial layer varies in different parts of the same joint (75); it can be fibrous, fibroareolar, areolar, or areolar–adipose (146). It is a loose fibrous connective tissue found in the synovial folds and is rich in blood vessels, lymphatics, and

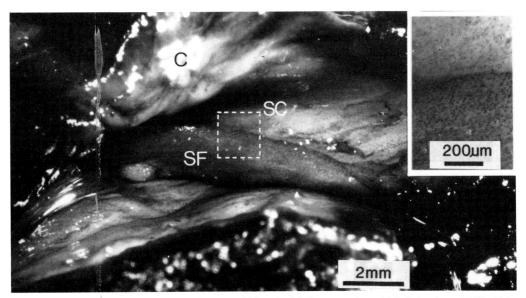

Figure 2.5. Fresh adolescent specimen (15-year-old female; L2–3 zygapophyseal joint) showing a fat-filled intra-articular synovial fold projecting from the posterior capsule into the joint cavity. The insert shows minute villi on the synovial fold and on the synovial lining of the joint cavity. C = joint capsule reflected; SC = synovial "cavity"; SF = synovial fold. (Immersed in 0.01% methylene blue.) (Reproduced with permission from Giles LFG, Taylor JR: Intra-articular synovial protrusions in the lower lumbar apophyseal joints. *Bull Hosp J Dis Orthop Inst* 42:248-255, 1982.)

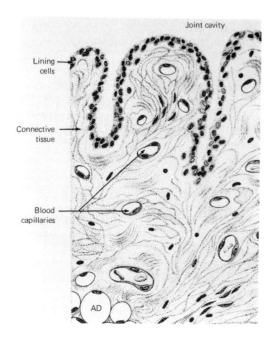

Figure 2.6. Histologic structure of synovial folds in general, with synovial lining cells in epitheloid arrangement. There is no basal lamina between the synovial lining cells and the underlying connective tissue, which is rich in capillaries and contains a variable amount of adipose cells (AD). (Modified from Cossermelli W: *Rheumatologia*. Basica, Sarvier, 1971, p 163.)

adipose tissue (64, 147), and the adipose cells form compact lobules, surrounded by vascular fibroelastic septa which impart firmness, deformability, and elastic recoil during joint movement (105). Sometimes it contains organized laminae of collagen and elastin fibers running parallel to the synovial lining surface (138). In addition to fibroblasts and lipocytes, the subsynovial tissue also contains macrophages (75) and mast cells (75, 147).

Compared with the synovial lining, the *subsynovial tissue* has received scant attention from electron microscopists apart from the studies by Ghadially and Roy (75), Giles et al (52), and Giles and Taylor (148) which showed two common types of subsynovial tissue, i.e, fibrous (characterized by innumerable bundles of collagen fibers) and fatty (made up of lipocytes interspersed with small amounts of fibrous tissue).

Synovial Folds

Synovial folds consist of a synovial lining layer with a subsynovial layer. The earliest appearance of a fold of synovial membrane in zygapophyseal joints is when the articular gap appears at the onset of ossification of the vertebral arches (in foetuses of 70-mm crown rump length) and a synovial fold is noted at the medial side of the joint, developing from a richly vascular interarticular mesenchyme (149).

Intra-articular synovial fold inclusions, which consist of various shapes and sizes and have numerous small blood vessels in fibrous connective tissue and adipose tissue, are described in all the zygapophyseal joints (12, 44, 47, 51, 98, 139, 149, 150–162) with maximum development in the mid-lumbar spine (149) and least frequency in the thoracic zygapophyseal joints. In addition to the synovial folds, intra-articular "mesenchymatous" menisci are also described, extending ventrally and dorsally into the zygapophyseal joints from the capsule (12, 163).

There is some controversy on the subject and nomenclature of "synovial folds" and "menisci" in zygapophyseal joints. According to Lewin et al (6), "true" mesenchymal intra-articular menisci are present in the zygapophyseal joints, and Engel and Bogduk (164, 165) refer to semi-lunar fibrous structures which remotely resemble menisci. According to Tondury (149), there are no "true" menisci in zygapophyseal joints and the embryologic development of a meniscus is quite different from that of synovial folds. Barnett et al (102) found "true" menisci or discs only in the knee, temporomandibular, sternoclavicular, wrist, and acromioclavicular joints in humans, while Fisher et al (166) found "fibrocollagenous" menisci in the finger joints of the hand.

Some confusion arises from variations in the histology of synovial folds themselves, related to their different functions. Areolar synovium is apparently adapted for greater movement, while "fibrous synovium" is generally seen in areas most subject to strain (144). The free irregular margins of the zygapophyseal joint synovial

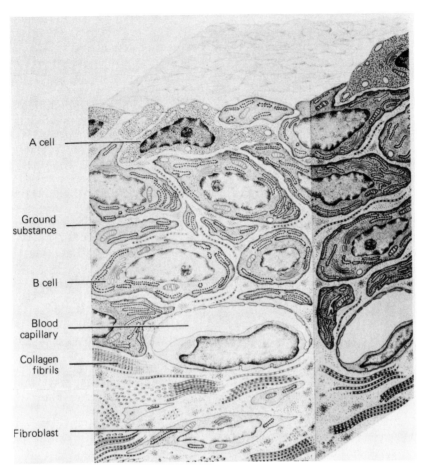

A cell

Ground
substance

B cell

Blood
capillary

Collagen
fibrils

Fibroblast

Figure 2.7.   Schematic representation of the ultrastructure of the synovial lining membrane in all synovial joints. A and B cell types are separated by a small amount of connective tissue ground substance. No basal lamina is seen separating the lining cells from the connective tissue. Blood capillaries are of the fenestrated type, which facilitates exchange of substances between blood and synovial fluid. (Reproduced with permission from Junqueira LC, Carneiro J, Long JA: *Basic Histology*, ed 5. Norwalk, CT, Appleton-Century-Crofts, 1986, p 164.)

folds may be quite long and thin (155) and frequently project between the articulating surfaces and are often fibrous at their tips (51, 139, 167, 168) or even "fibro-cartilaginous" (149, 169). Keller (152) could not find any cartilaginous metaplasia in the intra-articular synovial fold inclusions of intervertebral joints; however, he agreed that they may become fibrous as a result of being nipped within the joint (152). They are sometimes referred to as "meniscoid inclusions" (170).

Three types of intra-articular structures were identified by Engel and Bogduk (165)

in lumbar zygapophyseal joints, i.e., *adipose tissue pads* and *fibroadipose meniscoids* (both located at the superior and inferior poles of the joint) and *connective tissue rims* (located along the posterior and anterior ramus, when they examined human lumbar zygapophyseal joints, excluding the lumbosacral joints.

Function of the Synovial Folds

In addition to the general nutritive and lubricating functions of the synovial membrane, synovial folds have a packing or "space-filling" function which allows movement of adjacent structures (171). Thus, Tondury (149) maintains that the principal function of the synovial folds in zygapophyseal joints is to fill space between peripheral noncongruent parts of the articular surfaces, moving in and out of the joint freely in response to joint movement and forces. According to Hasselbacher (131), in synovial joints, the synovial membrane, with its villi and fat pads, is compressed by atmospheric pressure to conform to the outline of the articulating surfaces at all positions within the normal range of motion.

Wassilev (141) claims that, although the synovial membrane displays age-related changes, conditioning a reduction of the joint fluid elastoviscosity modulus in older individuals, it is endowed with regenerative potential for complete restoration of its ultrastructural and functional qualities.

Synovial Fluid

The synovial fluid (or synovia) is a viscous, pale yellow, clear fluid which consists of a dialysate of plasma, to which hyaluronate protein has been added as a result of secretion of the synovial lining cells (132). Nutrients flow through the synovial fluid to reach the articular cartilage, the source of the synovial fluid and its nutrients being the capillary bed surrounding the joint cavity and the capillaries occurring in the synovial membrane (172).

Only a film of synovial fluid separates the moving surfaces in joints, and the intra-articular cavity is primarily a potential space, containing so little free fluid (less than 1 ml in small joints), that none can be recovered from small joints by need aspiration (129, 132). The synovial fluid acts not only as a lubricant but also as an adhesive which helps to hold the articular cartilages in close apposition (129, 173).

Spinal Canal

In cross section, the lumbar spinal canal, which normally becomes progressively wider from L1 to L5, usually approximates to a triangular outline, but it can become trefoil in shape because incurved laminae and/or superior facets may encroach upon it (174). However, according to Eisenstein (175), a trefoil configuration is a common

nonpathologic condition, usually of the fifth lumbar vertebral canal, and is not necessarily dependent on or related to increasing age, osteophytosis, or spinal stenosis. The average transverse diameter of the spinal canal is 25 mm (107). The spinal canal encloses the spinal dural tube and its contents, the conus medullaris, cauda equina, and their blood vessels, bathed in cerebrospinal fluid (174). The extradural "space" is filled by varying amounts of fat, areolar tissue, and blood vessels (174), including the valveless extradural veins (176, 177). Hasue et al (178) also described an "epidural membrane," interposed between the dura and ligamentum flavum, as being continuous with an "epiradicular sheath" around the nerve roots. This has not been observed in other studies.

Intervertebral Canal

Standard anatomical textbooks such as *Gray's Anatomy* (105), *Cunningham's Textbook of Anatomy* (179), *A Colour Atlas of Human Anatomy* (180), and *Clinically Oriented Anatomy* (47) use the term "intervertebral foramina" to describe both the osseous nerve root canals and their medial and lateral "openings." However, Dommisse (107) suggests that the term "foramen" should only be used to describe the inner and outer boundaries of "intervertebral canals." The term "intervertebral canal" is used in this text since it appears to be a more accurate description of the structure.

The intervertebral canal length is approximately 9.1 mm at the L1–2 level and 21.9 mm at the L5–S1 level (110). The average superior-to-inferior diameter of the intervertebral canal at the lumbosacral level has been found to be 12 mm, while its average anteroposterior diameter is 7 mm (181) from the vertebral body to the ligamentum flavum. Postural changes result in variation of the size of this opening (121) which, in the lumbar area, is normally five to six times as large as the transverse area of the nerve passing through it (182), allowing for a generous reserve cushion (107, 183). However, Golub and Silverman (184), Bachop and Hilgendorf (185), and Bachop and Stern (186) described transforaminal ligaments, which are bands of tissue sometimes traversing lumbar intervertebral "foramina," which are commonest at L5 and which may encroach upon the nerve.

The spinal ganglion is located in the central or lateral part of the intervertebral canal (187–189).

References

1. Morris JM: Biomechanics of the spine. *Arch Surg (Chicago)* 107:418-423, 1973.
2. Hilton RC: Systematic studies of spinal mobility and Schmorl's nodes. In Jayson MIV (ed): *The Lumbar Spine and Back Pain*, ed 2. Kent, Pitman Medical, 1980, pp 115-134.
3. Taylor JR, Twomey L: Sagittal and horizontal plane movement of the human lumbar vertebral column in cadavers and in the living. *Rheumatology and Rehabilitation* 19:223-232, 1980.
4. Kraemer J, Kolditz D, Gowin R: Water and electrolyte content of human intervertebral discs under variable load. *Spine* 10:69-71, 1985.
5. Koreska J, Robertson D, Mills RH, Gibson DA, Albisser AM: Biomechanics of the lumbar spine and its clinical significance. *Orthop Clin North Am* 8:121-133, 1977.
6. Lewin T, Moffett B, Viidik, A: The morphology of the lumbar synovial intervertebral arches. *Acta Morphol Neerlando-Scandinavica* 4:299-319, 1961.
7. Hirsch C, Ingelmark BE, Miller M: The anatomical basis for low back pain. *Acta Orthop Scand* 33:1-17, 1963.
8. Lovett RW: The mechanism of the normal spine and its relation to scoliosis. *N Eng J Med* 153:349-359, 1905.
9. Shah JS: Structure, morphology and mechanics of the lumbar spine. In Jayson MIV (ed): *The Lumbar Spine and Back Pain*, ed 2. Kent, Pitman Medical, 1980, pp 359-406.
10. Nachemson AL: Advances in low-back pain. *Clin Orthop* 200:266-278, 1985.
11. Jenkins JPR, Hickey DS, Zhu XP, Machin M, Isherwood BA, Isherwood I: MR imaging of the intervertebral disc: a quantitative study. *Br J Rheumatol* 58:705-709, 1985.
12. Schmorl G, Junghanns H: *The Human Spine in Health and Disease*, ed 2. New York, Grune and Stratton, 1971, p 23, 28, 188.
13. Johnson EF, Berryman H, Mitchell R, Wood WB: Elastic fibres in the anulus fibrosus of the adult human lumbar intervertebral disc. A preliminary report. *J Anat* 143:57-63, 1985.
14. Pope MH: Biomechanical properties of the intervertebral disc. In Buerger AA, Greenman PE (eds): *Empirical Approaches to the Validation of Spinal Manipulation*. Springfield, IL, Charles C. Thomas, 1985, pp 30-41.
15. Taylor JR: Growth and development of the human intervertebral disc. Ph.D. thesis, Edinburgh University, Edinburgh, 1973.
16. Naylor A, Shentall RD, Nucklethwaite B: An electron microscopic study of the segment long spacing collagen from the intervertebral disc. *Orthop Clin* 8:217-223, 1977.
17. Eyre DR: Biochemistry of the intervertebral disc. In Hall DA, Jackson DS (eds): *International Review of Connective Tissue Research*. New York, Academic Press, 1979, Vol 8, pp 227-291.
18. Markolf KL: Stiffness and clamping characteristics of the thoraco-lumbar spine. In: *Proceedings of Workshop on Bioengineering Approaches to the Problems of the Spine*. Bethesda, MD, National Institutes of Health, 1970.
19. Markolf KL, Morris JM: The structural components of the intervertebral disc: a study of their contributions of the ability of the disc to withstand compressive forces. *J Bone Joint Surg* 56A:675-687, 1974.
20. Pritzker KPH: Aging and degeneration in the lumbar intervertebral disc. *Clin Orthop North Am* 8:65-77, 1977.
21. Naylor A, Horton WG: The hydrophilic properties of the nucleus pulposus of the intervertebral disc. *Rheumatism* 11:32-35, 1955.
22. Gower WE, Pedrini V: Age-related variations in proteinpolysaccharides from human nucleus pulposus, annulus fibrosus, and costal cartilage. *J Bone Joint Surg* 51A:1154-1162, 1969.
23. Lipson SJ, Muir, H: Proteoglycans in experimental intervertebral disc degeneration. *Spine* 6:194-218, 1981.
24. Kramer J: Pressure dependent fluid shifts in the intervertebral disc. *Orthop Clin North Am* 8:211-216, 1977.
25. Katz MM, Hargens AR, Garfin SR: Intervertebral disc nutrition. Diffusion versus convection. *Clin Orthop* 210:243-245, 1986.
26. Nachemson AL, Schulz AB, Berkson MH: Mechanical properties of human lumbar spine motion segments. Influences of age, sex, disc level and degeneration. *Spine* 4:1-8, 1979.
27. Adams MA, Hutton WC, Scott JRR: The resistance to flexion of the lumbar intervertebral joint. *Spine* 5:245-253, 1980.
28. Baddeley H: Radiology of lumbar spinal stenosis. In Jayson M (ed): *The Lumbar Spine and Back Pain*. London, Sector Publishing, 1976, pp 151-172.
29. Lutz G: Die Entwicklung der kleinen Wirbelgelenke. *Z Orthop* 104:19-28, 1967.
30. Pheasant HC: Sources of failure in laminectomies. *Orthop Clin North Am* 6:319-329, 1975.
31. Park WM: The place of radiology in the investigation of low back pain. *Clin Rheum Dis* 6:93-132, 1980.
32. Taylor JR, Twomey L: Age changes in lumbar zygapophyseal joints: observations on structure and function. *Spine* 11:739-745, 1986.
33. Cihak R: Variations of lumbosacral joints and their morphogenesis. *Acta Universitatis Carolinae Medica* 16:145-165, 1970.
34. Van Schaik JPJ, Verbiest H, van Schaik FDJ: The orientation of laminae and facet joints in the lower lumbar spine. *Spine* 20:59-63, 1985.
35. Weinstein PR, Ehni G. Wilson CB: Clinical features of lumbar spondylosis and stenosis. In Weinstein PR, Ehni G, Wilson CB (eds): *Lumbar Spondylosis, Diagnosis, Management and Surgical Treatment*. Chicago, Year Book Medical Publishers, 1977, pp 115-133.
36. Rauschning W: Computed tomography and cryomicrotomy of lumbar spine specimens. *Spine* 8:170-180, 1983.
37. Farfan, HF: *Mechanical Disorders of the Low Back*. Philadelphia, Lea and Febiger, 1973, pp 21.
38. Gardner E, Gray DJ, O'Rahilly R: *Anatomy and Regional Study of Human Structure*. ed 4. Philadelphia, W.B. Saunders, 1975.
39. Bogduk N: The lumbar mamillo-accessory ligament: its anatomical and neurological significance. *Spine* 6:162-167, 1981.
40. Francois RJ, Bywaters EGL, Aufdermaur M: Illustrated glossary for spinal anatomy. *Rheumatol Int* 5:241-245, 1985.
41. Bradley KC: The anatomy of backache. *Aust NZJ Surg* 44:227-232, 1974.
42. Koehler A, Zimmer EA: *Borderlands of the normal and*

early pathologic skeletal radiology. ed 3. Translated and edited by Wilk SP. New York, Grune and Stratton, 1968.

43. Bogduk N, Wilson AS, Tynan W: The lumbar dorsal rami. *J Anat* 134:383-397, 1982.
44. Hadley LA: Anatomico-roentgenographic studies of the posterior spinal articulations. *AJR* 86:270-276, 1961.
45. Keim HA: Low back pain. *Ciba Clinical Symposia* 25:4, 9, 1973.
46. Hadley LA: *Anatomico-Roentgenographic Studies of the Spine*. Springfield, IL, Charles C. Thomas, 1964, p 179.
47. Moore KL: *Clinically Oriented Anatomy*, ed 2. Baltimore, Williams & Wilkins, 1985, pp 35-36.
48. Giles LGF: Lumbar apophyseal joint arthrography. *J Manipulative Physiol Ther* 7:21-24, 1984.
49. Giles LGF, Taylor JR: The effect of postural scoliosis on lumbar apophyseal joints. *Scand J Rheumatol* 13:209-220, 1984.
50. Giles LGF, Taylor JR: Osteoarthrosis in human cadaveric lumbo-sacral zygapophyseal joints. *J Manipulative Physiol Ther* 8:239-243, 1985.
51. Giles LGF: Lumbo-sacral and cervical zygapophyseal joint inclusions. *Manual Medicine* 2:89-92, 1986.
52. Giles LGF, Taylor JR, Cockson A: Human zygapophyseal joint synovial folds. *Acta Anat* 126:110-114, 1986.
53. Adams MA, Hutton WC: The mechanical function of the lumbar apophyseal joints. *Spine* 8:327-330, 1983.
54. Putz R: The functional morphology of the superior articular processes of the lumber vertebrae. *J Anat* 143:181-187, 1985.
55. Hakim NS, King AI: Static and dynamic articular facet loads. In: *Proceedings, 20th STAPP Car Crash Conference*. 1976, pp 609-637.
56. Prasad P, King I, Denton RA, Begeman PC: Intervertebral force transducer. In: *Proceedings of the 10th International Conference of Medical Biological Engineers*. Dresden, Medical Biological Engineers, 1973, p 137.
57. Yang KH, King AI: Mechanism of facet load transmission as a hypothesis for low back pain. *Spine* 9:559-565, 1984.
58. Hutton WC, Adams MA: The forces acting on the neural arch and their relevance to low back pain. In: *Engineering Aspects of the Spine*. London, Mechanical Engineering Publications, 1980, pp 49-55.
59. Gregersen GG, Lucas DB: An in vivo study of axial rotation of the human thoracolumbar spine. *J Bone Joint Surg* 49A:247, 1967.
60. Farfan HF: Biomechanics of the lumbar spine. In Kirkaldy-Willis (ed): *Managing Low Back Pain*, New York, Churchill Livingstone, 1983, pp 9-21.
61. Tencer AF, Mayer TG: Soft tissue strain and facet face interaction in the lumbar intervertebral joint. II: Calculated results and comparison with experimental data. *J Biomech Eng* 105:210-215, 1983.
62. Smeathers JE, Biggs WD: Mechanics of the spinal column. In: *Engineering Aspects of the Spine*. London, Mechanical Engineering Publications, 1980, pp 103-109.
63. Walmsley R: Joints. In Romanes GJ (ed): *Cunningham's Textbook of Anatomy*, ed 11. London, Oxford University Press, 1972, p 211.
64. Rhodin JAG: *Histology: A Text and Atlas*. London, Oxford University Press, 1974, pp 200, 340-362.
65. Mankin HJ: Localization of Tritiated thymedine in articular cartilage of rabbits. III. Mature articular cartilage. *J Bone Joint Surg* 45A:529, 1975.
66. Bullough PG: Pathologic changes associated with the common arthritides and their treatment. *Pathol Ann* 2:14, 69-83, 1979.
67. Stockwell RA: *Biology of Cartilage Cells*. Cambridge,

Cambridge University Press, 1979, p 1.
68. Edwards CC, Chrisman OD: Articular cartilage. In Albright JA, Brand RA (ed): *The Scientific Basis of Orthopedics*. New York, Appleton-Century-Crofts, 1979, pp 315-347.
69. Bloebaum RD, Wilson AS: The morphology of the surface of articular cartilage in adult rats. *J Anat* 131:333-346, 1980.
70. Christensen SB: Osteoarthritis. *Acta Orthop Scand Sup* 214, 56:1-43, 1985.
71. Brower TD, Hsu W-Y: Normal articular cartilage. *Clin Orthop* 64:9-17, 1969.
72. Frost H: *The Physiology of Cartilaginous, Fibrous and Bony Tissue* (Orthopedic Lecures II). Springfield, IL, Charles C. Thomas, 1972, p 63.
73. Serafini-Fracassini MD, Smith JW: *The Structure and Biochemistry of Cartilage*. Edinburgh, Churchill Livingstone, 1974, p 21.
74. Ross MH, Reith EJ: *Histology: A Text and Atlas*. New York, Harper and Row, 1985, p 120.
75. Ghadially FN, Roy S: *Ultrastructure of Synovial Joints in Health and Disease*. London, Butterworths, 1969, p 1-48.
76. Ham AW, Cormack DH: *Histology*. ed 8. Philadelphia, J.B. Lippincott, 1979, pp 476, 642.
77. Mears DC: *Materials and Orthopedic Surgery*. Baltimore, Williams & Wilkins, 1979, pp 162-181.
78. Ghadially FN: Structure and function of articular cartilage. *Clin Rheum Dis* 7:3-28, 1981.
79. Malemud CJ, Moskowitz RW: Physiology of articular cartilage. *Clinc Rheum Dis* 7:29-55, 1981.
80. Kellgren JH, Samuel EP. The sensitivity and innervation of the articular capsule. *J Bone Joint Surg* 32B:84-92, 1950.
81. Simon A: Scale effects in animal joints. I. Articular cartilage thickness and compressive stress. *Arthritis Rheum* 13:244-256, 1970.
82. Gardner DL: Structure and function of connective tissue joints. In Scott JT (ed): *Copeman's Textbook of the Rheumatic Diseases*. ed 5. London, Churchill Livingstone, 1978, pp 78-124.
83. Fick R: *Handbuch der Anatomie und Mechanik der Gelenke, II.* Jena, Verlag G. Fischer, 1904, pp 77-89.
84. Woessner FF, Sapolsky AI, Nagase H, Howell DS: Role of proteolytic enzymes in cartilage matrix breakdown in osteoarthritis. *Arthritis Rheum* 20:116-123, 1977.
85. von der Mark K, Conrad G: Cartilage cell differentiation. *Clin Orthop* 139:185-205, 1979.
86. Kuettner KL, Harper E, Eisenstein R: Protease inhibitors in cartilage. *Arthritis Rheum* 20:124-132, 1977.
87. Benninghoff A: Form und Bau der Gelenk-knorpel in Ihren Beziehungen zur Funktion, *Z Anat Entwicklungsgesch* 76:43, 1925.
88. Goldwasser M, van der Rest M, Glorieux FH: The collagen composition in osteoarthritic human cartilage. In: *Transactives of the 24th Annual Meeting of the Orthopedic Research Society*. Dallas, TX, Orthopedic Research Society, 1978, Vol 3, p 139.
89. Kempson GE, Fregman MAR, Sevanson SAV: Tensile properties of articular cartilage. *Nature* 220: 1127, 1968.
90. MacConaill MA: The movement of bones and joints 4. The mechanical structure of articulating cartilage. *J Bone Surg* 33B:251, 1951.
91. Maroudas A: Balance between swelling pressure and collagen tension in normal and degenerate cartilage. *Nature* 260:808, 1976.
92. Weightman B: Tensile fatigue and human articular cartilage. *J Biomech* 9:133, 1976.
93. Kenzora JE, Yosipovitch Z, Glimcher MJ: The calcified cartilage zone of adult articular cartilages: a

viable functional entity. In: *Transactives of the 24th Annual Meeting of the Orthopedic Research Society*. Dallas, TX, Orthopedic Research Society, 1978, Vol 3, p 73.

94. Dintenfass L: Lubrication in synovial joints: a theoretical analysis. *J Bone Joint Surg* 45A:1241, 1963.

95. McCutchen CW: Animal joints and weeping lubrication. *New Scientist* 15:412, 1962.

96. Kopta JA, Blosser JA: Elasticity of articular cartilage. *Clin Orthop* 64:21-32, 1969.

97. Broom ND: Further insights into the structural principles governing the function of articular cartialge. *J Anat* 139:275-294, 1984.

98. Keller G: Die Bedeutung der Veranderungen an den kleinen Wirbelgelenken als Ursache des lokalen Ruckenschmerzes. *Z Orthop* 83:517-547, 1953.

99. Reilly J, Yong-Hing K, MacKay RW, Kirkaldy-Willis WH: Pathological anatomy of the lumbar spine. In Helfet AJ, Gruebel DM (ed): *Disorders of the Lumbar Spine*. Philadelphia, J.B. Lippincott, 1978, pp 26-50.

100. Prestar FJ: Morphologie and Funktion der Ligamenta interspinalia und des Ligamentum supraspinale der Lendenwirbelsaul. *Morphologia Medica* 2:53-58, 1982.

101. Cyron BM, Hutton WC: The tensile strength of the capsular ligaments of the apophyseal joints. *J Anat* 132:145-150, 1981.

102. Barnett CH, Davies DV, MacConaill MA: *Synovial Joints: Their Structure and Mechanics*. London, Longmans, 1961, pp 24, 48, 50.

103. Lewin T: Osteoarthritis in lumbar synovial joints. *Acta Orthop Scand* 72:1-111, 1964.

104. Bogduk N: *The Lumbar Zygapophysial Joints* (proceedings of low back pain symposium). Australia, Syndey, 1979, pp 32-40.

105. Williams PL, Warwick T: *Gray's Anatomy*. ed 36. London, Churchill Livingstone, 1980, pp 271, 427, 445, 545.

106. Quiring DP, Warfel JW: *The Head, Neck, and Trunk: Muscles and Motor Points*. London, Henry Kimpton, 1960, p 57.

107. Dommisse GF: Morhological aspects of the lumbar spine and lumbo-sacral region. *Ortho Clin North Am* 6:153-175, 1975.

108. Levine DB: The painful low back. In McCarthy DJ (ed): *Arthritis and Allied Conditions*, ed 9. Philadelphia, Lea and Febiger, 1979, pp 1044-1079.

109. Rolander SD: Motion of the lumbar spine with special reference to the stabilizing effect of posterior fusion. *Acta Orthop Scand Suppl* 90, 1966.

110. Twomey LT: *Age changes in the human lumbar vertebral column*. Ph.D. thesis, Department of Anatomy and Human Biology, University of Western Australia, Perth, 1981.

111. Horwitz T: Lesions of the intervertebral disc and ligamentum flavum of the lumbar vertebrae: anatomic study of 75 human cadavers. *Surgery* 6:410-425, 1939.

112. Heylings DJA: Supraspinous and interspinous ligaments of the human lumbar spine. *J Anat* 125:127-131, 1978.

113. Fairbank JCT, O'Brien JP: The abdominal cavity and thoraco-lumbar fascia as a stabiliser of the lumbar spine in patients with low back pain. In: *Engineering Aspects of the Spine*. London, Mechanical Engineering Publications, 1980, pp 83-88.

114. Brown HA: Enlargement of the ligamentum flavum. *J Bone Joint Surg* 20: 325-338, 1938.

115. Ramsey RH: The anatomy of the ligamenta flava. *Clin Orthop* 44:129-140, 1966.

116 Kapandji IA: The physiology of the joints. *The Trunk and the Vertebral Column*. Edinburgh, Churchill Livingstone, 1974, Vol 3, p 78.

117. Ellis H, Feldman S: *Anatomy for Anaesthetists*. ed 3.

118. Lee JA, Atkinson RS (ed): *Sir Robert Mackintosh's Lumbar Puncture and Spinal Analgesia, Intradural and Extradural*. ed 4. Edinburgh, Churchill Livingstone, 1978, pp 24-70.

119. Naffziger HC, Inman V, Saunders JB: Lesions of the intervertebral disc and ligamenta flava. *Surg Gynecol Obstet* 66:288-299, 1938.

120. Epstein B: *The Spine. A Radiological Text and Atlas,* ed 4, Philadelphia, Lea and Febiger, 1976.

121. Breig A: *Biomechanics of the Central Nervous System.* Stockholm, Almqvist and Wiksell, 1960.

122. Dockerty MB, Love JG: Thickening and fibrosis (so-called hypertrophy) of the ligamentum flavum: a pathological study of fifty cases. *Proc Staff Meet Mayo Clinic* 15:161-166, 1940.

123. Herzog W: Morphologie and pathologie des ligamentum flavum. *Frankfurter Zeitschrift fur Pathologie* 61:250-267, 1950.

124. Crawford JS: *Principles and Practice of Obstetric Anaesthesia*. ed 4. Oxford, Balckwell Scientific Publications, 1978, p 170.

125. Moir DD: *Obstetric Anaesthesia and Analgesia*. ed 2. London, Balliere Tindall, 1980, p 192.

126. Giles LGF: Leg length inequality with postural scoliosis: its effect on lumbar apophyseal joints. M.Sc. thesis, Department of Anatomy and Human Biology, University of Western Australia, Perth, 1982.

127. Parkin IG, Harrison GR: The topographical anatomy of the lumbar epidural space. *J Anat* 141:211-217, 1985.

128. Kirkaldy-Willis WH, Heithoff KB, Tchang S, Bowen CVA, Cassidy JD, Shannon R: Lumbar spondylosis and stenosis: correlation of pathological anatomy with high resolution computed tomographic scanning. In Post MJD (ed): *Computed Tomography of the Spine*. Baltimore, Williams & Wilkins, 1984, pp 495-505.

129. Simkin PA: Synovial Physiology. In McCarthy DJ (ed): *Arthritis and Allied Conditions*. ed 9. Philadelphia, Lea and Febiger, 1979, pp 167-178.

130. Simkin PA, Nilson KL: Trans-synovial exchange of large and small molecules. *Clin Rheum Dis* 7:99-129, 1981.

131. Hasselbacher P: Structure of the synovial membrane. *Clin Rheum Dis* 7:57-69, 1981.

132. Paget S, Bullough PG: Synovium and synovial fluid. In Owen R, Goodfellow J, Bullough P (eds): *Scientific Foundations of Orthopaedics and Traumatology*. London, William Heinemann Medical Books, 1980, pp 18-22.

133. Taylor T: Glucose metabolism and respiration. *Clin Rheum Dis* 7:167-175, 1981.

134. Collins DH: *The Pathology of Articular and Spinal Diseases*. London, Edward Arnold, 1949.

135. Dieppe P, Calvert P: *Crystals and Joint Disease*. London, Chapman and Hall, 1983, p 14.

136. Efskind I: Anatomy and physiology of the joint capsule. *Acta Orthop Scand* 12:214-260, 1941.

137. Liew M, Dick WC: The anatomy and physiology of blood flow in a diarthrodial joint. *Clin Rheum Dis* 7:131-148, 1981.

138. Davies DV: Structure and function of synovial membrane. *Br Med J* 1:92-95, 1950.

139. Giles LGF, Taylor JR: Intra-articular synovial protrusions in the lower lumbar apophyseal joints. *Bull Hosp* 42:248-255, 1982.

140. Barland P, Novikoff AB, Hamerman D: Electron microscopy of the human synovial membrane. *J Cell Biol* 14:207-220, 1962.

141. Wassilev W: Funktionelle struktur der synovial mem-

bran. *Verh Anat Ges* 75:221-234, 1981.
142. Hadler NM: The biology of the extracellular space. *Clin Rheum Dis* 7:71-97, 1981.
143. Cossermelli W: *Rheumatologia* Basica, Sarvier, 1971.
144. Schumacher HR: Ultrastructure of the synovial membrane. *Ann Clin* 5:489-498, 1975.
145. Junqueira LC, Carneiro J, Long JA: *Basic Histology*, ed 5. Norwalk, CT, Appelton-Century-Crofts, 1986, pp 201-303.
146. Castor CW: The microscopic structure of normal human synovial tissue. *Arthritis Rheum* 3:140, 1960.
147. Shaw NE, Martin BF: Histological and histochemical studies on mammalian knee joint tissues. *J Anat* 96:359, 1962.
148. Giles LGF, Taylor JR: Human zygapophyseal joint capsule and synovial fold innervation. *Br J Rheumatol* 26:93-98, 1987.
149. Tondury G: Anatomie fonctionelle des petites articulations de rachis. *Ann Med Physique* 15:173-191, 1972.
150. Schmincke A, Santo E: Zur normalen und pathologischen anatomie der halswirbelsaule. *Zbl allg Path path Anat* 55:369-372, 1932.
151. Tondury G: Beitrag zur Kenntniss der kleinen Wirbelgelenke. *Z Anat Entw Gesch* 110:568-575, 1940.
152. Keller G: Die Arthrose der Wirbelgelenke in ihrer Beziehung zum Ruckenschmerz. *Zeitschrift fur Orthopadie* 91:538-550, 1959.
153. Dorr W: Uber die Anatomie der Wirbelgelenke. *Arch Orthop Unfall Chir* 50:222-243, 1958.
154. Dorr W: Nochmals zu den Menisci in der Wirbelbogengelenken. *Z Orthop* 96:457-461, 1962.
155. Hadley LA: *Anatomico-Roentgenorgraphic Studies of the Spine.* Springfield, IL, Charles C. Thomas, 1976, pp 175, 186, 187.
156. Grant JCB: *Grant's Atlas of Anatomy.* ed 5. Baltimore, Williams & Wilkins, 1962, p 385.
157. DeMarchi FG: Le articolazioni intervertebrali studio anatomo-istologica. *Clinica Ortopedica* 15:26-33, 1963.
158. Penning L, Tondury B: Entstehung Bau and Funktion der meniscoiden Strukturen in den Halswirbelgelenken. *Z Orthop* 98:1-14, 1963.
159. Kos J: Contribution a l'etude de l'anatomie et de la vascularisation des articulations intervertebrales. *Bull Assoc Anat Berlin* 152:1.088-1.105, 1969.
160. Benini A: Das Kleine Gelenk der Lendenwirbelsaule. *Fortschr Med* 97:2103-2106, 1979.
161. Putz R: Funktionelle Anatomie der Wirbelgelenke. In: *Normale und Pathologische Anatomie* Stuttgart, George Thieme Verlag, 1981, Vol 43, pp 31, 32.
162. Rickenbacker J, Landolt AM, Theiler K: *Applied Anatomy.* Berlin, Springer-Verlag, 1985, pp 30, 31.
163. Lewin T: Anatomical variations in lumbosacral synovial joints with particular reference to subluxation. *Acta Anat* 71:229-248, 1968.
164. Engel RM, Bogduk N: The menisci of the lumbar zygapophyseal joints. Presented at the annual conference of the *Anatomical Society of Australia and New Zealand,* University of Sydney, Sydney, Australia, 1980.
165. Engel RM, Bogduk N: The menisci of the lumbar zygapophyseal joints. *J Anat* 135:795-809, 1982.
166. Fisher DM, Elliott S, Cooke TDV, Forrest WJ: Descriptive anatomy of fibrocartilaginous menisci in the finger joints of the hand. *J Orthop Res* 3:484-489, 1985.
167. Jee WSS: The skeletal tissues. In Weiss L (ed): *Histology: Cell and Tissue Biology,* ed 5. New York, Macmillan, 1983, p 254.
168. Kirkaldy-Willis WH: The relationship of structural pathology to the nerve root. *Spine* 9:49-52, 1984.
169. Kos J, Wolf J: Les Menisques Intervertebraux et leur Role Possible dans les Blocages Vetebraux. *Annals de Medecine Physique* 15:203-217, 1972.
170. Bourdillon JF: *Spinal Manipulation.* ed 2. London, William Heinemann Medical Books, 1973, pp 22-23.
171. Edwards JCW: The structure and function of normal synovial membrane. (Abstracts Supplement) 25:47, 1986.
172. Knight AD, Levick J: The density and distribution of capillaries around a synovial cavity. *Q J Exper Physiol* 68:629-644, 1983.
173. Semlak K, Ferguson AB: Joint stability maintained by atmospheric pressure. *Clin Orthop* 68:294-300, 1970.
174. McRae DL: Radiology of the lumbar spinal canal. In Weinstein PR, Ehni G, Wilson CB (eds): *Lumbar Spondylosis. Diagnosis. Management and Surgical Treatment.* Chicago, Year Book Medical Publishers, 1977, pp 92-114.
175. Eisenstein S: The trefoil configuration of the lumbar vertebral canal. *J Bone Joint Surg* 62B:73-77, 1980.
176. Batson OV: The vertebral vein system. *AJR* 78:195-212, 1957.
177. Shapiro R: *Myelography.* ed 3. Chicago, Year Book Medical Publishers, 1975, pp 77-94.
178. Hasue M, Kikuchi S. Sakuyama Y, Ito T: Anatomic study of the interrelation between nerve roots and their surrounding tissues. *Spine* 8:50-58, 1983.
179. Romanes CJ: *Cunningham's Textbook of Anatomy,* ed 12. Oxford, Oxford University Press, 1981, pp 207-257.
180. McMinn RHM, Hutchings RT: *A Colour Atlas of Human Anatomy.* London, Wolf Medical Publications, 1977, p 90.
181. Magnuson PD: Differential diagnosis of causes of pain in the lower back accompanied by sciatic pain. *Ann Surg* 179:878, 1944.
182. Epstein JA: Diagnosis and treatment of painful neurological disorders caused by spondylosis of the lumbar spine. *J Neurosurg* 17:991-1001, 1960.
183. Sunderland S: Mechanisms of cervical root avulsion in injuries of the neck and shoulder. *J Neurosurg* 51:705-714, 1974.
184. Golub B, Silverman B: Transforaminal ligaments of the lumbar spine. *J Bone Joint Surg* 51A:947-956, 1969.
185. Bachop W, Hilgendorf C: Transforaminal ligaments of the human lumbar spine. *Anat Rec* 199:144, 1981.
186. Bachop W, Stern H: Transforaminal ligaments and the straight leg raising test of Lasegue. In: *Twelfth Annual Biomechanics Conference on the Spine.* Boulder, CO, University of Colorado Biomechanics Laboratory, 1981, pp 281-294.
187. Haughton VM, Williams AL: *Computed Tomography of the Spine.* St. Louis, C.V. Mosby, 1982, p 88.
188. Rydevik B, Brown MD, Lundborg G: Pathoanatomy and pathophysiology of nerve root compression. *Spine* 9:7-15, 1984.
189. Vanderlinden RG: Subarticular entrapment of the dorsal root ganglion as a cause of sciatic pain. *Spine* 9:19-22, 1984.

CHAPTER **3**

Studies of the L4–5 and L5–S1 Zygapophyseal Joints and Their Associated Structures

In order to further investigate the detailed anatomy of the L4–5 and L5–S1 zygapophyseal joints, the anatomical studies I have conducted are discussed in this and following chapters.

Examination of the Synovial Folds from Lumbar Zygapophyseal Joints of Dissecting Room Cadavers

Appearance of Synovial Folds in Situ

Five embalmed cadavers, (aged 33–90 years; mean = 71 years) were used for this gross dissection study. Each of the posterolateral fibrous capsules from five lumbosacral zygapophyseal joints was vertically incised from the superior recess to the inferior recess, and then the facets were reflected laterally, so that the synovial fold inclusion

within each inferomedial joint recess was demonstrated in situ (Fig. 3.1). The synovial folds were then excised. A synovial fold, following excision, is shown in Figure 3.2.

The fat-filled synovial folds project from the inferior joint recesses up into the joint cavity. These appear, in fixed cadaver specimens, as white, glistening, and partly translucent folds. At the lumbosacral joint they are about 2.7 mm in width and depth at their bases, tapering along their intracapsular 8–10 mm length to a fine narrow tip which usually lies between the articular surfaces.

The inferomedial joint recess, from which the synovial fold in Figure 3.2 was removed, is shown in Figure 3.3

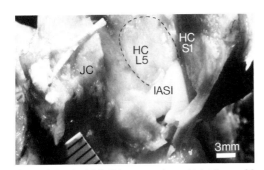

Figure 3.1. Left L5–S1 zygapophyseal joint from a 33-year-old male subject opened out to display the synovial fold in situ in the inferior recess. HCL5 = hyaline articular cartilage on the L5 inferior articular process which has been reflected so as to show the intra-articular synovial fold inclusion IASI; HCS1 = hyaline articular cartilage on the superior articular process of the sacrum; JC = posterolateral fibrous joint capsule.

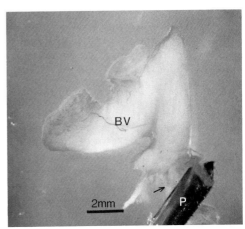

Figure 3.2. The synovial fold seen in Figure 3.1 following its excision. BV = blood vessel; P = probe. Arrow shows part of the synovial fold's region of attachment to the extracapsular recess.

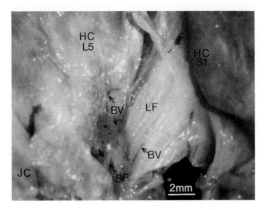

Figure 3.3. The same left L5–S1 inferior joint recess as in Figure 3.1 following removal of the synovial fold. The stump of the synovial fold is shown (SF). The outlines of the hyaline articular cartilage (HC) covered facets of L5 and S1 can be seen, as well as the vascularity (BV) of the synovium, lining the inner aspect of the capsule inferior to the L5 facet. Some of the vessels pass into the synovium which lines the ligamentum flavum (LF). The posterolateral fibrous joint capsule (JC) is reflected.

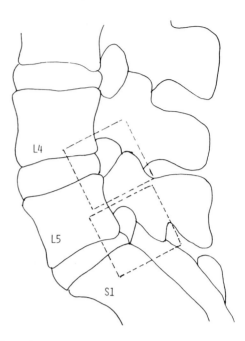

Figure 3.4. The "blocks" of spinal tissue at L4–5 and L5–S1 which are used for horizontal histologic sectioning are shown diagrammatically as squares. They look like squares in this projection but are actually rectangular blocks.

Appearance of Synovial Folds in Histologic Sections

Cadaveric paired L4–5 and L5–S1 zygapophyseal joints cut in (*a*) the horizontal plane and (*b*) the sagittal (vertical) plane were examined. The procedures used to obtain the histologic sections were as follows:

Horizontal Sections

Large blocks of tissue were cut from five embalmed spines (aged 36–80 years; mean = 60.4 years) by means of a band saw to include paired left and right L4–5 and L5–S1 zygapophyseal joints, respectively, with their ligamenta flava and other adjacent soft tissues (Fig. 3.4). The posterior parts of the vertebral bodies and intervening discs were also included to maintain zygapophyseal joint stability.

The spinal blocks were processed through stages of post fixation, decalcification, dehydration, and embedding in low-viscosity nitrocellulose with celloidin (LVNC), using the method of Giles (1) and Giles and Taylor (2). The spinal blocks were then cut in the horizontal plane at a section thickness of 100 μm using a Jung Tetrander (model K) microtome. One in seven sec-

tions, beginning from the top of the joint capsule and progressing downwards, were stained in Ehrlich's hematoxylin and light green, then dehydrated (2), cleared in Histoclear, and mounted in DePex or Eukitt. These large histologic sections (70 × 40 mm in size) were photographed using a 35-mm camera in conjunction with the Bolex Paillard camera and specimen support, using background illumination. The specimens were then examined and photographed by light microscopy, including dark-field illumination, using a Wild M400 photomacroscope.

Sagittal Sections

Five embalmed spines (aged 56–92 years; mean = 74.4 years) were used to investigate the origin, structure, and extent of the L4–5 and L5–S1 zygapophyseal joint inferior recess synovial fold inclusions and their blood supply by the following procedure.

The spinal blocks were cut by means of a

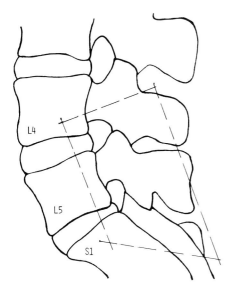

Figure 3.5. The "block" of spinal tissue (L4–S2) which is used for sagittal histologic sectioning.

plane to facilitate processing for histologic examination.

The large blocks were then processed for histology as described for the horizontal sections. The spinal blocks were cut in the sagittal plane, at a thickness of 150 μm, using a Jung Tetrander microtome. One in seven sections, from the median plane progressing laterally, were stained in Ehrlich's hematoxylin and light green, then dehydrated (2), cleared in Histoclear, and mounted in Eukitt. These large histologic sections (70 × 55 mm in size) were photographed using a 35-mm camera in conjunction with the Bolex Paillard camera and specimen support (with a 1-cm scale which was shown on each photograph) using background illumination. The specimens were then examined and photographed by light microscopy, including dark-field illumination, using the Wild M400 photomacroscope.

Figures 3.6 and 3.7 illustrate the paired L4–5 zygapophyseal joints and their associated soft tissues. Figure 3.6 shows a section from the upper half of each L4–5 joint, and Figure 3.7 shows a section from the inferior joint recess of an L4–5 zygapophyseal joint. As a comparison, Figures 3.8 and 3.10 illustrate paired lumbosacral joints and their

band saw, as shown in Figure 3.5, to include the L4–5 and L5–S1 zygapophyseal joints with their adjacent soft tissues and the posterior parts of the vertebral bodies and intervening discs, so as to maintain zygapophyseal joint stability. The spinal blocks were then bisected in the median sagittal

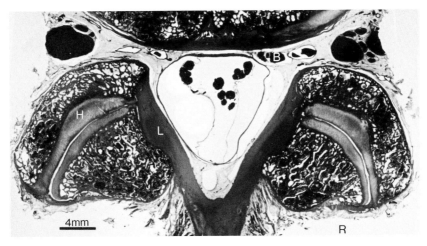

Figure 3.6. A 100-μm-thick horizontal section from the upper half of the L4–5 joint of a 54-year-old male is shown for comparison with the upper half of the L5–S1 zygapophyseal joint in Figure 3.8. B = Batson's venous plexus; H = hyaline articular cartilage on the superior articular process of L5; L = ligamentum flavum; R = right side. Note that the hyaline articular cartilage is thicker at the center of the concave and convex surfaces than it is peripherally, which is the usual pattern for lumbar zygapophyseal joints. (Ehrlich's hematoxylin stain with light green counterstain)

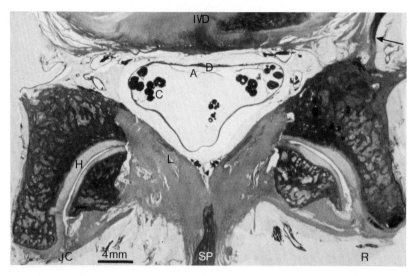

Figure 3.7. A 100-µm-thick horizontal section of the L4–5 joints at the level of the small inferior joint recesses from a 78-year-old female. Compare with the L5–S1 zygapophyseal joints in Figure 3.10. A = arachnoid membrane; C = cauda equina; D = dura mater; H = hyaline articular cartilage on the superior articular process of L5; IVD = intervertebral disc; JC = posterolateral fibrous capsule; L = ligamentum flavum; R = right side; SP = base of trimmed-off spinous process. The *arrow* shows part of a transforaminal ligament. (Ehrlich's hematoxylin stain with light green counterstain)

associated soft tissues. Figure 3.8 shows a section from the upper half of each lumbosacral joint, and Figure 3.10 shows a slightly oblique section from the lower end of each lumbosacral joint including the inferior joint recess. The right side of the section is lower than the left side, as shown by the ala of the sacrum on the right side, whereas the intervertebral canal is seen on the left side. It can be seen how the ligamentum flavum forms a thick medial capsule at both spinal levels. By contrast, the posterolateral part of the joint is closed by a thin lax fibrous capsule.

At the L4–5 joint level, the ligamentum flavum is usually firmly attached to most of

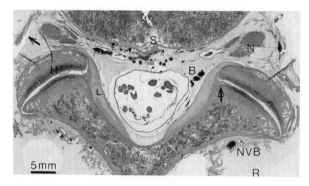

Figure 3.8. A 100-µm-thick horizontal section from the upper half of the lumbosacral zygapophyseal joint of a 54-year-old male. B = Batson's venous plexus; H = hyaline articular cartilage on the sacral superior articular process; L = ligamentum flavum; N = spinal ganglion with anterior and posterior nerve roots; NVB = neurovascular bundle; R = right side; S = sacrum. *Bisected arrow* shows a fibrous intra-articular inclusion projecting from the ligamentum flavum into the upper one-third of the right zygapophyseal joint, and *arrow* shows part of a transforaminal ligament. (Ehrlich's hematoxylin stain with light green counterstain) (Reproduced with permission from Giles LGF: Lumbo-sacral zygapophyseal joint tropism and its effect on hyaline cartilage. *Clin Biomech* 2:2-6, 1987. Copyright John Wright, London.)

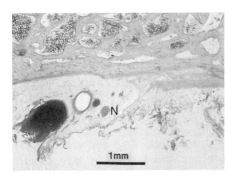

Figure 3.9. Enlargement of the right neurovascular bundle nerve (N) seen in Figure 3.8. The diameter of the nerve is 0.2 mm (200 μm). Section is cut at a thickness of 100 μm. (Ehrlich's hematoxylin stain with light green counterstain)

the medial surface of the inferior articular process. However, at the L5–S1 joint level, a space appears between the ligamentum flavum and the medial surface of the inferior articular process, in the lower half of the joint, which must be bridged by capsular material. This space accommodates the large intra-articular synovial fold (which consists of "white" fat covered by a synovial lining membrane) seen at the lumbosacral joint level. Such a large space is not found at the L4–5 joint level and there is usually not such a large intra-articular synovial fold at this level. Also, note the changes in the

orientation of the articular facets which are more coronal facing at the lumbosacral level than at the L4–5 level.

While the inferior recess is principally located inferior to the joint, each inferior recess at L5–S1, and to a lesser extent at L4–5, extends upwards between the inferior articular process and the ligamentum flavum.

In the region of the lumbosacral zygapophyseal joint inferior recess (Fig. 3.10), a large fat-filled synovial fold projects forwards (*arrow*) into the medial aspect of each joint. The inferior joint recess is enclosed by the ligamentum flavum medially and by fibrous capsular material posteriorly.

In Figures 3.8–3.11 parts of the course of the medial branch of the posterior primary ramus are illustrated. Figures 3.10 and 3.11 show the medial branch of L5 as it divides into three smaller branches. Figures 3.8 and 3.9 show the terminal branch of L4.

Figure 3.9 shows the neurovascular bundle including the medial branch of the posterior primary ramus, lateral to the superior articular process of the sacrum, as it divides into its three branches. As it descends obliquely from this point it will lie in close proximity to the left L5–S1 posterolateral joint capsule. One of the three branches can be traced in consecutive sections to the inferior joint recess posteromedial fibrous capsule. An enlarged view of the division of

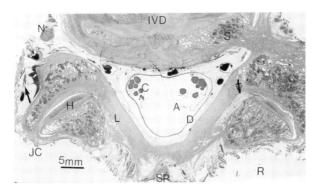

Figure 3.10. A 100-μm-thick horizontal section of the lumbosacral zygapophyseal joints at the level of the inferior joint recesses, from a 54-year-old male (the plane of section is slightly oblique). A = arachnoid membrane; C = cauda equina; D = dura mater; H = hyaline articular cartilage; IVD = intervertebral disc; JC = posterolateral fibrous capsule; L = ligamentum flavum; N = spinal ganglion; R = right side; S = sacrum; SP = base of trimmed-off spinous process. The intra-articular synovial fold inclusion is shown by the *bisected arrow*. A neurovascular bundle is shown by the *arrow*. (Erhlich's hematoxylin stain with light green counterstain) (Reproduced with permission from Giles LGF, Taylor JR: Intra-articular synovial protrusions in the lower lumbar apophyseal joints. *B Hosp J Dis Orthop Inst* 42(2):248-255, 1982.)

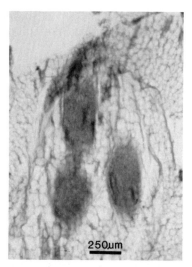

Figure 3.11. Enlargement of the "nerve bundle" showing division into three branches (from an adjacent section to the section seen in Fig. 3.10). Each fasciculus is 200–250μm in diameter and the average diameter of each nerve fasciculus is 240 μm. Sections are cut at a thickness of 100 μm. (Ehrlich's hematoxylin stain with light green counterstain)

the medial branch of the dorsal ramus into its three branches is shown in Figure 3.11.

The Zygapophyseal Joint Inferior Recess

There are no adequate descriptions of the lower lumbar inferior joint recesses in the literature, apart from brief descriptions by Lewin et al (5) and Giles and Taylor (4). Since the morphology of the lumbosacral inferior joint recess is quite different in several respects compared with the L4–5 level, it will be described in detail here.

The L4–5 zygapophyseal joint is usually almost entirely closed inferiorly by a joint capsule where the posterolateral fibrous capsule sweeps around an intracapsular inferior recess to fuse with the ligamentum flavum, which forms the anteromedial capsule (Fig. 3.7). Inferior to this, a small fat pad outside the joint capsule occupies a small fossa on the dorsal aspect of the lamina of L5 at the root of the L5 superior articular process; this fat pad communicates with an "intracapsular" synovial fold through a small opening in the inferior part of the joint capsule.

In contrast, at the lumbosacral joint the posterolateral fibrous capsule continues only part of the way around the inferior recess, where it ceases, leaving a gap of about 2 × 5 mm between it and the ligamentum flavum at the inferior margin of the anteromedial part of the joint capsule. An "accessory capsule," which will be described later, forms the posteromedial capsule (Figs. 3.10 and 3.12).

Through this gap, a *large*, fat-filled, "intracapsular" synovial fold communicates freely with a very large "extracapsular" fat

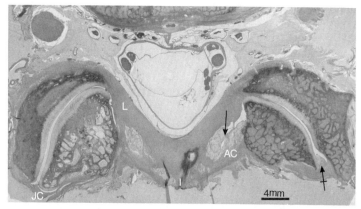

Figure 3.12. A 100-μm thick horizontal section of the lumbosacral zygapophyseal joints showing the "accessory" fibrous capsule, from a 36-year-old female. AC = posteromedial fibrous ("accessory") capsule; *bisected arrow* = intra-articular articular synovial fold inclusion at the lateral region of the zygapophyseal joint; *arrow* = intracapsular synovial fold inclusion in the inferomedial joint recess; I = interspinous ligament and spinous process remains; JC = posterolateral fibrous joint capsule; L = ligamentum flavum. Note the extension of the ligamentum flavum into the intervertebral canals. (Ehrlich's hematoxylin stain with light green counterstain)

pad in the fossa on the dorsum of the first sacral segment (Fig. 3.10). The large gap in the fibrous capsule of the lumbosacral inferior recess, which is a constant feature, makes it difficult to define exactly the junction of the "intracapsular" and "extracapsular" parts of this complex. The only structures which "close" the joint in this region are (*a*) the synovial membrane lining the intracapsular synovial fold, and (*b*) the "plug" of subsynovial fat passing from the intracapsular synovial fold to the extracapsular fat pad.

The Extracapsular Part of the Inferior Recess

The boundaries of the lumbosacral recess will be described graphically, initially with the use of osteologic landmarks, followed by drawings made from dissection, and finally with a description based on horizontal and vertical histologic sections.

A slightly oblique view of the posterior surface of the sacrum and the L5 vertebra is shown in Figure 3.13. The small bony fossa

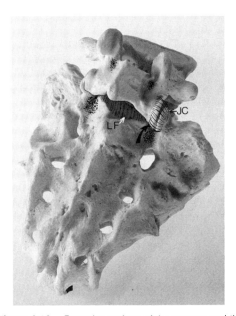

Figure 3.13.   Posterior surface of the sacrum and the L5 vertebra. JC = posterolateral fibrous joint capsule; LF = ligamentum flavum (there is some distance between the ligamentum flavum and the joint capsule, which is not apparent in this view). Dots highlight the L4–5 and L5–S1 bony fossae. *Curved arrow* shows the approximate region of entry of the extracapsular adipose pad into the inferomedial joint recess.

inferior to the L4–5 zygapophyseal joint and the large bony fossa inferior to the L5–S1 zygapophyseal joint are indicated by dots. In contrast to the L4–5 level, the L5–S1 zygapophyseal joint has a much larger bony fossa which has a deeper depression medially, occupied by a large extracapsular fat pad. An artist's impression of the osseous and soft tissue boundaries of the fossa at the L5–S1 level shows that it contains a very large extracapsular adipose pad (Fig. 3.14). This extracapsular fat pad has an upward extension from its medial aspect, through an opening in the capsule, into the joint.

The large lumbosacral extracapsular fat pad is limited as follows:

- inferiorly—by the attachment of the flat tendon of multifidus to the dorsum of the sacrum at the articular crest,
- medially—by the sacral spinous crest and the supraspinous ligament,
- posteriorly—by the tendinous sheet forming the deep surface of the multifidus muscle, and
- superiorly—by the inferior surface of the lumbosacral joint including the articular process of L5, by the root of the articular process of S1, and by the posteromedial fibrous "accessory" capsule.

The apex of the large triangular adipose pad projects upwards through the gap in the inferior joint capsule, beneath the "accessory" capsule, which bridges over from the medial margin of the L5 inferior articular process to the ligamentum flavum (Fig. 3.14**B**). The extracapsular pad is thus connected to the zygapophyseal joint intracapsular synovial fold inclusion which may project between the articular margins for a considerable distance. The intracapsular "fat pad" of the synovial fold is illustrated in Figure 3.14**C**. The "accessory" capsule is not shown in Figure 3.14**C** since it would obscure the intracapsular synovial fold inclusion, but it can be seen in Figure 3.15**B**.

The "Accessory Capsule"

A small accessory fibrous capsule, quite distinct from the posterolateral fibrous capsule (JC in Figs. 3.10 and 3.15**A**), bridges across from the medial surface of the inferior ar-

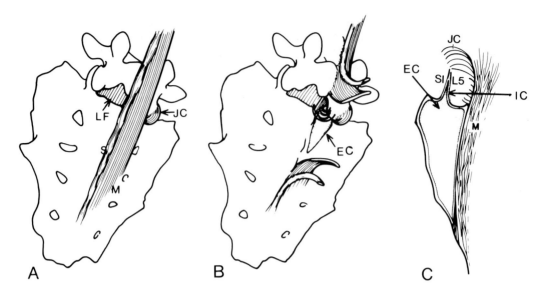

Figure 3.14. Artist's diagram of the anatomy of the lumbosacral inferior joint recess. **A**, Part of the multifidus muscle (M) covering the joint and its extracapsular recess; the posterolateral fibrous joint capsule (JC); the ligamentum flavum (LF); and the supraspinous ligament (S). **B**, The multifidus muscle and the supraspinous ligament reflected to show the morphology and extent of the extracapsular fat pad (EC) and the position of the inferior joint recess "accessory" capsule bridging from the inferior articular process of L5 to the ligamentum flavum. **C**, The joint recess in sagittal section and the communication of the extracapsular fat pad (EC) with the intracapsular "fat pad" (IC) of the synovial fold. L5 = inferior articular process of the L5 vertebra; S1 = superior articular process of the sacrum.

ticular process, some distance behind the articular margin, to the lateral aspect of the ligamentum flavum. It is unique to the lumbosacral joint, since the ligamentum flavum is usually directly attached to the inferior articular process at higher levels. Some fibers of the accessory capsule may be traced, arching posteromedially, to join with the interspinous ligament (see Figs. 3.10 and 3.12).

The Intracapsular Part of the Lumbosacral Inferior Recess and the "Opening" in the Accessory Capsule

From histologic studies, using horizontal and sagittal sections, the L5–S1 zygapophyseal joint is also shown to have a much larger intracapsular inferomedial joint recess than the L4–5 joint. The L5–S1 intracapsular recess is bounded by the ligamentum flavum medially, the accessory capsule posteriorly, and the L5 inferior articular process laterally, as shown in the horizontal histologic sections (Fig. 3.15A, B). The posterolateral fibrous joint capsule blends with the periosteum at the posterior

margin of the L5 inferior articular process. The quite separate and distinct fibers of the accessory capsule appear again at the posteromedial margin of the zygapophyseal joint, to mesh with the ligamentum flavum (Fig. 3.15A, B). The constant opening, beneath the accessory capsule, measures about 2.5 mm in horizontal width (an average), and about 5 mm in vertical extent. A "sequential" horizontal section (Fig. 3.1C), cut at a lower level of the lumbosacral joint, demonstrates that the fibrous joint capsule posteriorly is separated by a considerable distance from the ligamentum flavum; it also shows the continuity of the intra-articular synovial fold with the extracapsular recess.

The intracapsular synovial fold in Figure 3.15A is approximately 10 mm in length; some intracapsular synovial folds were 13 mm in length. Some synovial folds extended for a distance of up to 9 mm between the zygapophyseal joint facet surfaces (see Fig. 9.4).

At L5–S1, the tendinous sheet forming the deep surface of the multifidus muscle forms the posterior and posterolateral borders of

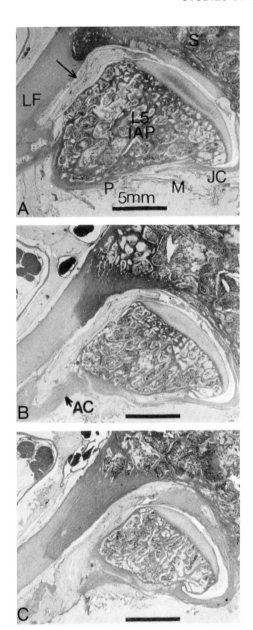

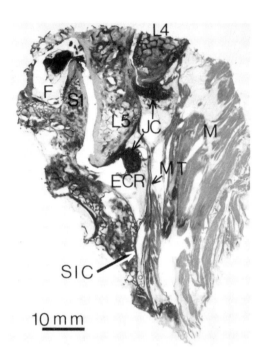

Figure 3.16. Sagittal section of the L4-5 and L5-S1 zygapophyseal joints. A 150-μm-thick sagittal section through the medial part of the zygapophyseal joint of a 92-year-old female showing the L4-5 and L5-S1 inferior joint recesses. ECR = extracapsular recess adipose pad; F = intervertebral canal; JC = fibrous capsule which appears to close the inferior recess at L4-5 (in this cadaver) and part of the incomplete capsule at L5-S1; L4 = inferior articular process of the L4 vertebra; L5 = inferior articular process of the L5 vertebra; M = multifidus muscle fibers; MT = multifidus muscle tendon inserting into the intermediate (articular) crest of the sacrum (SIC); S1 = superior articular process of the sacrum. Note the subluxation (imbrication) of the apposing lumbosacral facets (this is due to advanced thinning of the L5-S1 intervertebral disc as seen radiographically; there is no extension of L5 on S1, since the facet surfaces are parallel). Compare with Figure 4.3. (Ehrlich's hematoxylin stain with light green counterstain)

Figure 3.15. Three "sequential" horizontal sections of the lower end of the right lumbosacral zygapophyseal joint of a 54-year-old male, showing the opening in the accessory capsule. AC = inferior joint recess accessory capsule; JC = posterolateral fibrous joint capsule; LF = ligamentum flavum; L5IAP = inferior articular process of L5; M = mutifidus muscle fibers; P = periosteum; S = sacral superior articular process; *arrow* = intra-articular synovial fold inclusion. *Black line* represents 5 mm. *A-C* cephalad to caudal sections. (Ehrlich's hematoxylin stain with light green counterstain) (Reproduced with permission from Giles LGF; Lumbar apophyseal joint arthrography. *J Manipulative Physiol Ther* 7(1):21-24, 1984. Copyright National College of Chiropractic, Chicago.)

the lumbosacral extracapsular joint recess, as shown in the following sagittal sections (Figs. 3.16 and 3.17). Compare this with the artist's impression of a typical sagittal histologic section (Fig. 3.18).

The lumbosacral extracapsular recess from a 74-year-old male is shown in Figure 3.17.

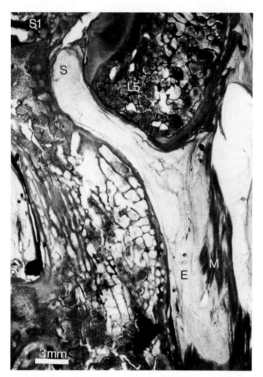

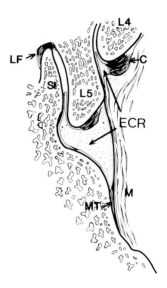

Figure 3.18. Artist's diagram of average L4–5 and L5–S1 inferior joint recesses, with synovial fold inclusions, cut in the sagittal plane. ECR = extracapsular recess adipose pad; C = fibrous capsule of L4–5 (which normally has a small opening in it); L4 = inferior articular process of the L4 vertebra; L5 = inferior articular process of the L5 vertebra; LF = ligamentum flavum; M = multifidus muscle fibers; MT = multifidus muscle tendon inserting into the intermediate (articular) crest of the sacrum; S1 = superior articular process of the sacrum.

Figure 3.17. Sagittal section of an L5–S1 zygapophyseal joint extracapsular recess. A 150-μm-thick sagittal section through the medial part of the zygapophyseal joint of a 74-year-old male showing the extracapsular recess adipose pad (E) and its continuity with the intra-articular synovial fold (S). The adipose pad is limited posteriorly and inferiorly by the multifidus (M). L5 = inferior articular process of the fifth lumbar vertebra; S1 = superior articular process of the sacrum. (Ehrlich's hematoxylin stain with light green counterstain)

The Extent and Cross-Sectional Area of the Synovial Folds from Five Sagitally Sectioned Cadaveric Joints

Measurement of Cross-Sectional Area of the Inferior Recess at L4–5 and L5–S1

The whole histologic sagittal sections were projected at a magnification of ×4.5. At the lumbosacral joint a ruler (calibrated in millimeters) was used to measure the distance from the tip of the inferior articular process of L5 to the point of attachment of the multifidus tendon to the sacrum, for each section (see dotted line on Fig. 3.19). The section with the longest distance between these two anatomical landmarks was then traced for each of the five processed

blocks. A similar method was used at the L4–5 joint. Using the standardized reference points shown on Figure 3.19, the cross-sectional area of each inferomedial recess was measured using an image analyzer for the tracings around the area of each recess, following the outlines of the bones, the posteromedial fibrous joint capsule and the deep margin of the multifidus muscle.

The image analyzer was a Reichert Kontron Manual Optical Analysis image analyzer system (MOP-3). This image analyzer incorporates a flat pad containing magnetized steel wires arranged as a network in X- and Y- directions through which pulses of current are passed. The pad is connected to a computer, and the measurements are made from the tracings by following the structure outlines using a stylus containing a receiver coil which is also connected to the computing device (7). On each occasion, prior to using the MOP-3 system, it was checked for accuracy by using the

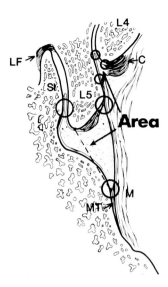

Figure 3.19. Sagittal section of the L5–S1 and L4–5 zygapophyseal joint inferior recesses showing the reference points (*encircled*) used for each spinal level. The cross-sectional area was measured for (a) each L5–S1 inferior recess (*large circles*) and (b) each smaller L4–5 inferior recess (*small circles*). The *large circles* are shown at the inferior margins of the hyaline cartilages, the multifidus tendon attachment to the L5 inferior articular process, and the multifidus attachment to the sacral median crest. The *small circles* are shown at the inferior margins of the hyaline cartilages, the posteromedial fibrous joint capsule attachment to the L4 inferior articular process, and the posteromedial fibrous joint capsule attachment to the L5 inferior articular process. C = fibrous joint capsule which is open at the L4–5 and L5–S1 levels; L4 = inferior articular process of L4; L5 = inferior articular process of L5; LF = part of the ligamentum flavum; M = multifidus muscle fibers; MT = multifidus muscle tendon; S1 = superior articular process of the sacrum.

Table 3.1.
Histologic Measurements of the Cross-Sectional Area of the L4–5 and L5–S1 Inferomedial Joint Recess in the Sagittal Plane

Measurement	L4–5 Zygapophyseal Joint		L5–S1 Zygapophyseal Joint	
	M	SD	M	SD
Length of the inferomedial joint recess (mm)	4.6	2.0	39.4	7.6
Cross-sectional area of the inferomedial joint recess (mm^2)	7.8	7.9	183.6	70.2

"Menisci" and Inclusions

In this investigation, using gross dissection and histologic sections to examine the interior of the zygapophyseal joint, no evidence was found to support the presence of any significant circumferential "menisci" referred to by Lewin et al (5) and Engel and Bogduk (9, 10). My findings are in accord with those of Tondury (11), who found no true "menisci" in zygapophyseal joints. The presence of occasional small dense fibrous intra-articular inclusions projecting from the ligamentum flavum between the facets in the medial upper one-third of the lumbosacral zygapophyseal joints was noted (Fig. 3.20). These may represent the structures referred to as "menisci" by Lewin et al (5) and Engel and Bogduk (9, 10). However, they were not examined further in this study.

Functional Significance of the Large Lumbosacral Inferior Recess

The vertical extent of the L5–S1 inferior articular recess, at its region of maximum sagittal cross-sectional area, is shown to be greater than at the L4–5 level by a factor of about 23.5 (Table 3.1). This supports the observation of Giles (6) that the L5–S1 inferior articular recess is much larger than the L4–5 inferior articular recess, as seen during zygapophyseal joint arthrography, where the radiopaque medium was seen to extend well below the level of the lumbosacral fi-

method of standardization suggested by the manufacturer (8).

Data of the dimensions of the L4–5 and L5–S1 inferomedial joint recesses are given in Table 3.1.

It can be seen from Table 3.1 that the mean cross-sectional area of the inferomedial joint recess at the L5–S1 level is larger than at the L4–5 level by a factor of 23.5. The volume of the fat pads has not been directly measured in this study, but it is suggested, on the basis of the data (Table 3.1), that the volume of the extracapsular inferior recess of L5–S1 would exceed that of L4–5 by a factor of approximately 200.

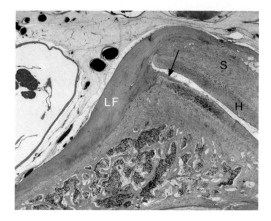

Figure 3.20. Horizontal section from the upper medial part of a lumbosacral zygapophyseal joint. *Arrow* indicates a dense fibrous intra-articular inclusion arising from the ligamentum flavum (LF) and projecting between the hyaline articular cartilages (H) of the joint. S = superior articular process of the sacrum. (Ehrlich's hematoxylin stain with light green counterstain) (Reproduced with permission from Giles LGF, Taylor JR: Intra-articular synovial protrusions in the lower lumbar apophyseal joints. *Bull Hosp Jt Dis Orthop Inst* 42(2): 248-255, 1982.)

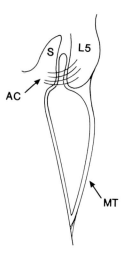

Figure 3.21. Large lumbosacral extracapsular fat pad communicating with the intracapsular synovial fold. AC = accessory capsule; L5 = inferior articular process of L5 vertebra; MT = multifidus muscle tendon; S = superior articular process of the sacrum.

brous joint capsule. This may explain the apparent "leakage" of radiographic contrast medium from the inferior aspect of the lumbosacral zygapophyseal joint capsule noted by Dory (12) and Maldague et al (13). The situation of these recesses, caudal to the joints on the dorsal aspect of the spine, suggests a function in relation to joint movements, particularly extension.

The large lumbosacral extracapsular fat pad, which communicates with the intracapsular synovial fold by passing beneath the accessory capsule, may be considered as having an "hour glass" arrangement (Fig. 3.21).

The hour glass arrangement of fat may allow for an exchange of fat through the opening beneath the accessory capsule in either direction during movement at the lumbosacral joint. The transition at this joint from a mobile segment (L5) to a stiff segment (the sacrum) has the potential to throw high stresses on the lumbosacral joints. The lumbosacral zygapophyseal joints in particular would therefore benefit from the exchange of fat between the intra- and extracapsular recesses which would

function, in conjunction with the accessory capsule, as a "pressure valve" or a hydraulic cushioning arrangement, tending to equalize intracapsular and extracapsular pressures and buffer the forces produced by sudden movements and extreme ranges of movement. The similar, but much smaller, intra- and extracapsular adipose structures, which communicate through a small opening in the L4-5 inferior recess capsule, probably serve a comparable function between two mobile spinal segments.

The range of sagittal motion at each lumbar mobile segment has been measured on radiographs by a number of authors, and at L4-5 the range is 12-18° while at L5-S1 it is 12-19° (14-17). Bakke (18) showed the mean range of sagittal movement at L4-5 to be 13.9° (flexion was 3.7° and extension 10.2°). He found the mean range at L5-S1 to be 18.6° (flexion was 2.2° and extension 16.4°). The particularly large degree of extension at the lumbosacral joint, where the flexible spine is attached to the sacrum, may explain the particular anatomy of the inferior recess of the lumbosacral zygapophyseal joint. In normal spinal extension the inferior articular process of L5 would be cushioned by the large extracapsular fat pad in the extracapsular recess (held in place by the contracting multifidus). In spinal flexion, stretching and tightening of the multifidus tendon as the L5 vertebra flexes on the sacrum may cause some of the fat to be propelled up through the opening beneath the accessory capsule to fill the synovial fold to enable it to occupy any incongruities in the joint.

The larger extra- and intracapsular adipose "pads" may be necessary at the L5–S1 level to accommodate other movements, such as axial rotation.

A greater range of axial rotation takes place at the lumbosacral joint than at higher levels (19), because the lumbosacral joints have an orientation closer to the coronal plane than do the upper lumbar zygapophyseal joints (20, 21). A range of approximately 6° of axial rotation was found to occur at the lumbosacral joint in vivo (22). This rotation can be increased to 13° in vivo when lateral bending and twisting to one side (23), but the iliolumbar ligaments may restrict excessive rotational motion (24, 25). Again, the synovial folds and fat pads may play a role in accommodating movement by filling potential spaces and irregularities within the lumbosacral zygapophyseal joint "cavity" during rotational joint movements.

Multifidus

The multifidus muscle is said to cover the zygapophyseal joints (5, 26, 27) while part of its tendon attaches to the posterior surface of the joint capsule (28, 30). This study confirms the intimate functional relationship of the multifidus muscle with the fibrous capsule (Figs. 3.16 and 3.17). The deeper tendinous sheet of the multifidus muscle forms the posterior boundary of the extracapsular part of the inferior recess adipose "pads" (Figs. 3.16 and 3.17). According to Lewin et al (5) and Taylor and Twomey (31), the multifidus muscle also has some control over the tension within the fibrous capsule and therefore must affect the potential spaces of the intra- and extracapsular recesses and their adipose pads as the zygapophyseal joint goes through various ranges of movement.

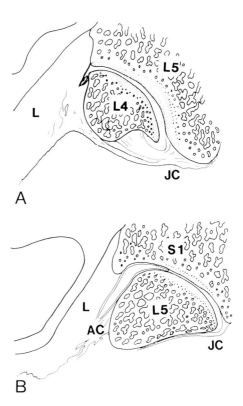

Figure 3.22. Comparison of the L4–5 and L5–S1 zygapophyseal joints at the level of the inferior joint recesses, based on photographs and tracings of various horizontally cut sections (see Figs. 3.7 and 3.10). Note that the L5–S1 zygapophyseal joint plane is more coronal than the L4–5 joint plane. **A,** The right L4–5 zygapophyseal joint. The thick ligamentum flavum (L) is firmly attached to the medial surface of the inferior articular process of L4. There is a small medial recess but there is usually no large intra-articular synovial fold. The posterolateral fibrous joint capsule (JC) sweeps around the L4 inferior articular process to mesh with the ligamentum flavum, almost entirely closing the inferior joint recess. **B,** The right L5–S1 zygapophyseal joint. The accessory capsule (AC) bridges the gap between the medial surface of the inferior articular process of L5 and the ligamentum flavum (L). The large intra-articular synovial fold inclusion fills the remainder of the large joint recess anterior to the accessory capsule. There is a relatively thin posterolateral fibrous joint capsule (JC) which blends with the periosteum at the posterior margin of the L5 inferior articular process.

Accessory Capsule and the Lumbosacral Inferior Recess

The accessory capsule, which bridges from the medial surface of the inferior articular process to the ligamentum flavum, is sometimes part of a larger ligament passing from the inferior articular process to the interspinous ligament. Such a ligament was described by Putz (32) as a "transverse ligament" of the joint capsule which could be up to 1 mm thick, and he ascribed to it the function of strengthening the fibrous capsule of the zygapophyseal joints.

The existence of an accessory capsule at the lumbosacral joint is most likely related to the change in plane of the L5–S1 joint to a more coronal orientation and the increased transverse distance between the paired lumbosacral zygapophyseal joints, compared with L4–5. These changes are associated with a marked change in the orientation of the medial surface of the inferior articular process.

As a consequence, while the ligamentum flavum is firmly attached to most of the medial surface of the inferior articular process of L4, a space appears between the ligamentum flavum and the medial surface of the inferior articular process of L5 that must be bridged by the accessory capsule (Fig. 3.22). This space accommodates the very large intra-articular synovial fold seen at the lumbosacral joint level. This series of changes in the orientation of the articular processes and associated ligaments is the principal reason for the much larger and differently situated inferior recess at the lumbosacral joint compared with higher levels.

References

1. Giles LGF: Leg length inequality with postural scoliosis: its effect on lumbar apophyseal joints. M.Sc. thesis, University of Western Australia, Perth, 1982.
2. Giles LGF, Taylor JR: Histological preparation of large vertebral specimens. *Stain Technol* 58:45-49, 1983.
3. Giles LGF: Lumbo-sacral zygapophyseal joint tropism and its effect on hyaline cartilage. *Clin Biomech* 2:2-6, 1987.
4. Giles LGF, Taylor JR: Intra-articular synovial protrusions in the lower lumbar apophyseal joints. *Bull Hosp Jt Dis* 42:248-255, 1982.
5. Lewin T, Moffett B, Viidik A: The morphology of the lumbar synovial intervertebral arches. *Acta Morphol Neerlando-Scandinavica* 4:299-319, 1961.
6. Giles LGF: Lumbar apophyseal joint arthrography. *J Manipulative Physiol Ther* 7:21-24, 1984.
7. Fraher JD: On methods of measuring nerve fibers. *J Anat* 130:139-151, 1980.
8. Reichert Kontron Messgerate GMBH. MOP4-AM03 Quantitative Bildauswertung, March 1979.
9. Engel RM, Bogduk N: The menisci of the lumbar zygapophyseal joints (abstract). Presented at the annual conference of the Anatomical Society of Australia and New Zealand, University of Sydney, Sydney, Australia, 1980.
10. Engel RM, Bogduk N: The menisci of the lumbar zygapophyseal joints. *J Anat* 135:795-809, 1982.
11. Tondury G: Anatomie fonctionelle des petites articulations de rachis. *Ann Med Physique* 15:173-191, 1972.
12. Dory MA: Arthrography of the lumbar facet joints. *Radiography* 140:23-27, 1981.
13. Maldague B, Mathurin P, Malghem J: Facet joint arthrography in lumbar spondylolysis. *Radiology* 140:29-31, 1981.
14. Begg AG, Falconer MA: Plain radiographs in intraspinal protrusion of lumbar intervertebral discs: a correlation with operative findings. *Br J Surg* 36:225-239, 1949.
15. Tanz SS: Motion of the lumbar spine: a roentgenologic study *AJR* 69:399-412, 1953.
16. Allbroook D: Movements of the lumbar spinal column. J Bone Joint Surg 39B: 339-345, 1957.
17. Froning EC, Frohman B: Motion of the lumbo-sacral spine after laminectomy and spine fusion. *J Bone Joint Surg* 50A:897-918, 1968.
18. Bakke SN: Rontgenologische Beobachtungen uber die Beweglichkeit der Wirbelsaule. *Acta Radiol* (Suppl) (Stockh) 13:1-75, 1931.
19. White AA III, Pinjabi MM: The basic kinematics of the human spine. A review of past and current knowledge. *Spine* 3:12, 1978.
20. Cihak R: Variations of lumbosacral joints and their morphogenesis. *Acta Universitatis Carolinae Medica* 16:145-165, 1970.
21. Farfan HF: *Mechanical Disorders of the Low Back.* Philadelphia, Lea and Febiger, 1973.
22. Lumsden RM, Morris JM: An in vivo study of axial rotation and immobilization of the lumbo-sacral joint. *J Bone Joint Surg* 50A:1591-1602, 1968.
23. Gregersen GG, Lucas DB: An in vivo study of axial rotation of the human thoracolumbar spine. *J Bone Joint Surg* 49A:247, 1967.
24. Parke WW: Applied anatomy of the spine. In : Rothman RH, Simeone FA (eds): *The Spine.* Philadelphia, W.B. Saunders, 1975, Vol 1, pp 19-52.
25. Luk KDK, Ho HC, Leong JCY: The iliolumbar ligament. A study of its anatomy, development and clinical significance. *J Bone Joint Surg* 68B:197-200, 1986.
26. Hirsch C, Ingelmark BE, Miller M: The anatomical basis for low back pain. *Acta Orthop Scand* 33:1-17, 1963.
27. Lewin T: Osteoarthritis in lumbar synovial joints. *Acta Orthop Scand* 72:1-111, 1964.
28. Barnett CH, Davies DV, MacConaill MA: *Synovial Joints: Their Structure and Mechanics.* London, Longmans,1961, p 47.
29. Cyron BM, Hutton WC: The tensile strength of the capsular ligaments of the apophyseal joints. *J Anat* 132:145-150, 1981.
30. Adams MA, Hutton WC: The mechanical function of the lumbar apophyseal joints. *Spine* 8:327-330, 1983.
31. Taylor JR, Twomey LT: Age changes in lumbar zygapophyseal joints: observations on structure and function. *Spine* 11:739-745, 1986.
32. Putz R: The functional morphology of the superior articular processes of the lumbar vertebrae. *J Anat* 143:181-187, 1985.

CHAPTER 4

Motion Segment Blood Vessels and Their Innervation

Blood Supply of Lumbar Vertebrae

It is necessary to describe the anatomy of the blood supply of lumbar vertebrae, including some aspects of paravascular nerve distribution to small blood vessels, since the relevance of this subject will be discussed in relation to pain of vascular origin in Chapter 5 of this text.

The blood supply of human vertebrae has been described by many authors (1–13). However, most of these are gross anatomical descriptions, with emphasis on the blood supply of the vertebral body. The extensive blood supply of the zygapophyseal joints has also been described (8, 14, 15).

The lumbar arteries, of which there are usually four pairs, arise from the posterior wall of the abdominal aorta, opposite the bodies of the upper four lumbar vertebrae; each pair of lumbar arteries passes laterally around the side of the vertebral body to a position immediately lateral to the intervertebral canal (8, 16). From this position each lumbar artery divides into three main sets of branches to (*a*) the posterior spinal elements, (*b*) the spinal canal, and (*c*) the abdominal body wall (8) (Fig. 4.1). The fifth pair of lumbar arteries, smaller in size, arise from the iliolumbar branch of the internal iliac artery, or occasionally arise from the median sacral artery (8, 17).

Blood Supply of the Posterior Spinal Elements

Since this text relates to the zygapophyseal joints in particular, only the posterior spinal and posterior spinal canal branches will be reviewed in detail here.

ABDOMINAL AORTA

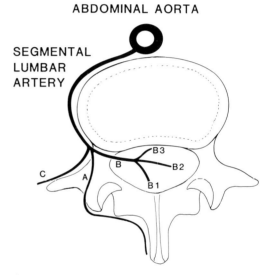

SEGMENTAL LUMBAR ARTERY

Figure 4.1. The arterial blood supply to a lumbar vertebra. A = posterior spinal branch; B = spinal canal branch; B1 = posterior spinal canal branch; B2 = nervous system branch; B3 = anterior spinal canal branch; C = abdominal body wall branch. (Reproduced with permission from Crock HV, Yoshizawa H: *The Blood Supply of the Vertebral Column and Spinal Cord in Man.* New York, Springer-Verlag, 1977.)

As the posterior spinal branch artery arches around the zygapophyseal joints, it gives off small branches which penetrate the outer surfaces of the zygapophyseal joints, the laminae, and the spinous process (8) (see Fig. 4.2). Numerous small branches of the posterior spinal branch artery supply the joint capsule, the adipose tissue in the superior recess, the fat in the inferior recess of the next higher joint, and the associated synovial folds (14, 15).

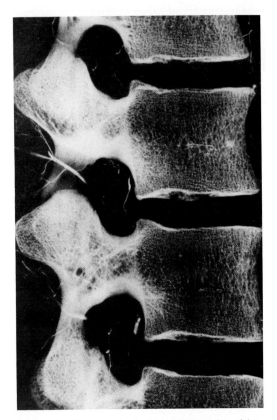

Figure 4.2. Radiograph of a thin sagittal section of the lumbar spine, showing the relations of the posterior branches of two lumbar arteries as they course backward behind the intervertebral "foramina." These arteries are constant lateral relations of the pars interarticularis of each lamina. In the lowest intervertebral "foramen" shown, the anterior and posterior spinal canal branches of the lumbar artery can be seen, separated by a clear band, this area being occupied by the nerve root at that level. Note also the branches which encircle the facet joint system to supply it. (Reproduced with permission from Crock HV, Yoshizawa H: The blood supply of the lumbar vertebral column. *Clin Orthop* 115:6-21, 1976, copyright J.B. Lippincott, Philadelphia; Crock HV, Yoshizawa H: *The Blood Supply of the Vertebral Column and Spinal Cord in Man.* New York, Springer-Verlag, 1977, p 20.)

The vessels divide and anastamose freely within the joint tissues to form a complex network around the joint between the capsule and the synovial membrane (18). From this network, branches supply the capsule, subsynovial tissue, synovial lining membrane, and the entheses (tendinous and ligamentous attachments to the periarticular bone). The superficial vessels of the ligaments and capsule communicate with those of the periosteum, while the deeper vessels terminate either as tufted loops at the bony or cartilaginous surface (18). Davies and Edwards (19) have shown that arteries enter the synovial membrane directly via the base of the fat pads and at the fringes of the articular margin (20). In general, the veins follow the arteries (18).

Distribution of Spinal Canal Branches

The spinal canal branches have three subdivisions, i.e., the posterior spinal canal branch (B1 in Fig. 4.1), the nervous system branch (B2 in Fig. 4.1), and the anterior spinal canal branch (B3 in Fig 4.1) (8).

The posterior spinal canal branches ultimately supply the cancellous bone of the lamina and the subchondral bone plates of the superior and inferior zygapophyseal joints, respectively (B). A small branch enters the anterior surface of the ligamentum flavum, close to its lateral border, and may contribute to the supply of the soft tissue elements of the anterior aspect of the zygapophyseal joint (14, 21).

The nervous system (radicular) branches accompany the nerve roots toward the spinal cord (7).

The anterior spinal canal branches bifurcate into ascending and descending branches, which anastomose with those above and below forming an arcade system (8).

Venous Drainage

The veins of the spine have been described by several authors, e.g., Bergmann and Alexander (22), Dommisse and Grobler (9), Gargano (23), Vogelsang (24), Clemens (25) and Crock and Yoshizawa (8).

Two groups of venous plexuses are found on the vertebral column outside the vertebral canal: (*a*) The anterior group, in front of the vertebral bodies, receives veins from vertebral bodies and communicates with the basivertebral and intervertebral veins. (*b*) The posterior group forms a network over the zygapophyseal joints, laminae, spinous processes, and adjacent deep musculature (2). The veins of the zygapophyseal joints, laminae, spinous processes, and vertebral bodies have been demonstrated his-

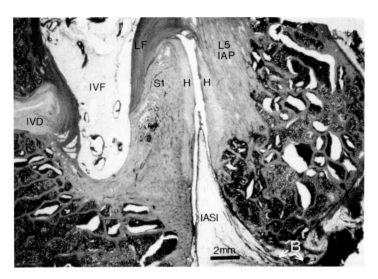

Figure 4.3. Large, highly vascular intra-articular synovial fold inclusion with a small fibrotic tip, within the inferior recess of the lumbosacral zygapophyseal joint from a 56-year-old male. The cartilage on the sacral superior process appears to have become "molded" adjacent to the fibrotic tip of the synovial fold, presumably as a result of pressure on the fibrotic tip. B = blood vessels; H = hyaline articular cartilage; IASI = intra-articular synovial fold inclusion; IVD = intervertebral disc of the lumbosacral joint; IVF = intervertebral foramen of the lumbosacral joint; LF = ligamentum flavum; L5 IAP = L5 inferior articular process; S1 = superior articular process of the sacrum. Note that there is no subluxation of the apposing facet surfaces. (Compare with Fig. 3.16, where there is subluxation of the L5–S1 zygapophyseal joint facets.) (Ehrlich's hematoxylin stain with light green counterstain) (Reproduced with permission from Giles LGF: Human lumbar zygapophyseal joint inferior recess synovial folds: a light microscope examination. *Anat Rec* 220:117-124, 1988. Copyright A.R. Liss, New York.)

tologically by Crock and Yoshizawa (8). The internal venous plexus on the inside of the vertebral canal lies between the dura and inner surfaces of the bony vertebral canal; it receives tributaries from the adjacent bony structures and the spinal cord (2).

Innervation of Small Blood Vessels

Small arteries open into muscular arterioles which branch into terminal arterioles forming the typical capillary bed arrangement of terminal arterioles, metarterioles (i.e., precapillary sphincter area; luminal diameter = 5–30 μm, capillaries (luminal diameter = 10–30 μm), and postcapillary venules (luminal diameter = 10–30 μm) (26, 27). The postcapillary venules are connected by collecting venules to the muscular venules (26).

The innervation of blood vessels includes both efferent and afferent nerve fibers (28). Arteries are supplied principally by unmyelinated nerve fibers which are mostly efferent vasomotor nerve fibers (17). Also,

near to the smooth muscle cells of the metarteriole (precapillary sphincter area), unmyelinated nerve fibers and denuded terminal axons with granular and agranular vesicles are present (26). Veins are supplied by postganglionic sympathetic efferent, and primary afferent, nerve fibers, but in much lesser numbers than in the case of arteries (17). These intrinsic nerve fibers of arteries and veins are arranged in three plexuses: an outer plexus in the adventitia, a deeper plexus at the border between the adventitia and the media, and a plexus in the media (28). The fibers in the adventitia are in part myelinated and in part unmyelinated; capillaries in the adventitia are commonly accompanied by one or more nerve fibers, but it is not possible, on the basis of histologic observations, to determine whether these fibers are functionally related to the capillaries or to the adventitia of the larger vessels (28).

Abraham (29) states that demonstration of the nerve fibers in capillary walls con-

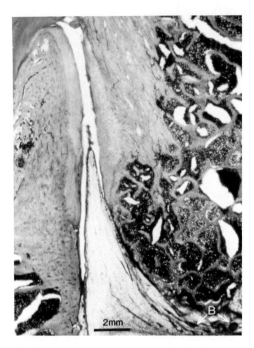

Figure 4.4. The large vascular intra-articular synovial fold inclusion from Figure 4.3. B = blood vessels.

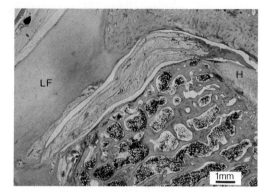

Figure 4.5. A large intra-articular synovial fold inclusion showing the extensive blood supply of a lumbosacral synovial fold inclusion from a 54-year-old male. Note the fibrotic tip of the synovial fold where it has been pinched between the hyaline articular cartilage surfaces. H = hyaline articular cartilage; LF = ligamentum flavum. (Ehrlich's hematoxylin stain with light green counterstain) (Reproduced with permission from Giles LGF, Taylor JR: Intra-articular synovial protrusions in the lower lumbar apophyseal joints. *Bull Hosp Jt Dis Orthop Inst.* 42(2): 248-255, 1982.)

stitutes one of the most difficult tasks of neurohistology. True capillaries, which have a luminal diameter of 3–10 μm (26), are composed only of endothelial cells, a surrounding basement membrane, and an occasional pericyte (26, 30). According to Cliff (31), capillaries are not innervated, and no definite proof has been obtained for a physiologic relationship between nerve endings and endothelial cells. However, a morphologic association between autonomic nerve fibers and capillaries has been revealed in the pancreas (32) and in the terminal hepatic arterial system (33).

Electron microscopy, histochemistry, and histology show sparse or no sympathetic nervous system innervation of the metarterioles (precapillary sphincters) which have a maximum luminal diameter of 30 μm (26, 34, 35). The possible relevance of these descriptions to pain of vascular origin will be reviewed in Chapter 5.

Blood Supply of the Synovial Folds

My findings support those of Lewin et al (14) and Kos (15) that the blood supply to the synovial fold is by means of arteries which pass through the multifidus muscle, i.e., branches of the posterior spinal branch, to enter the extracapsular recess. The blood vessels then supply and ramify within the synovial folds.

Two examples to show the possible extent of intra-articular synovial fold inclusions, with their blood supply, extending between the zygapophyseal joint hyaline cartilages are shown in Figures 4.3 and 4.4 (sagittal sections) and Figure 4.5 (a horizontal section), from the blocks of cadaveric spinal tissues embedded in low viscosity nitrocellulose with celloidin.

Examination of the synovial folds in fresh surgical specimens confirmed their highly vascular nature. Some fresh surgical specimens were silver impregnated and then stained with Verhoeff's (38) hematoxylin, and these specimens showed this vascularity as well as a high-elastic fiber component of the subsynovial tissue within interlocular fibrous septa. The elastic fibers appear to run in various directions throughout the subsynovial tissue. An example from the lumbosacral zygapophyseal joint of a 45-year-old female is shown in Figures 4.6–4.8.

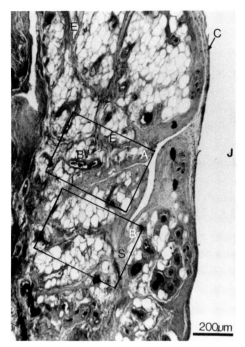

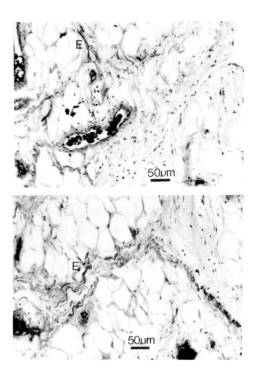

Figure 4.6.   This 30-μm-thick section shows part of a synovial fold from the lumbosacral zygapophyseal joint of a 45-year-old female. Note the synovial lining cells (C) in the synovial lining (intimal) layer. BV = blood vessels containing blood cells; E = elastic fibers; J = joint cavity; S = interlocular fibrous septum in the subsynovial (sub-intimal) layer. There is a rich blood supply, and the unilocular fat cells indicate that synovial folds consist of white adipose tissue in adults. The rectangles A and B are shown in Figures 4.7 and 4.8, respectively. (Modified Schofield's silver impregnation and Verhoeff's hematoxylin counterstain) (Reproduced with permission from Giles LGF: Human lumbar zygapophyseal joint inferior recess synovial folds: a light microscope examination. *Anat Rec* 220:117-124, 1988. Copyright A.R. Liss, New York.)

Figures 4.7 and 4.8.   High-power magnifications of parts of Figure 4.6 to show parts of the synovial fold from the lumbosacral zygapophyseal joint. The intralocular fibrous septa contain black-stained elastic fibers (E). Some of the blood vessels also show elastic fibers. (Reproduced with permission from Giles LGF: Human lumbar zygapophyseal joint inferior recess synovial folds: a light microscope examination. *Anat Rec* 220:117-124, 1988. Copyright A.R. Liss, New York.)

The villous formation increases the surface area of the synovial folds. The elastic fibers within the septa impart a contractile or recoil function to the synovial folds during joint movement. Figures 4.7 and 4.8 show the histology at a higher magnification.

The significance of the extensive blood supply of the synovial folds will be discussed in relation to low back pain in Chapter 5.

Blood Supply of the Ligamentum Flavum

Histologic examination of paired left and right zygapophyseal joint sections, cut in the horizontal plane, confirm the findings of Keller (39) Hirsch et al (16), and Reilly et al (40) that the posterolateral capsule of the zygapophyseal joint is fibrous, whereas the medial capsule is formed by the elastic ligamentum flavum.

This investigation supports the view that small midline intervals (Fig. 3.8) are present in the ligamentum flavum (17) but opposes the view of Brown (41), Ramsey (42), Kapandji (43), Ellis and Feldmen (44) and Lee and Atkinson (45) that the posterior margins completely fuse in the midline. The posterior margins completely fuse in the midline only in the area adjacent to the laminae and spinous process of the vertebra above and the vertebra below a given mobile segment.

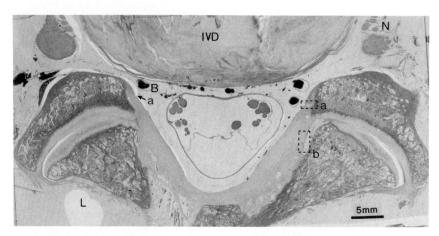

Figure 4.9.   A section cut in the horizontal plane from the lower region of the lumbosacral zygapophyseal joints of a 54-year-old male cadaver. B = Batson's venous plexus; IVD = intervertebral disc; N = spinal ganglion with nerve roots; a = bilateral vascular channels; b = blood vessels in the ligamentum flavum adjacent to an intra-articular synovial fold inclusion; L = left side of specimen. (Ehrlich's hematoxylin stain with light green counterstain) (Reproduced from Giles LGF: The anatomy of human lower lumbar and lumbosacral zygapophyseal joint inferior recesses with particular reference to their synovial fold innervation. Ph.D. thesis, Department of Anatomy and Human Biology, University of Western Australia, Nedlands, Western Australia, 1987.)

Horizontal section views from the lower part of a zygapophyseal joint, cut at a thickness of 100 μm, are shown in Figures 4.9–4.11. The paired lumbosacral zygapophyseal joints in Figure 4.9 are essentially normal. Bilateral vascular channels pass into the ligamentum flavum, a short distance anterior to the joints. These bilateral vascular channels are a constant finding in all specimens examined.

Figures 4.10 and 4.11 represent magnifications of the vascular channel and blood vessels, respectively, in Figure 4.9 and show

that the ligamentum flavum has a limited vascular supply. A few small vessels, with an average diameter of 10 μm, are seen in the superficial part of the posterolateral surface of the ligamentum flavum. The vessels

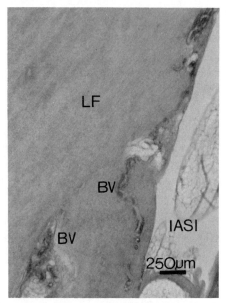

Figure 4.10.   Vascular channel in the ligamentum flavum shown in rectangle a in Figure 4.9. BV = blood vessel; VC = vascular channel; LF = ligamentum flavum.

Figure 4.11.   Vessels in the posterolateral part of the ligamentum flavum shown in rectangle b in Figure 4.9. BV = blood vessels; IASI = intra-articular synovial fold inclusion; LF = ligamentum flavum.

could be followed for only a short distance within the ligamentum flavum. Large parts of the ligamentum flavum appear to be avascular.

This study confirms the finding of Ramsey (42) that capillaries and very small blood vessels are seen irregularly dispersed in the ligamentum flavum; small blood vessels, with an average diameter of 40 µm, were frequently noted in the posterolateral regions of the ligamentum flavum (Figs. 4.9 and 4.11). A further finding was that bilaterally and symmetrically located vascular channels pass through the ligamentum flavum to supply the adjacent part of the zygapophyseal joint, as noted by Dorr (21). Thus the ligamentum flavum was found not to be as poorly vascularized as suggested by Herzog (47).

References

1. Ferguson WR: Some observations on the circulation in foetal and infant spines. *J Bone Joint Surg* 32A:649:656, 1950.
2. Kaplan A: Anatomy of the spine. In: *Ciba Collection of Medical Illustrations: Volume 1. Nervous System.* New York Ciba, 1962, pp 53, 54.
3. Guida G, Cigala F, Riccio V: The vascularization of the vertebral body of the human foetus at term. *Clin Orthop* 65:229-234, 1969.
4. Schmorl G, Junghanns H; *The Human Spine in Health and Disease,* ed 2. New York, Grune and Stratton, 1971, p 29.
5. Parke WW: Applied anatomy of the spine. In Rothman RH, Simeone FA (eds): *The Spine.* Philadelphia, W.B. Saunders, 1975, Vol 1, pp 19-52.
6. Arnoldi CC: Intraosseous Hypertension. *Clin Orthop* 115:30-34, 1976.
7. Crock HV, Yoshizawa H: The blood supply to the lumbar vertebral column. *Clin Orthop* 115:6-21, 1976.
8. Crock HV, Yoshizawa H: *The Blood Supply of the Vertebral Column and Spinal Cord in Man.* New York, Springer-Verlag, 1977, pp 4-21, 87-99.
9. Dommisse GF, Grobler L: Arteries and veins of the lumbar nerve roots and cauda equina. *Clin Orthop* 115:22-29, 1976.
10. Ratcliffe JF: Microarteriography of the cadaveric human lumbar spine. *Acta Radiologica Diagnosis* 19:656-668, 1978.
11. Ratcliffe JF: The arterial anatomy of the adult human lumbar vertebral body. *J Anat* 131:57-79, 1980.
12. Ratcliffe JF: The arterial anatomy of the developing human dorsal and lumbar vertebral body. A microarteriographic study. *J Anat* 133:625-638, 1981.
13. Ratcliffe JF: Arterial changes in the human vertebral body associated with aging. The ratios of peripheral to central arteries and arterial coiling. *Spine* 11:235-240, 1986.
14. Lewin T, Moffett B, Viidik A: The morphology of the lumbar synovial intervertebral arches. *Acta Morphol Neerlando-Scandinavica* 4:299-319, 1961.
15. Kos J: Contribution a l'etude de l'anatomie et de la vascularisation des articulations intervertebrales. *Bull Assoc Anat Berlin* 142:1.088-1.105, 1969.
16. Hirsch C, Ingelmark BE, Miller M: The anatomical basis for low back pain. *Acta Orthop Scand* 33:1-17, 1963.
17. Williams PL, Warwick T: *Gray's Anatomy,* ed 36. London, Churchill Livingstone, 1980, pp 445, 625-630, 719.
18. Liew M, Dick WC: The anatomy and physiology of blood flow in a diarthrodial joint. *Clin Rheum Dis* 7:131-148, 1981.
19. Davies DV, Edwards DAW: The blood supply of the synovial membrane and intra-articular structures. *Ann R Coll Surg* 1:142-156, 1948.
20. Davies DV: Synovial membrane and synovial fluid of joints. *Lancet* 2:815-818, 1946.
21. Dorr W: Uber die Anatomie der Wirbelgelenke. *Arch Orthop Unfall Chir* 50:222-243, 1958.
22. Bergmann L, Alexander L: Vascular supply of the spinal ganglia. *Arch Neurol Psychiatry* 46:761-782, 1941.
23. Gargano FP: Extradural venography. In Post MJD (ed): *Radiographic Evaluation of the Spine.* New York, Masson Publishers, U.S.A., 1980, pp 579-592.
24. Vogelsang H: *Intraosseous Spinal Venography.* Amsterdam, Excerpta Medica, 1970, p 13.
25. Clemens HJ: *Die Venesysteme der menschlichen Wirbelsaule (Morphologie und funktionelle Bedeutung).* Berlin, Walter de Gruyter, 1961.
26. Rhodin JAG: *Histology: A Text and Atlas.* London, Oxford University Press, 1974, pp 340-362.
27. Guyton AC: *Textbook of Medical Physiology,* ed 7. Philadelphia, W.B. Saunders, 1986, p 348.
28. Kuntz A: *The Autonomic Nervous System.* Philadelphia, Lea and Febiger, 1953, pp 157, 161.
29. Abraham A: *Microscopic Innervation of the Heart and Blood Vessels in Vertebrates Including Man.* Oxford, Pergamon Press, 1969.
30. Wolf JR: Ultrastructure of the terminal vascular bed as related to function. In Kaley G, Altura BM (eds): *Microcirculation.* Baltimore, University Park Press, 1977, Vol 1, pp 95-130.
31. Cliff WJ: *Blood Vessels.* Cambridge, Cambridge University Press, 1976, pp 133-140.
32. Lever JD, Spriggs TLB, Graham JD: A form of fluorescence: fine structural and autoradiographic study of the adrenergic innervation of the vascular tree in the intact and sympathectomized pancreas of the cat. *J Anat* 103: 15-34, 1968.
33. Burkel WE: The fine structures of the terminal branches of the hepatic arterial system of the rat. *Anat Rec* 167:329–350, 1970.
34. Burnstock G: Innervation of vascular smooth muscle: histochemistry and electron microscopy. *Clin Exp Pharmacol Physiol Suppl* 2:7, 1975.
35. Altura BM: Pharmacology of venular smooth muscle: new insights. *Microvasc Res* 16:91, 1978.
36. Giles LGF: Human lumbar zygapophyseal joint inferior recess synovial folds: a light microscope examination. *Anat Rec* 220:117-124, 1988.
37. Giles LGF, Taylor JR: Intra-articular synovial protrusions in the lower lumbar apophyseal joints. *Bull Hosp Jt Dis Orthop Inst* 42:248-255, 1982.
38. Verhoeff FH: Some new staining methods of wide applicability, including a rapid differential stain of elastic tissue. *JAMA* 50:876, 1908.
39. Keller G: Die Bedeutung der Veranderungen an den kleinen Wirbelgelenken als Ursache des lokalen Ruckenschmerzes. *Z Orthop* 83:517-547, 1953.
40. Reilly J, Yong-Hing K, MacKay RW, Kirkaldy-Willis WH: Pathological anatomy of the lumbar spine. In Helfet AJ, Gruebel DM (eds): *Disorders of the Lumbar Spine.* Philadelphia, J.B. Lippincott, 1978, pp 26-50.
41. Brown HA: Enlargement of the ligamentum flavum. *J Bone Joint Surg* 20:325-338, 1938.
42. Ramsey RH: The anatomy of the ligamenta flava. *Clin*

Orthop 44:129-140, 1966.

43. Kapandji IA: The physiology of the joints: *The Trunk and the Vertebral Column.* Edinburgh, Churchill Livingstone, 1974, p 78.

44. Ellis H, Feldman S: *Anatomy for Anaesthetists,* ed 3. Oxford, Blackwell Scientific Publications, 1979, pp 138-143.

45. Lee JA, Atkinson RS (ed): *Sir Robert Macintosh's Lumbar Puncture and Spinal Analgesia, Intradural and Extradural,* ed 4. Edinburgh, Churchill Livingstone, 1978, pp 24-70.

46. Herzog W: Morphologie und pathologie des ligamentum flavum. *Frankfurter Zeitschrift fur Pathologie* 61: 250-267, 1950.

CHAPTER 5

Brief Review of Peripheral Nerve Anatomy and Physiology Associated with Pain in Synovial Joints

In order to provide a background to some of the histologic neuroanatomy and the neurophysiology of pain which may be involved in the lumbosacral spine, a brief review of these topics, which are pertinent to this text, follows.

General Review of the Anatomy of Peripheral Nerves

Nerves, whether peripheral or spinal, are made up of axons traveling between different parts of the nervous system, usually the central nervous system and the peripheral end organ (1; S. Haldeman, personal communication, 1987).

Since the term "nerve fiber" is used in different senses in the literature, it will be briefly defined for the purpose of this text. Each *nerve fiber* consists of the axon or axis cylinder, the myelin sheath (when present), and the neurolemmal sheath (of Schwann) (2) (Fig. 5.1).

The *axons* consist of (*a*) the axon membrane, or axolemma, and (*b*) the axoplasm which contains mitochondria, microtubules, microfilaments, and neurofilaments. (1).

The *endoneurium* is the connective tissue framework which encircles each axon with its myelin sheath; it consists of fine collagen fibrils. The *perineurium* is the thin dense lamellated layer, composed of specialized perineurial cells, interspersed with fine collagen fibrils, which encircle each fasciculus. The *epinerium* is the areolar connective tissue which encloses and forms a protective packing for the nerve fasciculi (3).

The nerve fibers within each fascicle are of both myelinated and unmyelinated types

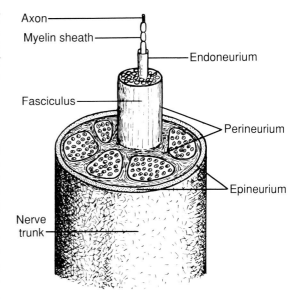

Figure 5.1. Structure of a peripheral nerve. (Reproduced with permission from Wilkinson JL: *Neuroanatomy for Medical Students.* Bristol, John Wright, 1986.)

and there is considerable variability in their diameter (5).

Classification of Peripheral Nerve Fibers

Classification of nerve fibers is based on (*a*) the size of the fibers, i.e. their overall diameter including the axon and its coverings; (*b*) their conduction velocity, and (*c*) their threshold for excitation by electric impulses (6).

The axons of *myelinated fibers* travel singly within individual myelin sheaths, and in adults myelinated axons are almost always larger than unmyelinated axons, ranging in diameter from less than 1 μm to 15 (7, 8) or up to 20 μm (1). The myelinated axons are ensheathed by numerous layers of the cell membrane of Schwann cells (9, 10). The myelin sheath is interrupted at regular intervals along the course of the fiber by the nodes of Ranvier which represent the boundaries of the individual cells that constitute the Schwann cell sheath (8).

X-ray diffraction studies have shown the fundamental repeating unit of peripheral myelin to be about 10% higher than that of central myelin (11). In electron micrographs of peripheral myelin sections, compact myelin presents as a series of light (intraperiod) and dark (major dense) lines in a repeating pattern of about 120 Ångstroms (12, 13). The major dense line is about 30 Ångstroms thick (13), whereas the intraperiod line can be resolved into a pair of lines 20 Ångstroms apart (14).

An *unmyelinated nerve* consists of a collection of small axons, 0.2–3.5 μm in diameter (8, 15), each invaginated within a separate recess in the surface of the Schwann cell; the apposed cell membranes connecting this recess to the superficial surface of the satellite cell are known as the *mesaxon* (8, 16)) (Fig. 5.2). The axons of an unmyelinated nerve are so slender as to be barely visible in the light microscope (8).

General Review of Nerve Receptors

Peripheral Receptors of Sensory Neurons

Microscopically, it is possible to distinguish between (*a*) *free nerve endings*, which form plexuses or are otherwise spread freely without any particular association with other cell types; and (*b*) *encapsulated endings*, where specialized nonnervous cells completely invest the neural process with several or many layers (17).

Although there is controversy surrounding "modality specificity" (18; D. Sinclair, personal communication, 1987), sensory receptors take various forms and can be classified by the particular modalities to which they are especially sensitive. For example, *mechanoreceptors*, which are particularly responsive to mechanical disturbances such as touch and pressure; *chemo-*

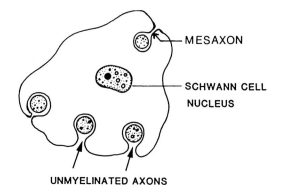

Figure 5.2. Unmyelinated nerve. (Modified from Daube JR, Reagan TJ, Sandok BA, Westmoreland BF: *Medical Neurosciences. An Approach to Anatomy Pathology and Physiology by Systems and Levels*, ed 2. Boston, Little, Brown, 1986, p 52)

receptors, which are sensitive to chemical changes; *nociceptors*, which transmit irritation or pain; and *proprioceptors* (16). Proprioceptors respond to stimuli in the deeper tissues, particularly of the locomotor system. They are concerned with reaction to movement or pressure and changes in position and include, for example, the neurotendinous organs of Golgi, the neuromuscular spindles, deeply placed Pacinian corpuscles, and joint proprioceptors (19).

Free Nerve Endings

Free nerve endings are found in all types of connective tissue, including joint capsules; the afferent fibers from free terminals are both myelinated and unmyelinated (19), and the sparse free nerve endings placed within and around the articular capsules and ligaments of synovial joints are of great importance in providing sensory information about these joints (20). All pain and temperature receptors, and a majority of touch receptors, have free nerve endings (21).

Encapsulated Nerve Endings

In encapsulated nerve endings the termination of the nerve is enveloped by a capsule which exhibits great variety in size and shape (19, 22). Histologists have identified a large number of sensory receptors based on differences in the morphology of the capsules surrounding the sensory axon, but only a few of these differences in structure are believed to have physiologic significance (21).

General Distribution of Nerves in Large Synovial Joints

In this text, particular attention is given to sensory nerves in zygapophyseal joints since the study is concerned with nociception in these joints and there is relatively little information in the literature on this topic. However, there are a number of published studies on large synovial joints and since all synovial joints probably have a common pattern of innervation, innervation of large synovial joints will be reviewed here.

The innervation of the joint capsules of large synovial joints has been extensively investigated (23–34). According to Gardner (24), in spite of variation in its origin, an articular nerve supplies a relatively constant region, with some overlap into areas supplied by adjacent articular nerves. There are regional differences in the density of nerve distribution to the capsule within a joint, since certain parts are more heavily supplied than others; the regions most subject to compression or deformation during movement are those with the more plentiful innervation (25).

Nerve Receptors in Joint Tissues

Each sensory nerve fiber arises as one or several peripheral arborizations; some nerve fibers ramify as free endings among the nonnervous tissue cells, while others attach to tissue cells by means of specialized "terminations" (13). Three groups of nerve terminals can be distinguished: (a) those in connective tissue, (b) those in epithelium, and (c) those in muscle (13).

The fibrous capsule is richly supplied with nerves which may conduct pain (31, 33–35), and there is no doubt that joint capsules are sensitive to painful stimuli (26). Ham and Cormack (35) claim that small myelinated fibers supply the joint capsule where they terminate as free endings but there are very few free endings in the synovial membrane; however, this is unsup-

ported by histologic evidence. According to Gardner (25), most evidence indicates that synovial tissue is also sensitive. A histologic examination of normal human articular capsule and synovial membrane shows a plexus of unmyelinated nerve fibers and a nerve bundle in the capsule, and fine nerve fibers ending in beadlike terminals in the synovial membrane (26). According to Ralston et al (36), who examined the synovial membrane in human joints from amputated upper and lower limbs, free fiber endings were present. Samuel (37) described myelinated and unmyelinated nerves, distributed in a plexiform manner, in the synovial membrane of human knee joints; these nerves ended in "various types of free nerve endings." Halata et al (34), using transmission electron microscopy, found three types of sensory nerve endings in human knee joint capsules: (a) free nerve endings, (b) Ruffini corpuscles, and (c) Pacinian corpuscles, confirming the findings of Ham and Cormack (35), who examined joint capsules.

Usually, nerve fasciculi in joints are closely associated with blood vessels; they accompany the vessels throughout the capsule and into the synovial tissue of these large joints, decreasing in size as the vessels decrease (25). Curtiss (38) described occasional myelinated and unmyelinated fibers in the synovial membrane, but it is generally claimed that nervous elements are very scarce in synovial tissue (25, 39). Hagen-Torn (23) could not find any unmyelinated fibers in the synovial membrane. On the other hand, Barr and Kiernan (2) claim that free nerve endings are abundant in the synovial membrane as well as in the capsule and periarticular connective tissue.

Pain Arising from the Fibrous Capsule and Synovial Membrane

In a clinical and physiologic study using human patients, Lennander (40) found the synovial membrane to be highly sensitive to pricking and pressure. In a further clinical and physiologic study, Kellgren and Samuel (26) described pain production and pressure sensibility in the fibrous capsule and synovial membrane of the knee joint under direct visual control in human volunteers and patients undergoing diagnostic arthrotomy under local anesthesia. They used a hypodermic needle to prick and pressurize the capsule, then inject it with 6% saline, and to prick and scratch the synovial membrane, then to inject it with 6% saline. The synovial membrane was also crushed and tractioned by means of artery forceps. They concluded that (a) the fibrous capsule is a highly sensitive structure giving rise to the sensation of pain and/or pressure when stimulated mechanically or chemically, and (b) the synovial membrane is relatively insensitive, with only occasional pain-sensitive spots.

Although Lennander (40) and Kellgren and Samuel (26) did not agree about the relative sensitivity of the synovial membrane in large synovial joints, both concur that this tissue is sensitive to stimulation by pricking and pressure.

Investigation of the innervation of zygapophyseal joints is undertaken on the hypothetical basis that they resemble the large joints in these respects.

Pain: Its Anatomical and Physiologic Basis with Reference to the Low Back

General Introduction

Since this text is primarily concerned with the anatomical basis of pain, in particular structures in the lower lumbar spine, the general topic of the pathophysiology of pain will now be considered. It is not within the scope of this text to consider the controversial phenomenon of "behavioral pain" which has been discussed at length in the literature (41–43).

Pain is a complex experience (21, 44) which normally occurs when tissue is damaged (45). It has important protective functions; normal persons are prevented by pain from persisting in activity which is injurious or damaging to themselves (46), for example, bending and twisting the low back with or without lifting.

Pain Sensation

While all pain is perceived "centrally" in the cerebral cortex, it is a sensation which normally results from noxious stimulation of peripheral nociceptive nerve endings by chemical or physical agents (e.g., pressure, tension, heat and cold) (47–49). Although the morphologic ultrastructure of pain receptors has not yet been identified unequivocally (50; D. Sinclair, personal communication, 1987), the particular nerve terminal which is considered to act as the pain receptor is the free nerve ending (1, 51). These endings are by far the most common of all the general sensory end organs (52), and some of these free nerve endings arise from small myelinated fibers (53).

Free endings respond to abnormal conditions by setting up impulse discharges which travel over specific or alternative afferent pathways to the sensory cortex where the activity evoked is interpreted as pain (54). Two types of pain are recognized: (a) the sharp well-localized sense of pain induced by a pin prick or laceration (i.e., *fast pain*, which is carried peripherally by small myelinated fibers), and (b) a more diffuse aching type of discomfort or pain, which may outlast the actual stimulus (i.e., *slow pain*, which is carried by slower conducting unmyelinated fibers) (1).

Somatic pain is produced by the stimulation of nociceptors in any intrinsic structures of the vertebral column (55); peripheral nociceptive afferent fibers (less than 5 μm in diameter) transmit the sensation centripetally (56).

Sensory Nerve Receptors

The receptors for pain are found on the ends of small myelinated (A-delta) and unmyelinated (C) sensory fibers (21), both of which carry pain impulses (57). Controversy still exists regarding the "specificity" of nerve *receptors* (D. Sinclair, personal communication, 1987). The peripheral nerve endings act as transducers, converting chemical, mechanical, and thermostimulation into electrical activity (53), and this excitation is transmitted to the central nervous system (53).

The Specificity of Sensory Nerve Receptors

The peripheral endings of the different types of sensory fibers are differently located, are differentially sensitive to different forms of energy, and have different properties such as adaptation, threshold refractoriness and after-discharge (58). Nonneural elements associated with nerve fiber terminals, such as encapsulating cells, are the structures which must be deformed to excite the nerve endings (59). Receptors can be divided into nociceptors, which only respond to noxious stimuli, and chemoreceptors, thermoreceptors, and mechanoreceptors (53), which may show more than one form of behavior, for example, both position and velocity detection (59).

According to Wang and Freeman (21), free nerve endings, i.e. pain receptors, (particularly those borne on the myelinated A-delta fibers), respond only to strong mechanical stimuli, while C-fibers respond to mechanical, thermal, and chemical stimuli. In all cases, the fibers which respond to pain stimuli are regarded as specialized for that purpose (21).

Fiber Types and Pain Pathways

Nerve fibers are classified in a number of ways (60, 61), but for practical purposes Wang and Freeman (21) suggest that primary afferent fibers be divided into two groups on the basis of different diameters and conduction velocities: (a) unmyelinated (C or Group 4) and small myelinated (A-delta or Group 3) fibers, which transmit pain when strongly stimulated (53, 58, 62); and (b) large myelinated fibers Group 2, which give rise to sensations of touch and pressure when stimulated (53). The large myelinated fibers have a lower threshold than do unmyelinated and small myelinated fibers (53) but conduct rapidly and transmit impulses from elaborate special receptors in the periphery. The small unmyelinated fibers and the small myelinated fibers conduct slowly and transmit impulses from less specialized receptors in the periphery (63).

Information relating to the nature, quality, and intensity of the sensation is transmitted along individual fibers as a pattern of activity or frequency code. This pattern is dependent in part on the velocity of conduction in the particular fiber; it is also determined by the time intervals between successive impulses and the total amplitude of the impulse discharge, which depends on the intensity of the stimulus (54).

Nociceptors are described as a distinct and separate class of peripheral nerve receptor. They can probably be divided into several subgroups, once again on the basis of fiber size and speed of transmission (46). The small diameter of pain fibers presents practical difficulties in physiologic research, making it difficult to be certain which fiber or fibers are being stimulated. This is one reason for many of the confusing reports on the responses of single units to painful stimuli (46).

Central Nervous System Connection

Temporal summation is documented for dull, delayed C-fiber pain, which is different in quality and less accurately projected than the fast, sharp pain from high-threshold A-delta nociceptors (64). However, although C-fibers have a "size disadvantage" they have great numerical predominance over others; e.g., in the phrenic nerve in cats there are approximately 750 myelinated fibers but 2000 or more unmyelinated fibers (A.S. Wilson, personal communication, 1986). Most small afferent fibers terminate in the more superficial laminae of the dorsal horn (65). The nocireceptive neurons in lamina I, which receive exclusively nociceptive inputs from myelinated and unmyelinated afferents, project, at least in part, to thalamic and brainstem regions (65).

The present evidence is that nociception can only clearly be identified as a property of the nocispecific neurons, such as those in lamina I of the cord (65). It is suggested that there are two parallel C-fiber primary afferent pathways carrying similar sensory information into different areas of the dorsal horn; the evidence supporting this hypothesis is largely derived from observations of the skin, but may equally apply to joints, muscles, and viscera (66). The central events and pathology that may underlie chronic pain states must take into account the different contribution made by the peptide- and non-peptide-containing C-fiber sensory pathways in nociception (66).

Experimental Correlation between Fiber Size and Pain

Theories of pain production and transmission in humans have been based partly on experiments in small mammals, performed to find out which fibers report stimulation when the stimuli cause "pain". The conclusion is that the fibers involved are small myelinated and unmyelinated fibers (67), although no description of the animal's response is given.

Vascular Pain

According to Gardner (25), the pattern of innervation of articular vessels is basically similar to that of other blood vessels, with both myelinated and unmyelinated fibers participating. According to Woollard (68), the myelinated fibers are regarded as afferent and the unmyelinated fibers as both afferent and postganglionic sympathetic efferent. The proximity of nerve fibers to a blood vessel does not necessarily imply vasomotor function since Hinsey (69) showed that after sympathectomy, a number of fine unmyelinated fibers persist in relation to the blood vessels in skeletal muscle. Similar results were obtained by Woollard et al (22) using the skin of rabbit ears. They showed that these remaining fibers are capable of mediating nociceptive responses when the fine unmyelinated (and myelinated) fibers are directly stimulated. This stimulation caused lightly anesthetized rabbits to struggle. Also, Woollard et al (22) found that pain was experienced when the point of a needle touched the capillary loop in human nail beds. Thus synovial blood vessels may conceivably be a source of pain. According to Kuntz (70), pain of vascular origin is a well-recognized clinical phenomenon, although the nature of the stimuli required to produce such pain is not fully understood. However, pain is associated with the contraction of vascular musculature, perhaps due either to the muscle spasm itself or to the resulting ischemia of tissues; it can be produced experimentally in arteries by the intra-arterial injection of irritating chemicals, such as barium chloride (70). There is good evidence that ischemic pain is transmitted along paravascular fibers (22). Thus, synovial fold blood vessels may be a source of pain, since pain of vascular origin is a well-recognized clinical phenomenon, although the stimuli for such pain are not fully understood (70).

Naturally occurring biologic substances have been implicated by Sicuteri et al (71) as producing pain in vascular disorders. These include bradykinin, 5-hydroxytryptamine, postassium, and adenosine triphosphate and are grouped under the term "vasoneuroactive substances."

Neurotransmission in Sensory Nerves

Many body tissues have the ability to react to noxious stimuli by releasing chemical compounds, such as substance P, histamine, acetylcholine, serotonin, or a series of kinins, or acids (49, 51, 72), and potassium ions (45). These chemicals are known to cause pain when applied to free nerve endings (73–75).

Substance P is a physiologically potent peptide discovered by von Euler and Gaddum (76); it has depolarizing excitatory effects on most neuronal membranes. According to Cuello et al (77), substance P is clearly related to primary sensory neurons. It has the following undecapeptide structure (*arrows* indicated points of cleavage by endogenous enzyme activity):

H-Arg-Pro-Lys-Pro-Gin-Phe-Phe-Gly-Leu-Met-NH/2 (78, 79).

Substance P is produced in the cell bodies of the spinal ganglion (80, 81) and is transported by axoplasmic flow to the central (82) and peripheral endings of sensory neurons (83) where it probably acts as a neurotransmitter or neuromodulator of pain signals (80, 81). The suggestion that its role is that of a sensory transmitter and potent muscle constrictor is also supported by the anatomical distribution of substance P, principally in the peripheral autonomic innervation (84) and in the central terminals of pain fibers (types AIII and C) where it probably acts as a primary transmitter in the pathway (4).

Immunohistochemical studies indicate that substance P is not confined to primary sensory neurons (85); it is concentrated in certain neurons of the posterior root ganglia, basal ganglia, hypothalamus, and cerebral cortex (86). It is present in 10–20% of spinal sensory neurons and is found within synaptic vesicles in the central terminals of sensory neurons located in laminae I and II of the posterior horn of the grey matter in the spinal cord (87).

Snow et al (88), who studied cat spinal ganglia, thought that substance P was not related to the nociceptive nature of neurons. Other authorities maintain that the presence of substance P in nerve fibers does indicate a probable nociceptive function in these fibers (81, 89). Salt et al (90) state that substance P may be involved in the mediation of mechanical nociception; the probable involvement of substance-P-containing fibers in conveying nociceptive information is reinforced by immunohistochemical observations following the application of the chemical desensitizing agent capsaicin (8-methyl-N-vanillyl-6-noneamide) (91). Further direct evidence of the role of substance P in nociception has been presented by Rossell (92), who administered a substance-P antagonist, (D-Pro/2,D-Trp/7,9)-SP, intrathecally to conscious rats and found it caused hypoalgesia in the hot-plate test. According to Korkala et al (93), substance P is known to participate in the sensory, especially nociceptive, transmission of neural impulses. Furthermore, in monkey spinal cords, substance P is present only in laminae of the dorsal horn which receive peripheral pain fibers (94).

Although it is not possible to associate substance P with certainty with any specific sensory modality (85), it is suggested that it is associated with input for pain (95, 96), and Liesi et al (89) suggest that it is involved in the primary pain transmission of low back pain.

References

1. Daube JR, Reagan TJ, Sandok BA, Westmoreland BF: *Medical Neurosciences. An Approach to Anatomy Pathology and Physiology by Systems and Levels.* ed 2. Boston, Little, Brown, 1986, pp 50, 119, 121, 262, 265.
2. Barr ML, Kiernan JA: *The Human Nervous System. An Anatomical Viewpoint.* ed 4. Philadelphia, Harper and Row, 1983, pp 38, 43.
3. Sunderland S: Advances in diagnosis and treatment of root and peripheral nerve injury. In Thompson RA, Green JR (eds): *Advances in Neurology* 22, New York, Raven Press, 1979, Vol 22, pp 271-305.
4. Wilkinson JL: *Neuroanatomy for Medical Students.* Bristol, John Wright, 1986, p 59.
5. Kessel RG, Kardon RH: *Tissues and Organs: A Text Atlas of Scanning Electron Microscopy.* San Francisco, W.H. Freeman, 1979, p 79.
6. Monnier M: *Functions of the Nervous System.* Amsterdam, Elsevier, 1970, vol 2, p 116.
7. Landon DN, Hall S: The myelinated nerve fibre. In Landon DN (ed): *The Peripheral Nerve.* London, Chapman and Hall, 1976, pp 1-105.
8. Landon DN: The structure of the nerve fibre. In Culp WJ, Ochoa J (eds): *Abnormal Nerves and Muscles as Impulse Generators.* Oxford, Oxford University Press, 1982, pp 27-53.
9. Crelin ES: Development of the Nervous System. *Clinical Symposia* (Ciba) 26:1-32, 1974.
10. Trapp BD, Quarles RH, Griffin JW: Myelin-associated glycoprotein and myelinating Schwann cell–axon interaction in chronic B,B′-iminodiproprionitrile neuropathy. *J Cell Biol* 98:1272-1278, 1984.
11. Finean JB: X-ray diffraction and electron microscope studies of nerve myelin. In Boyd JD, Johnson FR, Lever JD (eds): *Electron Microscopy in Anatomy.* London, Arnold, 1961, pp 114-125.
12. Karlsson U: Comparison of the myelin period of peripheral and central origin by electron microscopy. *J Ultrastruct Res* 15:451-468, 1966.
13. Angevine JB: The nervous tissue. In Bloom W, Fawcett DW (ed): *A Textbook of Histology.* ed 10. Philadelphia, W.B. Saunders, 1975, pp 333-385.
14. Peters A, Palay SL, Webster HdeF: *The Fine Structure of the Nervous System: The neurons and Supporting Cells.* Philadelphia, W.B. Saunders, 1976, p 225.
15. Ochoa F: The unmyelinated nerve fibres. In Landon DN (ed): *The Peripheral Nerve.* London, Chapman and Hall, 1976, pp 106-158.
16. Junqueira LC, Carneiro J, Long JA: *Basic Histology,* ed 5. California, Lange Medical Publications, 1986, pp 201-203.
17. Bannister LH: Sensory terminals of peripheral nerves. In Landon DN (ed): *The Peripheral Nerve.* London, Chapman and Hall, 1976, pp 396-463.
18. Chusid JG, McDonald JJ: *Correlative Neuroanatomy and Functional Neurology.* ed 13. California, Lange Medical Publications, 1967, p 192.
19. Williams PL, Warwick T: *Gray's Anatomy.* ed 36. London, Churchill Livingstone, 1980, pp 851-853.
20. Wyke BD: The neurology of joints. *Annals of the Royal College of Surgeons of England* 41:25, 1967.
21. Wang M, Freeman A: *Neural Function.* Boston, Little, Brown, 1987, p 66.
22. Woollard JJ, Weddell G, Harpman JA: Observations on the neurohistological basis of cutaneous pain. *J Anat* 74:413, 1939-1940.
23. Hagen-Torn O: Entwicklung und bau der synovialmembranon. *Archive fur Mikroskopische Anatomie* 21:591-663, 1882.
24. Gardner E: Conduction rates and dorsal root inflow of sensory fibers from the knee joint of the cat. *Am J Physiol* 152:436-445, 1948.
25. Gardner E: Physiology of movable joints. *Physiol Rev* 30:127-176, 1950.
26. Kellgren JH, Samuel EP: The sensitivity and innervation of the articular capsule. *J Bone Joint Surg* 32B:84-92, 1950.
27. Rossi F: Sur L'innervation fine de la Capsule Articulaire. *Acta Anat* 10:161-232, 1950.
28. Igari T: Histological study on innervation of joints especially of knee joint in adult human. *Arch Histol Jpn* 8:657-665, 1955.
29. Omori I: Comparative anatomical study on the nerve supply of the knee joint. *Acta Anatomica Nipponica* 31:446-452, 1956.
30. Hromada J: Beitrag zur kenntnis der entwicklung und der variabilatat der lamellen korperchen in der Gelenkkapsel und im periartikularen gewebe beim Menchlichen Fetus. *Acta Anat* 40:27-40, 1960.

56 ANATOMICAL BASIS OF LOW BACK PAIN

31. Polacek P: Differences in the structure and variability of encapsulated nerve endings in the joints of some species of mammals. *Acta Anat* 47:112-124, 1961.
32. Polacek P: Receptors of the joints: their structure, variability and classification. *Acta Facultalis Medical Universitalis Brunenis* 23:9-107, 1966.
33. Hirsch C, Ingelmark BE, Miller M: The anatomical basis for low back pain. *Acta Orthop Scand* 33:1-17, 1963.
34. Halata Z, Tettig T, Schulze W: The ultra-structure of sensory nerve endings in the human knee joint capsule. *Anat Embryol* 172:265-275, 1985.
35. Ham AW, Cormack DH: *Histology.* ed 8. Philadelphia, J.B. Lippincott, 1979, pp 476, 642.
36. Ralston HJ, Miller MR, Rasahara M: Nerve endings in human fasciae, tendons, ligaments, periosteum and joint synovial membrane. *Anat Rec* 136:137-139, 1960.
37. Samuel EP: The innervation of the articular capsule of the knee joint. *J Anat* 83:80, 1949.
38. Curtiss PH: Changes produced in the synovial membrane and synovial fluid by disease. *J Bone Joint Surg* 46A:873, 1964.
39. Barnett CH, Davies DV, MacConnaill MA: *Synovial Joints: Their Structure and Mechanics.* London, Longmans, 1961.
40. Lennander KG: Uber lokale Anasthesie und uber Sensibilitat in Organ und Gewebe, Weitere Beobachtung II. *Mitterlungem aus den grenggebieten der Medizin und Chirugie* 15:465-494, 1906.
41. Crown S: Psychological aspects of low back pain. *Rheumatology and Rehabilitation* 17:114-124, 1978.
42. Wood PHN, Badley EM: Back pain in the community. *Clin Rheum Dis* 6:3-16, 1980.
43. Campbell AJR, Shepel LF: Psychological assessment. In Kirkaldy-Willis WH (ed): *Managing Low Back Pain.* New York, Churchill Livingstone, 1983, pp 63-74.
44. Willis WD: Nociceptive pathways: anatomy and physiology of nociceptive ascending pathways. In Iggo A, Iversen LL, Cervero F (eds): *Nociception and Pain.* University Press, Cambridge, 1985, pp 35-50.
45. Wall PD: Physiological mechanisms involved in the production and relief of pain. In Bonica JJ, Procacci P, Pagni CA (eds): *Recent Advances in Pain: Pathophysiology and Clinical Aspects.* Springfield, IL, Charles C. Thomas, 1974, pp 36-63.
46. Iggo A: Pain receptors. In Bonica JJ, Procacci P, Pagni CA (eds): *Recent Advances in Pain: Pathophysiology and Clinical Aspects.* Springfield, IL, Charles C. Thomas, 1974, pp 3-35.
47. Sherrington CS: *The Integrative Action of the Nervous System.* New Haven, CT, Yale University Press, 1906.
48. Keele CA: The chemistry of pain production. *Proc R Soc Med* 60:419-422, 1967
49. Monnier M: *Functions of the Nervous System,* Amsterdam, Elsevier, 1975, vol 3, pp 85-135.
50. Andres KH, von During M: Morphology of cutaneous receptors. In Iggo (ed): *Handbook of Sensory Physiology: II. Somatosensory System.* New York, Springer-Verlag, 1973, pp 3-28.
51. Haldeman S: The neurophysiology of spinal pain syndromes. In Haldeman S (ed): *Modern Developments in the Principles and Practice of Chiropractic.* New York, Appleton-Century-Crofts, 1980, pp 119-141.
52. Arey LB: *Developmental Anatomy: A textbook and Laboratory Manual of Embryology.* Philadelphia, W.B. Saunders, 1965, p 521.
53. Lipton S: Pain relief: international anesthesiology clinics. *Recent Advances in Anesthesia and Analgesia* 16:224-260, 1978.
54. Sunderland S: *Nerves and Nerve Injuries.* London, Churchill Livingstone, 1968, p 368.
55. Bogduk N: The rationale for patterns of neck and back pain. *Patient Management* 8:13-21, 1984.
56. Wyke BD: Neurological mechanisms in the experience of pain. *Acupunct Electrother Res* 4:27-35, 1979.
57. Wyke BD: The pain pathway. *Bulletin of the Postgraduate Committee in Medicine.* University of Sydney 3(1):1-21, 1947.
58. Bishop GH: Neural mechanisms of cutaneous sense. *Physiol Rev* 26:77-102, 1946.
59. Burgess PR, Perl ER: Cutaneous mechanoreceptors and nociceptors. In Iggo A (ed): *Somatosensory System.* New York, Springer-Verlag, 1973, pp 29-78.
60. Gasser HC, Erlanger J: The role played by the sizes of the constituent fibers of a nerve trunk in determining the form of its action potential wave. *Am J Physiol* 80:522-547, 1927.
61. Lloyd DPC: Neuron patterns controlling transmission of ipsilateral hind limb reflexes in cat. *J Neurophysiol* 6:293-326, 1943
62. Loeser JD: Pain due to nerve injury. *Spine* 10:232-235, 1985.
63. Schaumburg HH, Spencer PS: Pathology of spinal root compression. In Goldstein M (ed): *The Research Status of Spinal Manipulative Therapy* (Monograph No. 15). Bethesda, MD, National Institute of Neurological and Communicative Disorders and Stroke, 1975, pp 141-148.
64. Torebjork E: Nociceptor activation and pain. In Iggo A, Iversen LL, Cervero F (eds): *Nociception and Pain.* Cambridge, Cambridge University Press, 1985, pp 9-16.
65. Iggo A, Steedman WM, Fleetwood-Walker S: Spinal processing: anatomy and physiology of spinal nociceptive mechanisms. In Iggo A, Iversen LL, Cervero F (eds): *Nociception and Pain.* Cambridge, Cambridge University Press, 1985, pp 17-34.
66. Hunt SP, Rossi J: Peptide- and non-peptide-containing unmyelinated primary afferents: the parallel processing of nociceptive information. In Iggo A, Iversen LL, Cervero F (eds): *Nociception and Pain.* Cambridge, Cambridge University Press, 1985, pp 65-72.
67. Nathan PW: Pain. *Br Med Bull* 33:149-156, 1977.
68. Woollard HH: The innervation of the heart. *J Anat* 60:345-373, 1926.
69. Hinsey JC: Some observations on the innervation of skeletal muscles of the cat. *J Comp Neurol* 44:87, 1927.
70. Kuntz A: *The Autonomic Nervous System.* Philadelphia, Lea and Febiger, 1953, pp 157, 161.
71. Sicuteri F, Franchi G, Anselm B, Del Bianco PL: Headache and cardiac pain. Physiopathologic and therapeutic perspectives. In Bonica JJ, Procacci P, Pagni CA (eds): *Recent Advances on Pain: Pathophysiology and Clinical Aspects.* Springfield, IL, Charles C. Thomas, 1974, pp 148-167.
72. Arcangeli P, Galletti R: Endogenous pain producing substances. In Bonica JJ, Procacci P, Pagni CA (eds): *Recent Advances on Pain: Pathophysiology and Clinical Aspects.* Springfield, IL, Charles C. Thomas, 1974, pp 82-104.
73. Keele CA, Armstrong D: *Substances Producing Pain and Itch.* London, Edward Arnold, 1964, pp 21-23.
74. Keele CA, Armstrong D: Mediators of pain. In Lim RKS (ed): *Pharmacology of Pain.* Oxford, Pergamon Press, 1968.
75. Lim RKS: Pain. *Annual Review of Physiology* 32:269-288, 1970.
76. von Euler US, Gaddum JM: An unidentified depressor substance in certain tissue extracts. *J Physiol (Lond)* 72:74-87, 1931.
77. Cuello AC, Priestley JV, Milstein C: Immunocytochemistry with internally labeled monoclonal antibodies. *Proc Natl Acad Sci USA* 79:665-670, 1982.
78. Chang MM, Leeman SE: Isolation of a sialogic peptide

from bovine hypothalamus tissue and its characterization as substance P. *J Biol Chem* 245:4784-4790, 1970.

79. Leeman SE, Mroz EA: Substance P. *Life Sci* 15:3287-3291, 1974.

80. Marx JL: Brain peptides: Is substance P a transmitter of pain signals? *Science* 205:886-889, 1979.

81. Henry JL: Relation of substance P to pain transmission: neurophysiological evidence. In Porter R, O'Connor M, (eds): *Substance P in the Nervous System* (Ciba Foundation Symposium). London, Pitman, 1982, pp 206-224.

82. Takahashi T, Otsuka M: Regional distribution of substance P in the spinal cord and nerve roots of the cat and the effect of dorsal root section. *Brain Res* 87:1-11, 1975.

83. Gamse R, Petsche U, Lembeck F, Jancso G: Capsaicin applied to peripheral nerve inhibits axoplasmic transport of substance P and somatostatin. *Brain Res* 239:447-462, 1982.

84. Polak JM, Bloom SR: Peripheral localization of regulatory peptides as a clue to their function. *J Histochem Cytochem* 28:918-924, 1980.

85. McGeer PL, Eccles JC, McGeer EG: *Molecular Neurobiology of the Mammalian Brain*. New York, Plenum Press, 1979.

86. Schwartz JH: Chemical basis in synaptic transmission. In Kandel ER, Schwartz JH (eds): *Principles of Neural Science*. New York, Elsevier/North-Holland, 1981, p 111.

87. Jessell TM: Pain. *Lancet* 2:1084-1088, 1982.

88. Snow PJ, Cameron AA, Leah JD: Pain transmission in identified pathways. *Neurosci Lett* Supp 19:S17, 1985.

89. Liesi P, Gronblad M, Korkala O, Karaharju E, Rasanen M: Substance P: neuropeptide involved in low back pain. *Lancet* 1:1328-1329, 1983.

90. Salt TE, Crozier CS, Hill RG: The effects of capsaicin pre-treatment on the responses of single neurons to sensory stimuli in the trigeminal nucleus caudalis of the rat: evidence against a role for substance P as the neurotransmitter serving thermal nociception. *Neuroscience* 7:1141-1148, 1982.

91. Cuello AC: Experimental studies on neurotransmitter immunoreactivity in the central and peripheral nervous system: studies with monoclonal antibodies. In Behan P, Spraefilo F (ed): *Neuroimmunology*. New York, Raven Press, 1984, pp 37-45.

92. Rossell S: Discussion. In: *Substance P in the Nervous System* (Ciba Foundation Symposium 91). London, Pitman, 1982, p 219.

93. Korkala O, Gronblad M, Liesi P, Karaharju E: Immunohistochemical demonstration of nociceptors in the ligamentous structures of the lumbar spine. *Spine* 10:156-157, 1985.

94. Carpenter MB: *Neuroanatomy*. ed 3. Baltimore, Williams & Wilkins, 1985.

95. Henry JL: Effects of substance P on functionally identified units in cat spinal cord. *Brain Res* 114:435-451, 1976.

96. Jessell TM, Iversen LL: Opiate analgesics inhibit substance P release from rat trigeminal nucleus. *Nature (Lond)* 268:549-551, 1977.

CHAPTER 6

Innervation of the Zygapophyseal Joints and Associated Structures (from L3 to S1)

Each spinal nerve is formed by the union of the anterior and posterior roots, each of which arises from the spinal cord as several rootlets; the spinal nerves pass from the spinal canal through the intervertebral canal then immediately divide to form anterior and posterior primary rami (1–3). The roots of each spinal nerve are collectively protected by a sleeve of dura mater which extends as far as the intervertebral "foramen," where it blends with the epineurium of the spinal nerve (4). The "intraspinal" segment of a lumbar spinal nerve root is anatomically different from the "extraspinal" one in that only the former has a dural sleeve, arachnoid covering, and is bathed in cerebrospinal fluid (5).

The posterior root carries sensory fibers whose cell bodies lie in the spinal ganglion (2). This is alternatively described as located in the "central" part of the intervertebral canal (6, 7) or in the lateral portion of the intervertebral canal (8). The anterior root is predominantly motor, but there is some controversy regarding the contribution made by different fiber types; Dripps et al (9) have shown that some afferent fibers enter the cord via this pathway. According to Coggeshall et al (10), who examined rat anterior roots, the anterior nerve roots contain both myelinated and unmyelinated nerve fibers, but according to Schaumburg and Spencer (11), the anterior roots are composed only of myelinated fibers. The nerve roots, spinal nerves, and their branches compose the various parts of long cellular extensions from nerve cell bodies, located in the anterior horn of the spinal cord or in the posterior nerve root ganglion (7).

Pain-Sensitive Structures in the Lumbosacral Spine

Some spinal structures, e.g., the nucleus pulposus, cartilage plates, and articular cartilages, have not been shown to have nerves despite repeated attempts to demonstrate them (12–14). However, most anatomical structures in the spine have a sensory innervation, including the zygapophyseal joint capsules, the outer anulus fibrosus, the major ligaments, the vertebral body, and all the posterior osseous structures (15). Sensory nerves are described in the periosteal covering of the vertebrae (16–19) and in parts of the dura mater and epidural adipose tissue (17, 20–24). Nerve fibers are seen in the walls of arteries and arterioles supplying spinal and paraspinal tissues (12), adventitial sheaths of the epidural and paravertebral veins (17, 21), cancellous bone of the vertebral bodies and their arches (20, 25), and the paraspinal muscles (26, 27).

It has frequently been claimed that in the adult, no nerve endings can be found in the intervertebral disc except for some free nerve endings located at the point where the superficial posterior fibers of the anulus fibrosus blend with the fibers of the posterior longitudinal ligament (12, 16–18, 25, 28–39). It seems likely from clinical experience involving the injection of hypertonic saline (11%) under fluoroscopic control into the L4–5 and L5–S1 intervertebral discs in patients with low back pain (12) that the disc is a source of pain. This view is supported by the observation that a patient's pain may be reproduced by discography (40) and that such pain is eliminated by injections of local anesthetic into the disc (41). This may provide evidence of the presence of nociceptors in the intervertebral disc if the hypertonic saline does not leak out of the disc and irritate other pain-sensitive structures, such as the posterior longitudinal ligament, which is rich in nociceptors (42) and has been shown to contain substance-P-positive profiles by Korkala et al (43). Holt (40) performed discography, using sodium diatrizoate, on asymptomatic volunteers and noted that severe back pain resulted in 15% of the examinations as a result of extravasation of the sodium diatrizoate into the epidural space from the nucleus in 37% of patients.

Similar evidence of the presence of nociceptors in zygapophyseal joints is provided by the observation that the injection of saline into zygapophyseal joints produces both local and referred pain (12), while local anesthetic injections eliminate this pain (44, 45).

According to Sherman (46), a rich nerve supply can be demonstrated in human bones of any age, but the nerve fibers, which are usually associated with arterial vessels, are mostly unmyelinated, are probably derived from the autonomic nervous system, and are concerned with the regulation of blood flow. Duncan and Shim (47) found that the intraosseous vessels in rabbits are richly supplied by adrenergic nerve fibers. In bone, there is a nerve supply to the endosteal surfaces of the medullary trabeculae and to the bone marrow, but none has been demonstrated in bone matrix (48, 49). Sherman (46) maintains that bone is relatively insensitive to painful "stimuli" and is not usually a source of pain. On the other hand, localized expanding tumors in vertebrae, e.g., osteoid osteomas, are associated with both pain and local muscle spasm (50–52).

Extracapsular Distribution of the Posterior Primary Ramus

In this text, the anatomy of the anterior primary ramus, which forms the lumbosacral plexus, is not reviewed; however, the distribution of the posterior primary ramus needs to be reviewed in detail.

The spinal nerve divides into an anterior

and a posterior primary ramus (Fig. 6.1).

As the posterior primary rami, which have a diameter of 2 mm or less and are quite small compared with the anterior primary ramus, pass from the intervertebral canal into the posterior compartment of the back, each is accompanied by an artery and its associated vein forming a neurovascular bundle. Each posterior primary ramus divides into a medial and a lateral branch, the finer medial branch being less than 1 mm in diameter (53, 54). The medial branch establishes important relationships with zygapophyseal joints (53, 54).

The medial branch of the posterior primary ramus descends obliquely on the fibrous capsule of the zygapophyseal joint. It gives branches to the lateral side of the capsule, and as it reaches the inferior aspect of the joint it may even be embedded in the capsule for a distance of 2–3 mm, at which point it lies directly superficial to the communication between the fat-filled inferior recess and the synovial cavity of the joint (55). Within the capsule, nerves break up into large numbers of diffusely ramifying branches containing sensory fibers (56, 57).

Most authors regard each zygapophyseal joint as supplied from only two spinal nerves (17, 53–55, 58–67). Each zygapophyseal joint fibrous capsule is innervated by medial branches of two posterior primary rami: The *superior portion of the joint capsule*

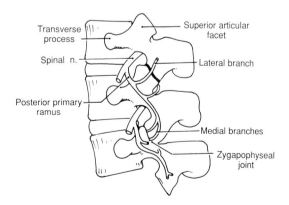

Figure 6.1. Two spinal nerves with some of their branches. (Reproduced with permission from Moore KL: *Clinically Oriented Anatomy*, ed 2. Baltimore, Williams & Wilkins, 1985.)

is innervated by "distal" branches arising from the nerve one level higher, and the *inferior portion of the joint capsule* is innervated by "proximal" branches arising from the nerve as it emerges from the intervertebral canal adjacent to the zygapophyseal joint in question. This gives an overlap of innervation. Bogduk et al (64) found the anatomy of the L1–4 posterior rami to be different from that of L5, in that the L1–4 posterior rami tend to form three branches (medial, lateral, and intermediate), whereas the L5 posterior ramus forms only a medial and an intermediate branch. According to Wyke (24, 57) and Paris (68), the zygapophyseal joint is innervated from no less than three successive posterior primary rami, i.e., the nerve emerging at the level of the joint, plus the spinal nerve above and the spinal nerve below.

In view of the controversy in the literature regarding the number of posterior primary rami, particularly in the innervation of each zygapophyseal joint, and whether a posterior primary ramus may innervate the fibrous joint capsule on both sides of the spine, I performed gross dissection studies of the extracapsular course of the posterior primary rami in five cadaveric lumbosacral spines (aged 33–90 years; mean 71 years).

This gross dissection found that each lumbar nerve emerges from the upper part of the intervertebral canal, immediately below the pedicle, and behind the vertebral body. As it emerges from the intervertebral canal, the nerve divides into anterior and posterior primary rami. The distribution of the anterior ramus is not explored in this text. Figures 6.2 and 6.3 show the course and branches of the posterior primary rami in simplified diagrams which are not drawn to scale.

The posterior primary ramus, which is much smaller than the anterior primary ramus, runs downward and backward across the lateral surface of the adjacent superior articular process of the zygapophyseal joint, then passes backward above the origin of the transverse process where it divides into medial and lateral branches. From its inferolateral aspect, before it passes beneath the mamilloaccessory ligament, the posterior primary ramus gives off

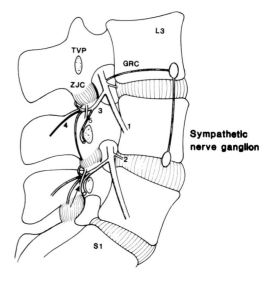

Figure 6.2. Part of the lower spinal innervation (lateral view). 1 = anterior primary ramus of the spinal nerve; 2 = anterior primary ramus branch to the intervertebral disc; 3 = posterior primary ramus of the spinal nerve: 4 = medial branch of the posterior primary ramus with an adjacent zygapophyseal joint capsule (articular) branch, and a descending branch to the zygapophyseal joint capsule (articular branch) one joint lower; 5 = lateral branch of the posterior primary ramus; GRC = grey ramus communicans; TVP ⊤ transverse process; ZJC = zygapophyseal joint capsule; *arrow* = mamilloaccessory ligament.

a lateral branch which passes obliquely over the transverse process to supply the iliocostalis lumborum muscle (Figs. 6.2 and 6.3). Only the medial branch supplies zygapophyseal joints.

The medial branch descends beneath the mamilloaccessory ligament. It then divides into the following branches:

1. The first branch goes to the adjacent zygapophyseal joint capsule in the region of the inferior recess. It appears to divide into several small twigs as it penetrates the capsule.
2. The second branch goes to the adjacent multifidus muscles.
3. The third branch goes to the superior aspect of the zygapophyseal joint capsule one segment caudad. Division of the branch into several terminal twigs may be observed where it penetrates the capsule.

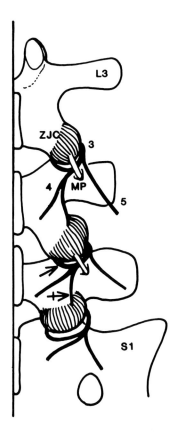

Figure 6.3. Part of the lower spinal innervation (posterior view). 3 = posterior primary ramus of the spinal nerve; 4 = medial branch of the posterior primary ramus with an adjacent zygapophyseal joint capsule (articular) branch (*arrow*), and a descending branch to the zygapophyseal joint capsule (articular) branch one joint lower (*bisected arrow*); 5 = lateral branch of the posterior primary ramus; MP = mamillary process with mamilloaccessory ligament; ZJC = zygapophyseal joint capsule.

No branches could be found crossing the midline, and there was no evidence that zygapophyseal joints on one side of the spine receive innervation from the contralateral posterior primary ramus.

It can be readily demonstrated that each posterior primary ramus supplies two zygapophyseal joint capsules, but no evidence could be found of any supply from one dorsal ramus to a third joint capsule. This supports the work of Lewin et al (55), Bradley (54, 66), Sunderland (53), and Bogduk (62). Despite a careful search, it was not possible to substantiate the claims of Wyke (24, 57)

and Paris (68) that each zygapophyseal joint is innervated from no less than three nerve roots. The medial branch of the posterior primary ramus lies directly superficial to the inferior recess and also gives branches to the lateral side of the capsule, but no trace of any branches ascending to the zygapophyseal joint above the level of origin of the posterior primary ramus could be found.

Distribution of Nerves within the Capsule, Ligamentum Flavum, and Synovial Folds

Joint Capsule

According to Resnick (69), human zygapophyseal joint fibrous capsules have a rich innervation. Immersion of human capsular material in methylene blue showed these nerves to consist of myelinated and unmyelinated fibers, with a "full triad" of nerve endings, i.e., (*a*) fine free fibers, (*b*) complex unencapsulated endings, and (*c*) small encapsulated endings (12). Nerve endings classified as "pain sensitive," on the basis of their histologic appearance, have also been described in (*a*) the fibrous capsule (16, 17), (*b*) the ligamentum flavum, and (*c*) the adjacent interspinous ligaments (12, 20, 21, 28).

Pedersen et al (17) combined their histologic studies with physiologic studies on decerebrate cats. They used mechanical (crushing) stimuli as well as injections of hypertonic saline to assess what effect these stimuli had on respiration and blood pressure. The cat's response varied from mild hyperpnoea to a "gasping" inspiratory shift, with or without minor blood pressure changes. From these experiments, Pedersen et al (17) concluded that the posterior primary rami, in addition to their cutaneous and muscular distribution, give sensory fibers to spinal ligaments and fasciae, vertebral periosteum, and all intervertebral joints. Pedersen et al's (17) view is generally applicable to all joints so far examined and is in accord with Hilton's law (70). This law states that the nerves supplying a joint also supply the muscles moving the joint and the skin covering the insertion of these muscles.

According to Lewinnek (71), only two

kinds of nerve endings are found in the fibrous joint capsule: (*a*) complex unencapsulated endings, and (*b*) smaller encapsulated endings. Other workers have found free nerve endings in the zygapophyseal joint capsule by histologic investigation (67, 72), and these endings are generally regarded as related to pain sensation (73–75).

According to Wyke and Polacek (76) and Wyke (57, 77), all the synovial joints of the body in mature individuals, including the zygapophyseal joints, are provided with four varieties of receptor nerve endings. Wyke (57) has classified these as follows:

Type I—Mechanoreceptors which consist of clusters of thinly encapsulated globular corpuscles embedded in the outer layers of the fibrous capsule.
Type II—Mechanoreceptors which are thickly encapsulated conical corpuscles embedded in the deeper layers of the fibrous capsule.
Type III—Mechanoreceptors which are much larger, thinly encapsulated corpuscles applied to the surfaces of joint ligaments, but which are absent from the spinal ligaments.
Type IV—A receptor system in the fibrous capsules of joints which is represented by a plexus of unmyelinated nerve fibers, which weave in three dimensions throughout the entire thickness of the joint capsule but are entirely absent from synovial tissue and intra-articular menisci. The irritation of this system is said to be responsible for evoking joint pain.

Wyke's statements, relating these four types of articular nerve receptor endings to particular function, are repeated in several of his papers (57, 77–80). He states that a correlation between fiber size and function does occur (81). He appears to base his statements on the results of "neurohistological studies considered in combination with oscillographic analyses of the impulse traffic in the articular nerves, electrical stimulation procedures, and other neurophysiological investigations" (82). However, it is unclear if his conclusions are based entirely on work with cats or also apply to humans.

Ligamentum Flavum

Accounts of innervation in the ligamentum flavum are variable, contradictory, and inconclusive. Doubt remains regarding both the source of its innervation and which parts of it are innervated. According to Bogduk (83), the medial branches of the posterior rami are the most likely source of innervation of the ligamenta flava because of their proximity to the posterior surfaces of the ligament. Fine free nerve fibers and endings were described by Pedersen et al (17) and Hirsch et al (12) on the outermost posterior surface of the ligamenta flava, but it is claimed that nerves have never been demonstrated in its deeper regions (12, 18, 67, 84, 85). On the other hand, Bridge (21) made the surprising observation that in a few cases, the ligamentum flavum, which is a highly elastic structure, contained many nerves in its deep region, as well as on its surface, in thoracolumbar specimens. According to Pedersen et al (17), the nerve filaments on the posterior surface are derived from the posterior rami, while the sinuvertebral nerves may supply the anterior surface. Korkala et al (43) found no immunoreactivity for substance P in small pieces of the ligamentum flavum and therefore concluded that no nociceptive-type nerves were present in the ligamenta flava.

Synovial Folds

The topic of innervation of the synovium in large synovial joints has already been reviewed in Chapter 5.

The subject of innervation of the lumbar zygapophyseal joint synovial folds is even more controversial than the innervation of the ligamentum flavum. The opinion of Mooney and Robertson (86) that the synovial membrane of human zygapophyseal joints contains a rich supply of nerves is unsupported by histologic or other evidence; neither is Hasselbacher's (87) suggestion that nerve fibers are rare in the synovium and are only paravascular unmyelinated autonomic nerve fibers, seen in the deeper synovium. Gardner (88) and Hadley (72) were unable to find any nerves in human zygapophyseal joint synovial folds. Wyke (157, 78) states categorically that there are no receptor nerve endings of any description in the synovial tissue or intra-articular "menisci" in the zygapophyseal joints of "mature individuals"; therefore he concludes that there is no mechanism whereby articular pain can arise directly from the synovial tissues (57). This is surprising in view of the previously mentioned physiologic experiments of Kellgren and Samuel (89) on knee joints, in which they found the synovial membrane to have occasional pain-sensitive spots due to pricking and scratching the synovial membrane in volunteer adults.

A clearly documented histologic description of nerves in joint synovium is provided by Goldie and Wellisch (90), who reported nerve fibers in pathologic specimens from 27 patients with well-established signs of rheumatoid arthritis. Nerve fibers were described in the synovium from knee, elbow, and wrist joints; the fibers were of 1–3 μm in diameter, with irregularly placed nodules along their course which often occupied a blood vessel wall.

Some histologic studies have been performed by Gardner (88), Hirsch et al (12), Hadley (72), Dee (91), Gardner (92), and Wyke (80), who reported myelinated and unmyelinated nerve fibers in normal human zygapophyseal joint capsules. No other reports can be found in the literature on the intracapsular innervation of healthy human zygapophyseal joint capsules, their synovium, and their intra-articular synovial fold inclusions, apart from those of this author (93–95). Therefore, this author's findings in fresh human surgical material will be described in detail in Chapter 7.

The pattern of innervation of articular vessels is basically similar to that of other blood vessels, with both myelinated and unmyelinated fibers participating (88). The myelinated fibers are afferent, and the unmyelinated fibers are both afferent and postganglionic sympathetic efferent (96).

Sinuvertebral Nerve Distribution

Although the sinuvertebral nerve distribution was not investigated in my study, it is briefly reviewed here because (a) it is possible that some branches may pass to the vertebral arches and to the zygapophyseal joints (54), and (b) the proximity of the sinuvertebral nerve to the zygapophyseal joints may permit its paravascular twigs to reach these joints "indirectly."

The sinuvertebral nerves, which are present at all vertebral levels (97, 98), contain autonomic and somatic sensory fibers (99). The sinuvertebral nerve was first described by von Luschka (100), and each nerve is described as arising by two roots: one from the anterior ramus, and another from the grey ramus communicans (4) (Fig. 6.4) at all spinal levels (101).

At this stage the sinuvertebral nerve is 0.5–1 mm thick (31, 67); it reenters through the intervertebral foramen (4, 17, 20, 21, 65, 100), before dividing into a series of short and long terminal branches which may ascend and descend in variable ways (17, 20–22, 39, 102). The short branches supply the walls of extradural veins (20) and the posterior longitudinal ligament up to two vertebral levels lower than the nerve's origin (102). The longer terminal branches pass into the epidural space. Some are described as penetrating bone on the posterior aspects

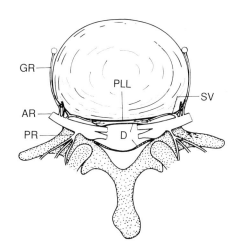

Figure 6.4 Transverse view of the distribution of a typical lumbar spinal nerve. AR = anterior primary ramus; D = dura mater; GR = grey ramus communicans; PLL = posterior longitudinal ligament; PR = posterior primary ramus; SV = sinuvertebral nerve. (Modified from Bogduk N: The rationale for patterns of neck and back pain. *Patient Management* 8:13-21, 1984.)

of the vertebral bodies and the adjacent outer layer of the anulus fibrosus, and the anterior aspects of the laminae (20); others are said to reach the flaval ligaments (23, 25), with free nerve endings which probably mediate pain sensation (67). In some cases a sinuvertebral nerve is said to join across the midline with the contralateral sinuvertebral nerve (17, 71, 97), but other investigators were unable to find such anastamoses (20, 31, 102).

References

1. Vick NA: The peripheral nervous system. In: *Grinker's Neurology.* ed 7. Springfield, IL, Charles C. Thomas, 1976, pp 101-111.
2. Moore KL: *Clinically Oriented Anatomy.* ed 2. Baltimore, Williams & Wilkins, 1985, p 649.
3. Tortora GJ, Anagnostakos NP: *Principles of Anatomy and Physiology.* ed 5. New York, Harper and Row, 1987, 292-294.
4. Bogduk N: The anatomy and physiology of lumbar back disability. *Bulletin of the Postgrad Committee In Medicine.* University of Sydney, 1980, pp 2-17.
5. El Mahdi MA, Abdel Latif FV, Janko M: The spinal nerve root "innervation" and a new concept of the clinicopathological inter-relations in back pain and sciatica. *Neurochirurgia* 24:137-141, 1981.
6. Haughton VM, Williams AL: *Computed Tomography of the Spine.* St. Louis, C.V. Mosby, 1982, p 88.
7. Rydevik B, Brown MD, Lundborg G: Pathoanatomy and pathophysiology of nerve root compression. *Spine* 9:7-15, 1984.
8. Vanderlinden RG: Subarticular entrapment of the dorsal root ganglion as a cause of sciatic pain. *Spine* 9:19-22, 1984.
9. Dripps RD, Eckenhoff JE, Vandam LD: *Introduction to Anesthesia: The Principles of Safe Practice.* Philadelphia, W.B. Saunders, 1977, pp 358-360.
10. Coggeshall RE, Emery DG, Ito H, Maynard CW: Unmyelinated and small myelinated axons in rat ventral roots. *J Comp Neurol* 172:601-608, 1977.
11. Schaumburg HH, Spencer PS: Pathology of spinal root compression. In Goldstein M (ed): *The Research Status of Spinal Manipulative Therapy* (Monograph No. 15). Bethesda, MD, National Institute of Neurological and Communicative Disorders and Stroke, 1975, pp 141-148.
12. Hirsch C, Ingelmark BE, Miller M: The anatomical basis for low back pain. *Acta Orthop Scand* 33:1-17, 1963.
13. Rhodin JAG: *Histology: A Text and Atlas.* London, Oxford University Press, 1974.
14. Stockwell RA: *Biology of Cartilage Cells.* Cambridge, Cambridge University Press, 1979, p 1.
15. White AA III, Pinjabi MM: *Clinical Biomechanics of the Spine.* Philadelphia, J.B. Lippincott, 1978, p 279.
16. Ikari C: A study of the mechanism of low back pain. The neurohistological examination of the disease. *J Bone Joint Surg* 36A:1272-1281, 1954
17. Pedersen HE, Blunck CFJ, Gardner E: The anatomy of lumbosacral posterior rami and meningeal branches of spinal nerves (sinu-vertebral nerves) with an experimental study of their function. *J Bone Joint Surg* 38A:377-391, 1956.
18. Jackson HC, Winklemann RK, Bickel WH: Nerve endings in the human lumbar spinal column and related structures. *J Bone Joint Surg* 48A:1272-1281, 1966.
19. Gronblad M, Liesi P, Korkala O, Karahurju E, Polak J: Innervation of human bone periosteum by peptidergic nerves. *Anat Rec* 209:297-299, 1984.
20. Hovelacque A: Le nerf sinuvertebral. *Ann d'Anat Path* 5:435-443, 1925.
21. Bridge CJ: Innervation of spinal meninges and epidural structures. *Anat Rec* 133:553-561, 1959.
22. Edgar MA, Nundy S: Innervation of the spinal dura mater. *J Neurol Neurosurg Psychiatry* 29:530-534, 1966.
23. Wyke BD: The neurological basis of thoracic spinal pain. *Rheumatology and Physical Medicine* 10:356-367, 1970.
24. Wyke BD: The neurology of low back pain. In Jayson MIV (ed): *The Lumbar Spine and Back Pain.* ed 2. Kent, Pitman Medical, 1980, pp 265-339.
25. Roofe PG: Innervation of annulus fibrosus and posterior longitudinal ligament. *Arch Neurol Psychiatry* 44:100-103, 1940.
26. Lim RKS, Guzman F, Rodgers DW: Note on the muscle receptors concerned with pain. In Barker D (ed): *Symposium on Muscle Receptors.* Hong Kong, Hong Kong University Press, 1961.
27. Iggo A: Non-myelinated afferent fibers from mammalian skeletal muscle. *J Physiol (Lond)* 155:52P, 1961.
28. Jung A, Brunschwig A: Recherches histologique des articulations des corps vertebraux. *Presse Med* 40:316-317, 1932.
29. Tsukada K: Histologische studien uber die zwischenwirbelscheibe des menschen altersvanderungen. *Mitt Akad Kioto* 25:1-29, 1939.
30. Lazorthes G, Poulhes J, Espagno J: Etude sur les nerfs sinu-vertebraux lombaires. Le Nerf de Roofe existe-t-il? *Compte Rendu de l'Association des Anatomistes* 34:317-320, 1947.
31. Wiberg C: Back pain in relation to the nerve supply of the intervertebral disc. *Acta Orthop Scand* 18-19:214, 1949.
32. Kuhlendahl H: Uber die Beziehungen zwischen anatomischer und funktioneller Laision der lumbalen Zwischenwirbelscheiben. *Artzl Wschr* 5:281, 1950.
33. Kuhlendahl H, Richter H: Morphologie und funktionelle Pathologie der Lendenbandischeiben. *Langenbecks arch klin Chir* 272:519, 1952.
34. Hirsch H, Schajowicz F: Studies on structural changes in the lumbar annulus fibrosis. *Acta Orthop Scand* 22:184-231, 1952.
35. Malinsky J: The ontogenetic development of nerve terminations in the intervertebral discs of man. *Acta Anat* 38:96-113, 1959.
36. Ferlic DC: The nerve supply of the cervical intervertebral disc in man. *Johns Hopkins Hospital Bulletin* 113:347-351, 1963.
37. Shinohara H: A study on lumbar disc lesions. *Journal of the Japanese Orthopedic Association* 44:553, 1970.
38. Kumar S, Davis PR: Lumbar vertebral innervation and intra-abdominal pressure. *J Anat* 114:47-53, 1973.
39. Bogduk N, Tynan W, Wilson AS: The nerve supply to the human lumbar intervertebral disc. *J Anat* 132:39-56, 1981.
40. Holt AP: A question of lumbar discography. *J Bone Joint Surg* 50A:720-725, 1968.
41. Bogduk N: The rationale for patterns of neck and back pain. *Patient Management* 8:13-21, 1984.
42. Dixon ASt: Diagnosis of low back pain—sorting the complainers. In Jayson M (ed): *The Lumbar Spine and Back Pain.* ed 2. Kent, Pitman Medical, 1980, pp 135-156.

43. Korkala O, Gronblad M, Liesi P, Karaharju E: Immunohistochemical demonstration of nociceptors in the ligamentous structures of the lumbar spine. *Spine* 10:156-157, 1985.
44. Kirkaldy-Willis WH: A comprehensive outline of treatment. In Kirkaldy-Willis WH (ed): *Managing Low Back Pain.* New York, Churchill Livingstone, 1983, pp 147- 160.
45. Aprill C: Lumbar facet joint arthrography and injection in the evaluation of painful disorders of the low back (abstract). Presented at a meeting of the International Society for the Study of the Lumbar Spine, Dallas, 1986.
46. Sherman MS: Nerves of bone. *J Bone Joint Surg* 45A:522-528, 1963.
47. Duncan CP, Shim SS: The autonomic nerve supply of bone. *J Bone Joint Surg* 59B:323-330, 1977.
48. Miller MR, Kasahara M: Observations on the innervation of human long bones. *Anat Rec* 145:13, 1963.
49. Reimann I, Christensen SB: A histological demonstration of nerves in subchondral bone. *Acta Orthop Scand* 48:345-352, 1977.
50. Keim HA: Low back pain. *Ciba Clinical Symposia* 25:4, 9, 1973.
51. Robbins SL: *Pathologic Basis of Disease.* Philadelphia, W.B. Saunders, 1974, 1451.
52. Parsons V: *A Colour Atlas of Bone Disease.* Holland, Wolfe Medical Publications, 1980, p 61.
53. Sunderland S: Anatomical perivertebral influences on the intervertebral foramen. In Goldstein (ed): *The Research Status of Spinal Manipulative Therapy.* (Monograph No. 15). Bethesda, MD, National Institute of Neurological and Communicative Disorders and Stroke, 1975, pp 129-140.
54. Bradley KC: The posterior primary rami of segmental nerves. In Dewhurst D, Glasgow EF, Tahan P, Ward AR, Idczak RM (eds): *Aspects of Manipulative Therapy. Proceedings of a Multidisciplinary International Conference on Manipulative Therapy.* Melbourne, Ramsay Ware Stockland, 1980, pp 56-59.
55. Lewin T, Moffett B, Viidik A: The morphology of the lumbar synovial intervertebral arches. *Acta Morphol Neerlando-Scandinavica* 4:299-319, 1961.
56. Sunderland S: Traumatized nerves, roots, and ganglia: musculoskeletal factors and neuro-pathological consequences. In Korr M (ed): *The Neurobiologic Mechanisms in Manipulative Therapy.* New York, Plenum Press, 1978, pp 137-166.
57. Wyke BD: The neurology of joints: a review of general principles. *Clin Rheum Dis* 7:223-239, 1981.
58. Fick R: *Handbuch der Anatomie und Mechanik der Gelenke.* Jena, Verlag G. Fischer, 1904, vol 2. pp 77-89.
59. Zukschwerdt L, Emminger E, Biedermann F, Zettel H: *Wirbelgelenk und Bandscheibe.* Stuttgart, Hippokrates-Verlag, 1955.
60. Lazorthes G: Les branches posterieures des nerfs rachidiens et le plan articulaire vertebral posterieur. *Ann Med Phys* 15:192- 202, 1972.
61. Sunderland S: Advances in diagnosis and treatment of root and peripheral nerve injury. In Thompson RA, Green JR (eds): *Adv Neurol* 22:271-305, 1979.
62. Bogduk N: The anatomy of the lumbar intervertebral disc syndrome. *Med J Aust* 1:878-881, 1976.
63. Bogduk N, Long DM: The anatomy of the so- called "articular nerve." *J Neurosurg* 51:172-177, 1979.
64. Bogduk N, Wilson AS, Tynan W: The lumbar dorsal rami. *J Anat* 134:383-397, 1982.
65. Edgar MA, Ghadially JA: Innervation of the lumbar spine. *Clin Orthop* 115:35-41, 1976.
66. Bradley KC: The anatomy of backache. *Aust NZ J Surg* 44:227-232, 1974.
67. Reilly J, Yong-Hing K, MacKay RW, Kirkaldy- Willis WH: Pathological anatomy of the lumbar spine. In Helfet AJ, Gruebel DM (ed): *Disorders of the Lumbar Spine.* Philadelphia, J.B. Lippincott, 1978, pp 26-50.
68. Paris SV: Anatomy as related to function and pain. *Orthop Clin North Am* 14:475-489, 1983.
69. Resnick D: Degenerative diseases of the vertebral column. *Radiology* 156:3-14, 1985.
70. Hilton J: *Rest and Pain. A Course of Lectures.* ed 2 (reprinted from the last London edition). Cincinnati, OH, P.W. Gardfield, 1891.
71. Lewinnek GE: Management of low back pain and sciatica. *Int Anesthesiol Clin* 21:61-78, 1983.
72. Hadley LA: *Anatomico- Roentgenographic Studies of the Spine.* Springfield, IL, Charles C. Thomas, 1976, pp 186, 189, 190.
73. Haldeman S: The neurophysiology of spinal pain syndromes. In Haldeman S (ed): *Modern Developments in the Principles and Practice of Chiropractic.* New York, Appleton-Century-Crofts, 1980, pp 119-141.
74. Kandel ER, Schwartz JH: *Principles of Neural Science.* New York, Elsevier/North-Holland, 1981, p 168.
75. Daube JR, Reagan TJ, Sandok BA, Westmoreland BF: *Medical Neurosciences. An Approach to Anatomy Pathology and Physiology by Systems and Levels.* ed 2. Boston, Little, Brown, 1986, p 119.
76. Wyke BD, Polacek P: Articular neurology: the present position. *J Bone Joint Surg* 57B:401, 1975.
77. Wyke BD: Articular neurology and manipulative therapy. *Aspects of Manipulative Therapy.* Melbourne, Lincoln Institute of Health, 1980, pp 67-74.
78. Wyke BD: Articular neurology: a review. *Physiotherapy* 58:94-99, 1972.
79. Wyke BD: Neurology of the cervical spinal joints. *Physiotherapy* 65:72-76, 1975.
80. Wyke BD: Neurological mechanisms in the experience of pain. *Acupunct Electrother Res* 4:27-35, 1979.
81. Wyke BD: *Principles of General Neurology.* Amsterdam, Elsevier, 1969, pp 48-49.
82. Wyke BD: The neurology of joints. *Annals of the Royal College of England* 41:25, 1967.
83. Bogduk N: The innervation of the lumbar spine. *Spine* 8:286-293, 1983.
84. Dockerty MB, Love JG: Thickening and fibrosis (so-called hypertrophy) of the ligamentum flavum: a pathological study of fifty cases. *Proc Staff Meet Mayo Clinic* 15:161-166, 1940.
85. Ramsey RH: The anatomy of the ligamenta flava. *Clin Orthop* 44:129-140, 1966.
86. Mooney V, Robertson J: The facet syndrome. *Clin Orthop* 115:149-156, 1976.
87. Hasselbacher P: Structure of the synovial membrane. *Clin Rheum Dis* 7:57-69, 1981.
88. Gardner E: Physiology of movable joints. *Physiol Rev* 30:127-176, 1950.
89. Kellgren JH, Samuel EP: The sensitivity and innervation of the articular capsule. *J Bone Joint Surg* 32B:84-92, 1950.
90. Goldie I, Wellisch M: The presence of nerves in original and regenerated synovial tissue in patients synovectomised for rheumatoid arthritis. *Acta Orthop Scand* 40:143-152, 1969.
91. Dee R: The innervation of joints. in Sokoloff L (ed): *The Joints and Synovial Fluid.* New York, Academic Press, 1978, vol 1, pp 177-204.
92. Gardner DL: Structure and function of connective tissue and joints. In Scott JT (ed): *Copeman's Textbook of the Rheumatic Diseases.* ed 5. London, Churchill Livingstone, 1978, pp 78-124.
93. Giles LGF, Taylor JR, Cockson A: Human zygapophyseal joint synovial folds. *Acta Anat* 126:110-114, 1986.
94. Giles LGF, Taylor JR: Human zygapophyseal joint capsule and synovial fold innervation *Bri J Rheumatol*

26:993-98, 1987.

95. Giles LGF, Taylor JR: Innervation of human lumbar zygapophyseal joint synovial folds. *Acta Orthop Scand* 58:43-46, 1987.

96. Woollard HH: The innervation of the heart. *J Anat* 60:345-373, 1926.

97. Kimmel DL: Innervation of spinal dura mater and dura mater of the posterior cranial fossa. *Neurology* 11:800-809, 1961.

98. Kimmel DL: The nerves of the cranial dura mater and their significance in dural headache and referred pain. *Chicago Medical School Quarterly* 22:16-26, 1961.

99. Allbrook D: The intervertebral disc. In Twomey LT (ed): *Low Back Pain: Proceedings of a Conference on Low Back Pain.* Western Australia, Institute of Technology, 1974, pp 14-19.

100. von Luschka H: *Die nerven des menschlichen wirbelkanales.* Tubingen, Laupp and Siebeck, 1850.

101. Williams PL, Warwick T: *Gray's Anatomy.* ed 36. London, Churchill Livingstone, 1980, p 1131.

102. Spurling RG, Bradford FK: Neurologic aspects of herniated nucleus pulposus. *JAMA* 113:2019-2022, 1939.

CHAPTER 7

Studies of the Intracapsular Distribution of Nerves Using Fresh Surgical Material

In order to further examine the intracapsular distribution of nerves, surgeons were asked to provide the author with fresh surgical laminectomy specimens.

Eighty adult patients from whom these specimens were obtained were healthy apart from nucleus pulposus extrusion; they either had no radiologic evidence of osteoarthritis or had minor osteoarthritis of the zygapophyseal joints. Patients who suffered from any other diseases of the lumbar spinal column and its soft tissues were excluded from this study.

Surgeons were asked to provide specimens including (*a*) the posteromedial fibrous joint capsule of the inferior recess, (*b*) the adjoining part of the ligamentum flavum, and (*c*) the synovial fold of the inferior joint recess (see Fig. 7.1). The superior joint recess was not examined since it is not involved in routine laminectomy procedures.

At the lumbosacral level the specimen frequently included part of a large extra-articular "fat pad."

Of these specimens, 50 had adequate portions of capsule, with sufficiently complete synovial folds, to be included in the nerve study. Their ages ranged from 20 to 70 years (mean- 37.6 years).

A typical specimen is illustrated in Figure 7.2. Some lumbosacral specimens, as in Figure 7.2, show a very large synovial fold projecting from the internal surface of the capsular material. Blood vessels can be seen coursing and branching within fibrous septa.

Figure 7.3 diagrammatically shows the regions which were examined for nerves: (*a*)

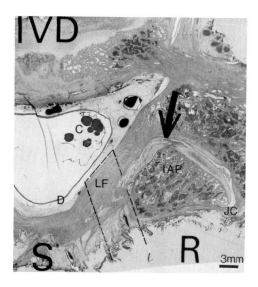

Figure 7.1. Horizontal section of the right L5–S1 zygapophyseal joint from a 54-year-old male. The rectangle represents the approximate extent of the surgical material removed during laminectomy, i.e., part of the inferior joint recess comprising the posteromedial (accessory) fibrous capsule and adjacent ligamentum flavum *with the adjoining synovial fold.* C = cauda equina; D = dura mater; IAP = inferior articular process of L5; IVD = intervertebral disc; JC = posterolateral fibrous joint capsule; LF = ligamentum flavum; S = the remains of the spinous process. The *black arrow* indicates a highly vascular connective tissue structure projecting between the right lumbosacral zygapophyseal joint facets, i.e., an intra-articular synovial fold inclusion. (Ehrlich's hematoxylin stain with light green counterstain) (Reproduced with permission from Giles LGF, Taylor JR, Cockson A: Human zygapophyseal joint synovial folds. *Acta Anat* 126:110-114; 1986. Copyright S. Karger AG, Basel.)

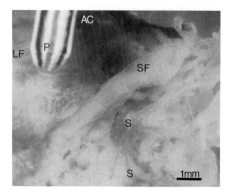

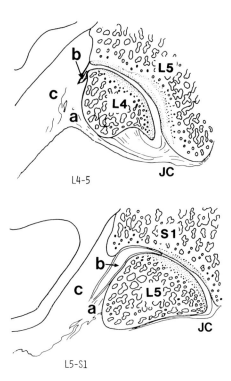

Figure 7.2. The capsular internal surface of a whole-mount unstained specimen, from the L5–S1 zygapophyseal joint of a 35-year-old female. Note the large synovial fold (SF) with its typical glistening fat cells, projecting from the accessory capsule (AC) of the inferior joint recess. LF = ligamentum flavum. The probe (P), of exactly 1.5 mm diameter, was used to stabilize whole-mount specimens during photography, and the diameter of the probe, closest to the plane of the specimen, was also used as a scale to check the scale of magnification shown on the Wild photomacroscope. Blood vessels are seen within fibrous septa (S). (Reproduced with permission from Giles LGF, Taylor JR, Cockson A: Human zygapophyseal joint synovial folds. *Acta Anat* 126:110-114, 1986. Copyright S. Karger AG, Basel.)

Figure 7.3 The zygapophyseal joint soft tissue regions which were examined for nerves. Region a = the posteromedial "accessory" fibrous capsule at L5–S1 and the posteromedial fibrous capsule at L4–5; region b = subsynovial and synovial lining membrane tissues; region c = ligamentum flavum. JC = posterolateral fibrous joint capsule; L4 = inferior articular process of the L4 vertebra; L5 = the superior and inferior articular processes respectively of the L5 vertebra; S1 = superior articular process of the sacrum. See Figures 3.7 and 3.10. (From Giles LGF: The anatomy of human lower lumbar and lumbosacral zygapophyseal joint inferior recesses with particular reference to their synovial fold innervation. Ph.D. thesis, Department of Anatomy and Human Biology, University of Western Australia, Nedlands, Western Australia, 1987.)

the accessory fibrous capsule of the inferior joint recess of L5–S1 and the posteromedial fibrous capsule of L4–5, (*b*) the synovial fold of the inferior joint recess—both the subsynovial and synovial lining membrane, and (*c*) the ligamentum flavum.

Electron Microscopy Studies of Nerves in Surgical Material

Preliminary light microscopy of 2-μm-thick epon/araldite sections from the joint capsule and synovial folds revealed numerous fat cells and small blood vessels (Fig. 7.4). The unperfused blood vessels are seen to contain many blood cells. The quality of fixation cannot be compared with that obtained from perfused animal tissue.

The subsynovial tissue has a fairly constant morphology (Fig. 7.5), with numerous capillaries in the interstices between the fat cells.

Nerves in Synovial Folds

Transmission electron microscopy showed that small blood vessels, such as arterioles, in the synovial folds have paravascular myelinated nerve fibers (see Figs. 7.6–7.8). Nerve fibers were demonstrated in 5 out of 13 specimens in the inferior joint recess synovial fold subsynovial tissue. The approximate situations of these nerve fibers within

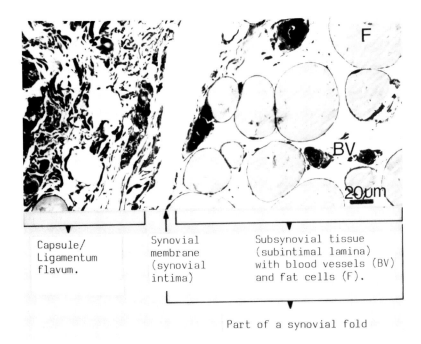

Figure 7.4.   Part of a synovial fold. This high-powered light photomicrograph (cut at a thickness of 2 μm) shows the capsule–ligamentum flavum junction area and part of a synovial fold from the lumbosacral joint of a 33-year-old female (specimen a; see Table 7.1). (Stained with 0.1% toluidine blue in 1% borax) (Reproduced with permission from Giles LGF, Taylor JR, Cockson A: Human zygapophyseal joint synovial folds. *Acta Anat* 126:110-114; 1986. Copyright S. Karger AG, Basel.)

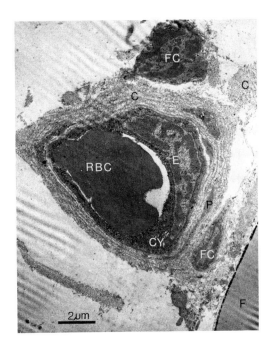

Figure 7.5.   This transmission electron photomicrograph from the lumbosacral joint synovial fold of a 33-year-old female (specimen b; see Table 7.1) shows a capillary (with a lumen of approximately 5.3 μm) and adjacent fibrocytes and collagen, in close proximity to a fat cell (F). Red blood cells (RBC) are seen in the lumen of the capillary. C = collagen fibers; CY = cytoplasm of the endothelial cell; E = endothelial cell nucleus; FC = fibrocyte; P = pericyte process. (Uranyl magnesium acetate and lead citrate stains) (Reproduced with permission from Giles LGF, Taylor JR, Cockson A: Human zygapophyseal joint synovial folds. *Acta Anat* 126:110-114, 1986. Copyright S. Karger AG, Basel.)

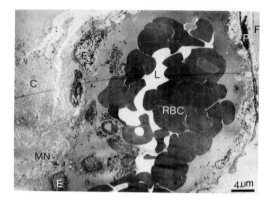

Figure 7.6. A small blood vessel, with a lumen (L) of 24 μm containing erythrocytes (RBC), with a small 0.2-μm-diameter paravascular myelinated nerve fiber (MN) within the subsynovial tissue (subintimal lamina) of the synovial fold of a 35-year-old female (L5–S1 level); (region b on Fig. 7.3). C = collagen fibers; E = endothelial cell nucleus; F = fat cell; M = macrophage; P = pericyte nucleus. Glutaraldehyde/osmium tetroxide fixation. (Uranyl magnesium acetate and lead citrate stains) (Reproduced with permission from Giles LGF, Taylor JR: Human zygapophyseal joint capsule and synovial fold innervation. *Br J Rheumatol* 26:93-98, 1987. Copyright Bailliere Tindall, London.)

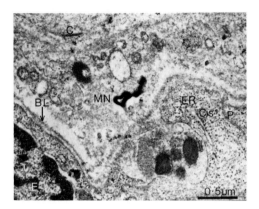

Figure 7.7 A transmission electron photomicrograph of the region of the myelinated nerve fiber shown in Figure 7.6. BL = basal lamina; C = collagen fibers; Cis = cisterna of the granular endoplasmic reticulum; E = endothelial cell nucleus; ER = endoplasmic reticulum; MN = myelinated nerve; P = plasmalemma. *Note:* It was necessary to underexpose the structure MN in order to show the myelin layers (see Fig. 7.8). (Reproduced with permission from Giles LGF, Taylor JR: Human zygapophyseal joint capsule and synovial fold innervation. *Br J Rheumatol* 26:93-98, 1987. Copyright Bailliere Tindall, London.)

the synovial folds are shown in Figure 7.3, region b.

Figures 7.7 and 7.8 show higher magnifications of the myelinated nerve fiber in Figure 7.6. This nerve followed the blood vessel for a distance of at least 8 μm before the blood vessel disappeared from the face of the block.

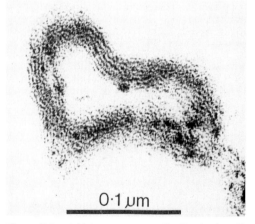

0·1 μm

Figure 7.8. A higher power magnification to show the myelin layers of the small myelinated nerve fiber shown in Figures 7.6 and 7.7. Each major dense line is approximately 25 Ångstroms thick.

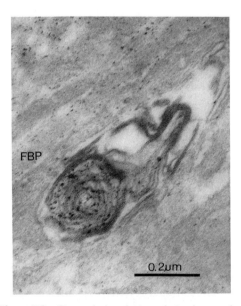

Figure 7.9. Transmission electron photomicrograph of part of a synovial fold showing a small myelinated nerve fiber among fibroblast processes (FBP). The nerve diameter is 0.3 μm. From a 42-year-old male, region b on Figure 7.3. Each major dense line is approximately 28 Ångstroms thick. (Uranyl magnesium acetate and lead citrate stains) (Reproduced with permission from Giles LGF, Taylor JR, Cockson A: Human zygapophyseal joint synovial folds. *Acta Anat* 126:110-114, 1986. Copyright S. Karger AG, Basel.)

A further example of a small paravascular myelinated nerve fiber from the inferior joint recess subsynovial tissue of a lumbosacral synovial fold is shown in Figure 7.9. There is some fragmentation of the myelin.

Nerves in the Accessory and Posteromedial Fibrous Capsules and the Ligamentum Flavum

No neural structures could be demonstrated in the ligamentum flavum tissue by transmission electron microscopy, despite a long and careful search. Nerve fibers were seen in the accessory (L5–S1) and/or posteromedial fibrous (L4–5) capsule in 3 out of 13 specimens. An example, shown in Figure 7.10, illustrates the poor fixation, characteristic of the nerve fibers seen in this tissue using this method.

Table 7.1 lists the average diameter of the myelinated nerve fibers demonstrated in the transmission electron microscopic study.

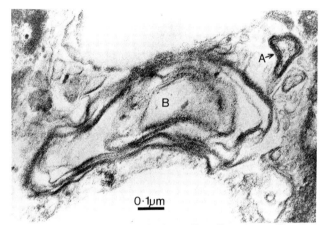

Figure 7.10. Transmission electron photomicrograph of a small myelinated nerve fiber (0.2 μm average diameter) (A) and a larger, apparently myelinated structure (B) (0.7 μm average diameter) in the joint capsule (region a on Fig. 7.3), adjacent to a synovial fold. From a 28-year-old male. (Uranyl magnesium acetate and lead citrate stains) (Reproduced with permission from Giles LGF, Taylor JR: Human zygapophyseal joint capsule and synovial fold innervation. *Br J Rheumatol* 26:93-98, 1987. Copyright Bailliere Tindall, London.)

Table 7.1.
Diameter of Nerve Fibers Found in the Transmission Electron Microscopy Study[a]

Age and Sex	Lumbar Level	Range of Nerve Fiber Diameters[b]	
		Synovial Fold	Inferior Joint Recess Accessory or Posteromedial Fibrous Capsule
		μm	μm
20F	L5–S1	—	0.8
28M	L5–S1	—	0.2 & 0.7
32M	L5–S1	0.2	—
35F	L5–S1	0.2	—
33F (a)	L5–S1	—	—
33F (b)	L5–S1	—	—
38M	L4–5	—	3.2
40M	L4–5	—	—
42M	L5–S1	0.3	—
43F	L4–5	—	—
45M	L4–5	0.2	—
45M	L5–S1	0.4	—
57M	L4–5	—	—

[a]None of the surgical specimens showed neural structures in the ligamentum flavum.
[b]These values may represent an underestimate of the true nerve fiber diameter because of contracture artifact which may be of the order of 5–10% for epon/araldite (4).

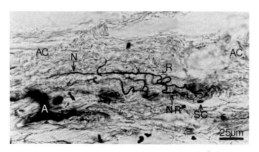

Figure 7.11. Montage made from a section (cut at a thickness of 30 μm) which shows an argyrophilic fibrous structure in close proximity to the inferior joint recess accessory capsule–synovial fold junction (region a on Fig. 7.3) of a 34-year-old male and exhibiting the features characteristic of a nerve receptor structure. AC = inferior joint recess accessory capsule; N = nerve fiber; NR = node of Ranvier; R = reticular fibers; SC = Schwann cell nucleus. Where the nerve fiber is marked by an N, its diameter is 1.5 μm. The coiled terminal part of the axon has a diameter of 0.5 μm. A = artefact. (Modified Schofield's silver impregnation) (Reproduced with permission from Giles LGF, Taylor JR: Human zygapophyseal joint capsule and synovial fold innervation. *Br J Rheumatol* 26:93-98, 1987. Copyright Bailliere Tindall, London.)

Demonstration of Nerves Using Silver Impregnation Studies

Fifteen out of 17 silver-stained specimens showed clearly defined nerve fibers (see Table 7.2). These were found in 8 of the synovial specimens and in 12 of the inferior joint recess accessory fibrous capsule (L5–S1) and/or posteromedial fibrous capsule (L4–5) specimens.

Nerves in the Accessory and Posteromedial Fibrous Capsules

In 3 of the 17 specimens, argyrophilic fibrous structures which appeared to be encapsulated nerve endings, were seen in the fibrous tissue of the zygapophyseal joint inferior recess accessory capsule (Figs. 7.11 and 7.12). In 12 specimens the nerve fibers were traced through serial sections to what appeared to be their unencapsulated "terminations" in the fibrous tissue of the capsule (Figs. 7.13 and 7.14).

In the capsular portions of the surgical specimens nerve fibers were seen entering

Table 7.2.
Diameter of Nerve Fibers and/or Fasciculi Found in the Silver Impregnation Study [a]

Age and Sex	Lumbar Level	Range of Nerve Fiber and/or Fasciculus Diameters	
		Subsynovial Tissue/Lining Membrane	Inferior Joint Recess Accessory or Posteromedial Fibrous Capsule
		μm	μm
27F	L5–S1	1.5–11.4	1.5–11.4
29F	L4–5	—	—
33F	L5–S1	—	13.0
34M	L5–S1	—	0.5 & 1.5
37M	L4–5	1.2 (M[b])	2.6–7.8
40M	L5–S1	0.8 & 2.6	—
41F	L4–5	0.5 (M)	10.4 & 18.2
42M	L4–5	—	5.7 & 13.0
43F	L5–S1	0.6 & 2.6	—
45F	L5–S1	1.3–13.0 0.8 (M)	2.6–45.0 —
47F	L4–5	0.9 (M)	4.0–10.0
48F	L5–S1	—	—
49F	L4–5	1.1 (M)	—
53F	L4–5	—	11.0
53F	L5–S1	—	7.0
54F	L4–5	—	0.5 & 2.6
61M	L5–S1	—	19.6

[a]None of the surgical specimens showed neural structures in the ligamentum flavum.
[b]Synovial lining membrane.

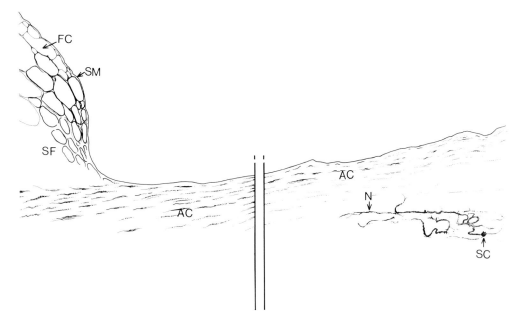

Figure 7.12. Artist's diagram of the encapsulated nerve fiber ending shown in Figure 7.11. AC = inferior joint recess accessory capsule; FC = fat cell; N = nerve fiber; SC = Schwann cell nucleus; SF = synovial fold; SM = synovial lining membrane.

the base of synovial folds from the accessory capsule (Fig. 7.15).

The anatomical relationship between the argyrophilic fibrous structure shown in Figure 7.11 and the base of its associated synovial fold is shown diagrammatically in Figure 7.12. The diagram is a composite picture of the information obtained from focusing through multiple focal planes. The distance between the nerve fiber in the inferior joint recess accessory capsule (Fig. 7.12) and the base of the synovial fold is 4.2 mm, as measured on the histologic section.

Figure 7.15 shows a silver-stained whole-mount specimen of part of the base of a synovial fold, adjacent to the inferior joint recess accessory capsule; two small nerves project from the capsule into the synovial fold; the microscope was focused on the nerves, one of which is shown in a montage in Figure 7.16.

Nerves in Synovial Folds

In 8 out of 17 of the silver-impregnated specimens, nerve fibers were demonstrated in the synovial fold, both in the subsynovial tissue (4) and/or in the synovial membrane (5).

Figure 7.17 shows a silver-impregnated whole mount of a totally resected zygapophyseal joint intra-articular synovial fold. A highly magnified view of the rectangle in Figure 7.17 is shown in Figure 7.18.

Part of a silver-impregnated synovial fold lining membrane, with a very small nerve fiber, which runs in a paravascular situation for part of its course, is demonstrated in Figure 7.19.

In five specimens nerve fibers were demonstrated actually in the surface of the synovial lining membrane, closely associated with blood vessels (Fig. 7.19.)

Nerves in the Ligamentum Flavum

None of the preparations showed any neural structures in the portions of ligamentum flavum included in the surgical specimens.

Summary Statement

Table 7.2 lists all examples of nerve fibers and/or fasciculi demonstrated by the silver impregnation technique.

Figure 7.13. A nerve fasciculus, which appears to "terminate" in the inferior joint recess capsule of a 42-year-old male (L4–5 level). The maximum diameter of the fasciculus, which contains several axons, is 13 μm (region a on Fig. 7.3). (Modified Schofield's silver impregnation.)

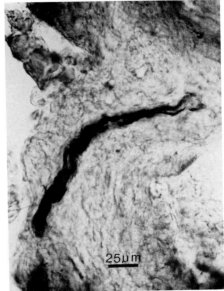

Figure 7.14. Montage made from a section (cut at a thickness of 30 μm) which shows what appears to be a nerve fasciculus in the inferior joint recess capsule of a 42-year-old male (L4–5 level). The maximum diameter of the nerve (N) is 5.7 μm (region a on Fig. 7.3). *Note:* The stained nerve fibers illustrated were traced to their termination as seen in serial sections. (Modified Schofield's silver impregnation.)

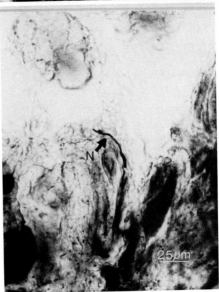

Figure 7.15. A whole-mount silver-impregnated specimen of the L5–S1 zygapophyseal joint from a 27-year-old female, showing the inferior joint recess accessory capsule (AC) with nerve fasciculi (N) projecting from it into the synovial folds (SF), adjacent to a fibrous septum (S) (region of the junction between a and b on Fig. 7.3). The average diameter of the nerve fasciculi is 11.4 μm. The nerve fasciculus in the rectangle, which was resected, then serially sectioned (at a thickness of 30 μm) is shown in Figure 7.16. (Modified Schofield's silver impregnation) (Reproduced with permission from Giles LGF, Taylor JR: Innervation of lumbar zygapophyseal joint synovial folds. *Acta Orthop Scand* 58:43-46, 1987. Copyright Munksgaard International Publishers, Denmark.)

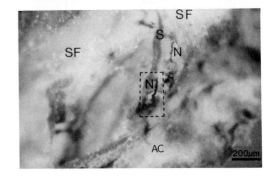

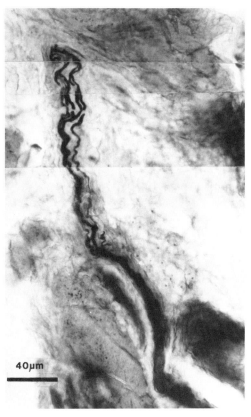

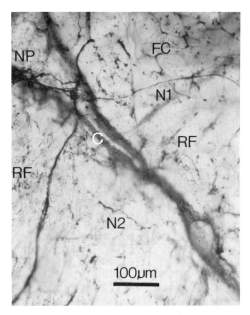

Figure 7.18. Highly magnified view of the rectangle on the whole mount shown in Figure 7.17. The following can be observed: the extensive paravascular nerve plexus (NP) on the capillary (C); the synovial fold fat cells (FC); the single nerve fiber (N1), with an average diameter of 1.7 μm, traversing the synovial fold and not related to any blood vessels; the silver-stained structure (N2) which consists of one or two nerve fibers; and the reticular fibers (RF) adjacent to the fat cells. (Reproduced with permission from Giles LGF, Taylor JR: Innervation of lumbar zygapophyseal joint synovial folds. *Acta Orthop Scand* 58:43-46, 1987. Copyright Munksgaard International Publishers, Denmark.)

Figure 7.16. Montage of the nerve fasciculus containing six axons in the rectangle on Figure 7.15; its average diameter is 11.4 μm. The average diameter of each axon is approximately 1.5 μm. (Reproduced with permission from Giles LGF, Taylor JR: Innervation of lumbar zygapophyseal joint synovial folds. *Acta Orthop Scand* 58:43-46, 1987. Copyright Munksgaard International Publishers, Denmark.)

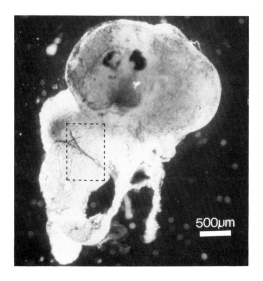

Figure 7.17. A whole-mount silver-impregnated intra-articular synovial fold from the L5–S1 zygapophyseal joint of a 40-year-old male (region b on Fig. 7.3). Numerous small blood vessels are noted, and the area within the rectangle is shown in Figure 7.18. (Modified Schofield's silver impregnation) (Reproduced with permission from Giles LGF, Taylor JR: *Acta Orthop Scand* 58:43-46, 1987. Copyright Munksgaard International Publishers, Denmark.)

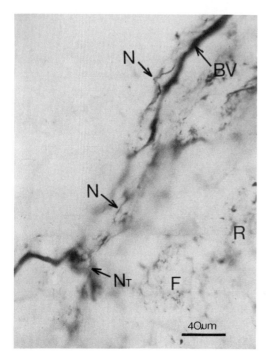

Figure 7.19. Montage of the L4–5 zygapophyseal joint synovial fold from a 49-year-old male, showing the extremely small nerve fiber (N) which appears to terminate as a "free ending" (NT) in the synovial lining membrane. The average diameter of the nerve fiber between N and N is 1.1 μm (region b on Fig. 7.3). BV = blood vessel; F = fat cell; R = reticular fibers. (Modified Schofield's silver impregnation) (Reproduced with permission from Giles LGF: Human zygapophyseal joint inferior recess synovial folds: a light microscope examination. *Anat Rec* 220:117-124, 1988. Copyright A.R. Liss, New York.)

In 8 out of the 17 silver-impregnated specimens, neural structures were demonstrated in the synovial fold, both in the subsynovial tissue (4) and/or in the synovial lining membrane (5). In 12 of the 17 cases, neural structures were found in parts of the accessory fibrous capsule (L5–S1) and/or posteromedial fibrous capsule (L4–5) adjacent to the inferior recess.

Nerve fiber and fasciculus diameters are listed in columns 3 and 4 of Table 7.2. A single figure indicates that only one nerve fiber and/or fasciculus was seen; a range of diameters indicates that several nerve fibers and/or fasciculi of different diameters were found. The neural structures in the synovial fold were paravascular as well as independ-

ent of blood vessels. In the silver technique it is not possible to distinguish between myelinated and unmyelinated longitudinal fibers since only the axons are impregnated and not the myelin.

Demonstration of Nerves Using Gold Chloride Impregnation Studies

Eight out of 16 specimens showed clearly defined nerve fibers. These were found in 7 of the synovial fold specimens and in 3 of the inferior joint recess accessory fibrous capsule (L5–S1) and/or posteromedial fibrous capsule (L4–5) specimens.

A low-power view of a whole-mount gold-chloride-impregnated synovial fold is demonstrated in Figure 7.20. It has not yet been cleared in glycerine.

Figure 7.21 shows a semi-whole-mount teased portion of an L4–5 inferior joint recess posteromedial fibrous capsule, with its adjacent synovial fold. A small nerve fasciculus, which is remote from blood vessels, is seen weaving through the synovial fold. The area in the rectangle of Figure 7.21 is

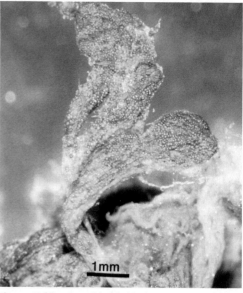

Figure 7.20. A gold-chloride-impregnated synovial fold from a 39-year-old female (L5–S1 level). (Modified gold chloride impregnation technique of Zinn DJ, Morln LP: The use of commercial citric juices in gold chloride staining of nerve endings. *Stain Technol* 37:380-382, 1962.)

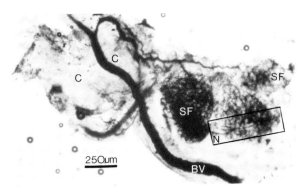

Figure 7.21. A gold-chloride-impregnated specimen, which has been cleared and mounted in glycerine, from a 25-year-old male (L4–5 level), showing a nerve fasciculus (regions a and b on Fig. 7.3). C = inferior joint recess posteromedial fibrous capsule: BV = blood vessel; N = nerve fasciculus; SF = synovial fold. (Modified gold chloride impregnation technique of Zinn DJ, Morin LP: The use of commercial citric juices in gold chloride staining of nerve endings. *Stain Technol* 37:380-382, 1962. (Reproduced with permission from Giles LGF, Taylor JR: Human zygapophyseal joint capsule and synovial fold innervation. *Br J Rheumatol* 26:93-98, 1987. Copyright Bailliere Tindall, London.)

shown enlarged in the form of a montage in Figure 7.22. This montage shows that the fasciculus contains approximately six axons, each ranging from 0.6 to 1.0 μm in diameter.

An example of a teased gold-chloride-impregnated whole-mount specimen, which has been cleared in glycerine, is shown in Figure 7.23. An extensive vascular plexus is seen in this inferior joint recess posteromedial fibrous capsule of L4–5. It extends into the synovial folds and consists of a number of blood vessels (BV) with cross communications which can be clearly recognized from their "hollow" nature and intermittent erythrocyte content. A single nerve fiber with what is possibly a mitochondrial swelling or "bead" is shown.

As with the transmission electron microscopy and silver impregnation techniques, small paravascular axons were demonstrated in the synovial folds using gold chloride impregnation. An example of a blood vessel with two paravascular axons accompanying it, as it courses through the synovial fold, is shown in Figure 7.24.

Summary Statement

Table 7.3 lists all examples of neural structures demonstrated by the gold chloride impregnation technique. In 7 out of 16 gold-chloride-impregnated specimens, neural structures were demonstrated in the syn-

ovial fold, both in the subsynovial tissue (5) and in the synovial lining membrane (2). In 3 of the 16 cases, neural structures were found in parts of the accessory fibrous capsule (L5–S1) and/or posteromedial fibrous capsule (L4–5) adjacent to the inferior recess. None of the preparations showed any neural structures in the portions of ligamentum flavum included in the surgical specimens.

Nerve fiber and fasciculus diameters are listed in columns 3 and 4 of Table 7.3. A single figure indicates that only one nerve fiber and/or fasciculus was seen; a range of diameters indicates that several nerve fibers and/or fasciculi of different diameters were found. The neural structures in the synovial fold were paravascular as well as independent of blood vessels. In the gold chloride technique it is not possible to distinguish between myelinated and unmyelinated longitudinal fibers since only the axons are impregnated and not the myelin.

Demonstration of Sensory Nerves by Substance P Immunohistochemical Studies

Substance P immunofluorescent profiles were observed in two out of four specimens in the lumbosacral inferior joint recess capsule and in three out of four adjacent synovial folds. The immunopositive profiles were easily distinguished from the diffuse

Figure 7.22. Enlargement of the rectangular area on Figure 7.21 showing the nerve fasciculus from near the tip of the synovial fold (region b on Fig. 7.3). (Reproduced with permission from Giles LGF, Taylor JR: Human zygapophyseal joint capsule and synovial fold innervation. *Br J Rheumatol* 26:93-98, 1987. Copyright Bailliere Tindall, London.)

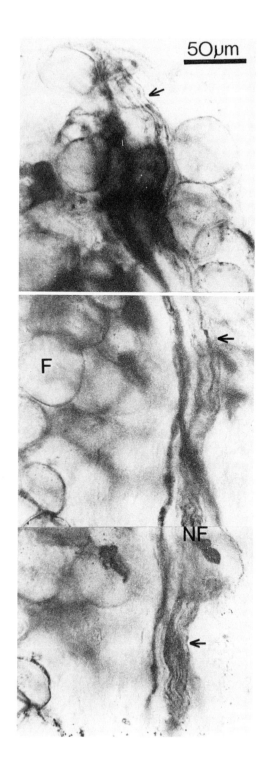

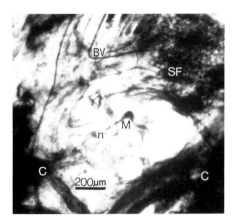

Figure 7.23. A small nerve fiber (n) (diameter-3.1 μm) is associated with a 31-μm-diameter mitochondrial swelling or "bead" (M), which is adjacent to a synovial fold (SF) amidst articular blood vessels, some of which leave the inferior joint recess posteromedial fibrous capsule (C) and enter the synovial folds (50-year-old female, L4–5 zygapophyseal joint; regions a and b on Fig. 7.3). BV = blood vessels. (Modified gold chloride impregnation technique of Zinn DJ, Morin LP: The use of commercial citric juices in gold chloride staining of nerve endings. *Stain Technol* 37:380-382, 1962.)

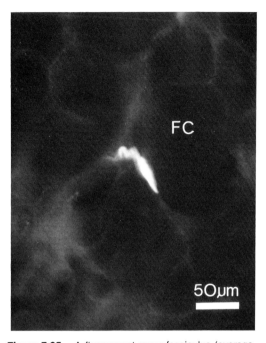

Figure 7.25. A fluorescent nerve fasciculus (average diameter approximately 6.3 μm) is seen within the synovial fold (region b on Fig. 7.3). From 25-year-old male (a); see Table 7.4. FC = fat cell. From Giles LGF, Harvey AR: Immunohistochemical demonstration of nociceptors in the capsule and synovial folds of human zygapophyseal joints. *Br J Rheumatol* 26:362-364, 1987. Copyright Bailliere Tindall, London.)

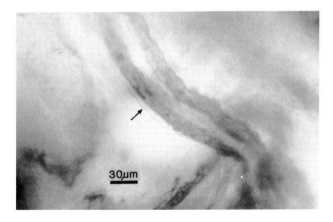

Figure 7.24. Two paravascular axons (region b on Fig. 7.3) can be seen (*arrow*) accompanying the blood vessel, which is seen as a nonuniformly stained structure, in the subsynovial tissue from a 50-year-old female (L4–5 level). The average diameter of the lumen of the blood vessel is 15 μm. This photomicrograph is from the synovial fold (SF) region in Figure 7.23. (Modified gold chloride impregnation technique of Zinn DJ, Morin LP: The use of commercial citric juices in staining of nerve endings: *Stain Technol* 37:380-382, 1962. Reproduced with permission from Giles LGF,: Human lumbar zygapophyseal joint inferior recess synovial folds: a light microscope examination. *Anat Rec* 220:117-124, 1988. Copyright A.R. Liss, New York.)

Table 7.3.
Diameter of Nerve Fibers and/or Fasciculi Found in the Gold Chloride Impregnation Study [a]

Age and Sex	Lumbar Level	Range of Nerve Fiber and/or Fasciculus Diameters	
		Subsynovial Tissue/Lining Membrane	Inferior Joint Recess Accessory or Posteromedial Fibrous Capsule
		µm	µm
20M(a)	L4–5	—	—
20M(b)	L4–5	—	—
25M(a)	L4–5	0.6–1.0	—
25M(b)	L4–5	—	—
29F	L4–5	1.1(M[b])	—
33M	L4–5	1.0(M)	—
36F	L5–S1	—	—
37F	L4–5	9.7	—
39F	L4–5	11.0	—
39F	L5–S1	—	25.0
48F	L5–S1	—	—
50F	L4–5	1.0–4.0	0.65–15.6
57M	L4–5	—	—
58M	L4–5	—	—
67M	L4–5	0.5	1.3 & 18.0
70M	L4–5	—	—

[a]None of the surgical specimens showed neural structures in the ligamentum flavum.
[b]Synovial lining membrane.

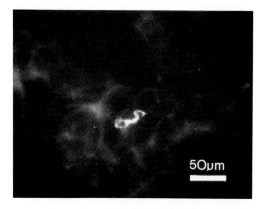

Figure 7.26. A fluorescent nerve fiber (average diameter approximately 3.1 µm) is seen within the synovial fold (region b on Fig. 7.3). From 25-year-old male (b); see Table 7.4.

Table 7.4.
Diameter of Nerve Fibers Found in the Immuno-histochemical Study [a]

Age and Sex	Lumbar Level	Range of Nerve Fiber and/or Fasciculus Diameters	
		Synovial Fold	Inferior Joint Recess Accessory Capsule
		µm	µm
25M(a)	L5–S1	6.3–7.6	27.0
25M(b)	L5–S1	3.1–11.0	3.0–20.0
30M	L5–S1	1.5–3.0	—
33M	L5–S1	—	—

[a]None of the surgical specimens showed neural structures in the ligamentum flavum.

background fluorescence of the collagenous tissue of the capsule and the background of the synovial fold adipose tissue (Figs. 7.25 and 7.26). The morphology of the fluorescent profiles shown is in keeping with the view that these are nerve fibers.

Nerve fiber and/or fasciculus diameters are listed in columns 3 and 4 of Table 7.4.

The diameter of the nerve fibers in the inferior joint recess accessory capsule fibrous tissue ranged from 3.0 to 27 µm. The diameter of the nerve fibers in the synovial folds ranged from 1.5 to 11 µm.

The immunopositive nerve fibers were sparsely scattered in both types of tissue, but their distribution was comparable to that

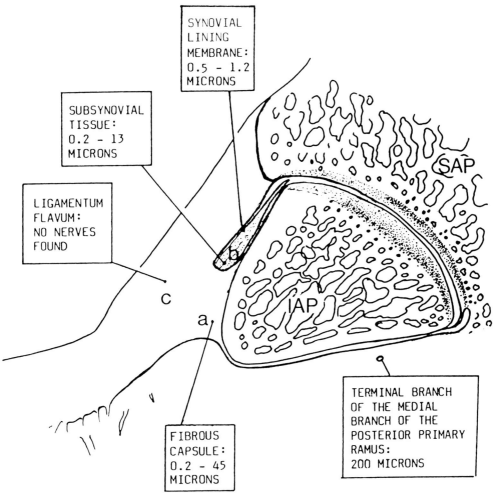

Figure 7.27. Artist's diagram of a composite drawing of the L4–5 and L5–S1 zygapophyseal joints, with particular reference to their soft tissue structures. This figure represents the approximate positions of the nerve fibers and/or fasciculi demonstrated, as well as their ranges in diameter. IAP = inferior articular process of the vertebra; SAP = superior articular process. Nerve fibers, fasciculi, and encapsulated endings were found in both the accessory capsule at L5–S1 and in the posteromedial fibrous capsule at L4–5 (a); nerve fibers and fasciculi were found in the subsynovial tissue of the intra-articular synovial fold, and nerve fibers were found in the synovial lining membrane (b). No neural structures were found in the ligamentum flavum (c).

found by silver and gold chloride impregnation techniques. The control sections did not show any immunofluorescent structures.

A summary of the approximate location and diameter of nerve fibers and/or fasciculi in the regions referred to in Figure 3.30 is shown in Figure 7.27.

It can be seen from Figure 7.27 that the diameters of the nerve fibers and/or fas-

ciculi found by the different histologic techniques were as follows:

- 0.5–1.2 µm in the synovial lining membrane;
- 0.2–13 µm in the subsynovial tissue;
- 0.2–45 µm in the accessory fibrous capsule (L5–S1) and/or posteromedial fibrous capsule (L4–5).

The diameter of the terminal branch of the medial branch of the posterior primary ramus is 200 µm.

The significance of the intracapsular nerve study techniques and their results are discussed in Chapters 8 and 14.

References

1. Giles LGF, Taylor JR, Cockson A: Human zygapophyseal joint synovial folds. *Acta Anat* 126:110-114, 1986.
2. Giles LGF: *The anatomy of human lower lumbar and lumbosacral zygapophyseal joint inferior recesses with particular reference to their synovial fold innervation.* Ph.D thesis, Department of Anatomy and Human Biology, University of Western Australia, Nedlands, Western Australia, 1987.
3. Giles LGF, Taylor JR: Human zygapophyseal joint capsule and synovial fold innervation. *Br J Rheumatol* 26:993-98, 1987.
4. Kushida H: A study of cellular swelling and shrinkage during fixation, dehydration and embedding in various standard media. *J Electron Microsc* 11:135, 1962.
5. Giles LGF, Taylor JR: Innervation of human lumbar zygapophyseal joint synovial folds. *Acta Orthop* 58:43-46, 1987.
6. Giles LGF: Human lumbar zygapophyseal joint inferior recess synovial folds: a light microscope examination. *Anat Rec* 220:117-124, 1988.
7. Zinn DJ, Morin LP: The use of commercial citric juices in gold chloride staining of nerve endings. *Stain Technol* 37:380-382, 1962.
8. Giles LGF, Harvey AR: Immunohistochemical demonstration of nociceptors in the capsule and synovial folds of human zygapophyseal joints. *Br J Rheumatol* 26:363-364, 1987.

CHAPTER **8**

Significance of the Nerve Study Techniques and Their Results

A limitation of gross dissection is that very small nerves cannot be distinguished from the capsular fibers. Therefore, a histologic correlation was essential to confirm the identity and position of nerves in relation to the capsule and its inferior recess. No single histologic method is ideally suited to the demonstration of nerves in connective tissues. Thus, several special histologic techniques were employed to demonstrate nerves and to distinguish between the nerves and other tissues in humans. Low back pain is appropriately studied in humans because of the particular morphology, posture, and susceptibility of the human lumbosacral spine to low back pain. Disadvantages associated with using human material are the difficulties in (*a*) obtaining material and (*b*) adequately fixing it for refined histologic techniques.

Techniques Required to Demonstrate Nerves in Connective Tissues

Ehrlich's hematoxylin and light green were used to stain the low-viscosity nitrocellulose and celloidin (LVNC) sections to illustrate the general anatomy of zygapophyseal joints, as well as the extracapsular course of the medial branches of the posterior primary ramus nerve bundles. This technique successfully demonstrated the anatomical structure of the joints, spinal ganglia, and large nerves (1, 2). However, once the small nerves entered the fibrous capsule, it was not possible to follow their course using this particular histologic technique.

The difficulty of demonstrating small-diameter nerves in embalmed cadaveric material by silver staining is well known,

and it is thought to be due to the fact that cadavers are not perfused until 24–48 hours after death, so that the small nerves degenerate (A. S. Wilson, personal communication, 1986). Therefore, special histologic methods had to be applied to fresh surgical material in order to demonstrate the nerves in human zygapophyseal joint capsules and synovial folds.

Evaluation of Techniques used to Demonstrate Nerves in Surgical Material

The routinely removed surgical material provided by various surgeons varied in size and in the proportions of ligamentum flavum and other capsular material provided, but the synovial folds were usually complete in the 50 specimens processed. The ligamentum flavum was also recognizable from its yellow color. Thus the tissue in which the neural structures were found was known to be synovial fold, ligamentum flavum, or accessory capsule, but the precise location of these structures within each of those tissue types could not always be accurately specified. The continuity of these structures between different parts of the specimen could not always be followed.

Fixation of Tissues

Workers in the field of neurohistology have always been greatly handicapped by difficulties in adequate fixation of neural structures to demonstrate the exact structure (3, 4). Bearing this in mind, the rationale behind the use of fixatives in this study was to try to maintain the tissue in a condition as near as possible to that existing in vivo. Surgery provides the best available method of obtaining human material for transmission electron microscopy, but the quality of immersion-fixed surgical material cannot be compared with that obtained from the perfused tissue of small mammals (5). In spite of the problems involved in fixing large human specimens by immersion, it has been possible to demonstrate nerves in the capsule and inferior recess synovial folds using the following techniques.

Silver Impregnation Studies: Modified Schofield's Method

With any impregnation staining technique it is necessary to clearly establish criteria for the identification of nerve fibers as opposed to other "fibers". *Nerve fibers or fasciculi* were identified as evenly stained black "ribbons," with occasional Schwann cell nuclei along their length. *Reticulin fibers* were identified by the fibrous wavy threads which leave them at irregular intervals, while *collagen fibers* were identified as brown fibers with a very regular wave pattern (6). Silver impregnation techniques allow identification and description of each of these three types of "fiber," but they are not suitable for demonstrating myelin (7). Such techniques have traditionally been the most usual methods used to trace the course of nerve fibers (8). According to Stone (9), the disadvantages of silver impregnation are that (*a*) it will not distinguish between myelinated and unmyelinated fibers, (*b*) it will not "stain" all the axons present, and (*c*) it does not necessarily impregnate all the terminals of an axon. In addition, large quantities of fat, as seen in the synovial folds, make the demonstration of endings difficult (10), and thus many techniques produce inconsistent results (11). An advantage of silver impregnation is that it can be used on freshly fixed tissues, whereas most other methods, e.g., the methylene blue techniques of "staining" fibers, are limited to living tissues (3). Also, silver techniques stain some other tissues, e.g., blood vessels, thus making it possible to relate the nerve fibers to blood vessels.

Some silver impregnation methods are notoriously capricious (12) and unreliable (10) and are plagued by inconstant staining

of fine terminals (7, 13–16). However, Schofield's (17) technique as modified by Wilson (A. S. Wilson, personal communication, 1986) was found to give mainly artifact-free results with minimal black precipitate formation (see Appendix 3). The physical-chemical basis of the reduction of some metallic compounds by small fibers is fully discussed by Drury and Wallington (10).

Gold Chloride Impregnation Studies

Gold chloride impregnation, followed by formic acid, produces a black impregnation of neural elements against a pink–grey background (10), depending on optimum staining. The gold chloride technique is designed to show peripheral nerve fibers and their endings (18). The technique was used in this investigation to confirm and support the evidence of silver impregnation. However, it was found to be less reliable than the silver impregnation method in that neural structures were shown in only 8 of the 16 specimens, whereas neural structures were shown in 15 of the 17 silver-impregnated specimens.

Evidence from Silver and Gold Chloride Impregnation Studies

Acceptable results were usually obtained with the silver and gold chloride impregnation studies of zygapophyseal joint synovial folds and the fibrous portions of the capsular material.

Nerves in the Fibrous Capsule

Both methods showed clearly defined nerve fibers and/or fasciculi within the fibrous part of the joint capsule, including the accessory capsule. The silver impregnation method also demonstrated nerve endings in this capsular material. Some nerve fibers appeared to end in mechanoreceptorlike structures (Fig. 7.11) with an appearance similar to the simple encapsulated corpuscles described in cats by Polacek (19) and Polacek and Peregrin (20). Polacek (21) refers to the great variation in the appearance and distribution of nerve endings in joints. This text supports his findings.

It has been shown that joint receptors discharge with changes in joint angle (22–24), and, according to Skoglund (25), location of joint receptors within the joint soft tissues suggests that they are activated at a particular position of the joint or by movements within a restricted angle. Therefore, it is suggested that the encapsulated argyrophilic fibrous end organs found in this study may relate to mechanoreception at the synovial fold–fibrous capsule junction. Other nerve fibers, which were presumed to have a myelinated axon in view of their diameter, appeared to terminate without end organs. No clearly defined unmyelinated fibers were found in the fibrous capsule, contrary to the findings of Hadley (26), who claimed to have found unmyelinated fibers in human zygapophyseal joint capsules using silver impregnation. However, the validity of Hadley's (26) finding of unmyelinated nerve fibers must be questioned in view of the fact that metallic impregnation does not "stain" myelin, so it is not possible to clearly distinguish between myelinated and unmyelinated axons using metallic impregnation alone for longitudinal axons.

Nerve fiber and/or fasciculus diameters in the inferior joint recess fibrous capsular material ranged from 0.5 μm per fiber to 45 μm per fasciculus.

Nerves in Synovial Folds

Nerve fibers and/or fasciculi also projected well beyond the inferior joint recess accessory capsule into the synovial folds. The diameters ranged from 0.5 μm per fiber to 13.0 μm per nerve fasciculus in the synovial folds as they weaved between the fat cells and occasionally in the synovial lining membrane. The only motor nerves in synovial folds would be vasomotor to the numerous blood vessels. However, most of the nerves shown in this study were independent of blood vessels, coursing at some distance from the blood vessels. They were, therefore, almost certainly sensory in function. No encapsulated nerve endings were observed in the synovial folds, in spite of the nerve fibers being carefully traced in serial sections to their apparent terminations where they appeared to end without any visible end organs. This appearance could be due to (a) lack of staining of specific endings (Q. Bone, personal communication, 1985) or (b) the possibility that the nerve fiber terminal may be too small for the resolving power of the microscope (A. S. Wilson, personal communication, 1986). Taking these two points into account, the nerve fiber "terminations" are more likely to be "free nerve fiber endings," since encapsulated endings "stain" in the *capsule* of surgical material using the same technique (see Fig. 7.11).

Transmission Electron Microscopy Studies

Transmission electron microscopy represents a substantially true and detailed picture of the morphology of cells and tissues in life (27), although all histologic fixation techniques may cause tissue shrinkage (F. C. Richmond, personal communication, 1986); different techniques result in different degrees of tissue shrinkage (28). The use of epoxy resins is considered to result in a linear contraction of 5–10% (28, 29). The main disadvantage of transmission electron microscopy techniques with human material is that perfusion cannot be used, and immersion fixation involves some delay in penetration of the fixative to deeper structures.

The surgical specimens were placed in Karnovsky's (30) fixative, containing 2 mM of calcium chloride to improve the stability of membranes. This is said to virtually eliminate myelinlike figures (8, 29, 31, 32). The transmission electron microscopy sections were adequate to demonstrate synovial fold ultrastructure, including small extracellular paravascular myelinated nerve fibers in the synovial folds. Some showed disintegrating myelin "fragments," similar to those demonstrated by Vaughn and Skoff (33), and by Adams et al (34) in their isolation of myelin fractions from adult rat brains. With the fresh surgical specimens, areas of disintegrating myelin reflect problems in dealing with immersion-fixed specimens, not with disease processes, since all the samples used were from healthy patients who suffered only from nucleus pulposus extrusion.

The use of calcium chloride ions in the fixation process and the observations that (a) the nerve fiber diameters were always of the same order (0.2 μm in synovial folds), (b) the major dense lines were of the normally accepted range (25–31 Ångstroms, which is in keeping with Angevine's [35] finding of approximately 30 Ångstroms for peripheral nerve fibers), and (c) the nerve fibers were always paravascular in location all support the conclusion that the structures are indeed myelinated axons and not myelinic figures.

Transmission electron microscopy did not demonstrate any unmyelinated nerve fibers in this study, although Schumacher (36), using various mammalian synovial folds, found unmyelinated "nerves" only, and then infrequently. Ralston et al (37) found only free-fiber endings in the synovial membrane of joints from human upper and lower limbs.

Although transmission electron microscopy shows the morphology of the nerve fibers, it does not indicate their physiologic behavior. The only certain method for determining the precise function of nerve fibers and receptors is direct electrophysiologic stimulation of identifiable nerve fibers. This is not practical or ethical in the investigation of human zygapophyseal joint synovial folds. Thus, an immunohistochemical technique was used to investigate the putative physiologic function of nerve fibers in the surgical material in this study.

Immunohistochemical Studies

Immunohistology utilizes the ability of an antibody to couple specifically with a corresponding antigen (38). Since the demonstration of specific antigens and antibodies in tissue sections and the localization of the exact sites of antigen–antibody reactions are now possible by the use of markers, either fluorescent dyes or enzymes (10), an immunohistochemical approach was used in an attempt to determine the possible function of the nerve fibers in the synovial folds. The antibodies (antisera) are conjugated with a fluorescent dye, while leaving their capacity to combine with an antigen unchanged; the degree of success of this technique depends on the high degree of contrast that can be obtained between the structures labeled and the surrounding tissues (10).

Immunohistology can be used to identify the probable function of nerve receptors in humans and has been used in the study of nociception. Substance P immunofluorescent nerve fibers, which are known to participate in the sensory, especially nociceptive, transmission of neural impulses (39), have been found in the posterior longitudinal ligament (39, 40), human periosteum (41), knee synovial membrane and menisci (42), and human tooth pulp (43).

The substance P nerve fibers demonstrated in this study strongly suggest the presence of putative nociceptive nerve fibers in the synovial folds and fibrous capsule.

The method of direct immunohistologic staining was used. Substance P immunofluorescent positive profiles were observed in two of the four specimens of inferior recess joint capsule, and in three of the four adjacent synovial folds. The immunopositive profiles were easily distinguished from the diffuse background fluorescence of the collagenous tissue of the capsule, and the nonfluorescent background of the synovial fold adipose tissue (see Figs. 7.25 and 7.26). The diameter of nerve fibers and/or fasciculi in the capsular tissue ranged from 3.0 to 27 µm and from 1.5 to 11 µm in the synovial folds. The control sections did not show any immunofluorescence.

The evidence presented by Henry (44) and Liesi et al (40) on the probable nociceptive significance of substance P (Chapter 5) emphasizes the potential physiologic and clinical significance of the demonstration of substance P positive profiles in the capsule and synovial folds (but not in the ligamentum flavum) in this study. This potential clinical significance relates to some cases of low back pain, which will be discussed in Chapter 14.

The Nature and Function of Nerves Demonstrated in the Joint Tissues

A limitation of the serial-sectioning method is that nerve endings without a specialized morphology may not be easily differentiated from other nervous structures (45). The relative paucity of neural structures found is in keeping with Wyke's (46) finding that "free nerve endings are sparse" in the fibrous capsule. According to Samuel (47), myelinated and unmyelinated nerves, which often accompany blood vessels in human knee joints, are distributed in a plexiform manner through the fibrous capsule and synovial membrane and terminate in "various types of nerve endings." Previous differences of opinion regarding the existence of nerves and their endings in human synovial joint fibrous capsules and synovial folds were the result of previous investigators' examining too small a series of specimens. While 20 of the 50 specimens examined in this present study showed neural structures in the fibrous joint capsule, and 23 showed nerve fibers and/or fasciculi in the synovial folds, a plexiform arrangement was not found in human zygapophyseal joints.

The external fiber diameter has been used by some authors to classify myelinated fibers into major functional groups since fiber diameter correlates well with physiologic properties, e.g., speed of conduction (48). Light microscopic inspection of a transverse section of human peripheral nerve reveals that it is composed of fibers of many different diameters, ranging from about 0.08 μm, or less, to 25 μm (49). The axons of myelinated fibers in adults range in diameter from less than 1 to 2 μm (50, 51); unmyelinated fibers (C-fibers), which also include postganglionic efferents (52), have a diameter of 0.2–1.0 μm (53, 54) and are nociceptive, as are small myelinated fibers (A-delta fibers) with a diameter of 1–4 μm (53). On the basis of this classification, the small-diameter fibers demonstrated in the present study are C-fibers and small-diameter myelinated A-delta fibers. Those which do not accompany blood vessels are most likely afferent fibers which may have a nociceptive function. The small 0.2-μm myelinated paravascular nerve fibers accompanying the small blood vessels within the synovial folds are considered to have an autonomic vasoregulatory function.

The Search for Nerves in the Ligamentum Flavum

The region of meshing of the fibrous "accessory" capsule and the elastic ligamentum flavum has small neural structures, but none were found in the elastic ligamentum flavum itself in spite of using various techniques. However, this does not disprove Bogduk's (55) speculative suggestion that

the ligamentum flavum may receive some innervation from the medial branch of the posterior primary ramus, or the findings of Pedersen et al (56) and Hirsch et al (57) that fine free-fiber endings are present on the "outermost layer" of the posterior surface of the ligamentum flavum, since the special methods used to demonstrate neural structures in this study were used on only relatively small portions of ligamentum flavum. The ventral surface of the ligamentum flavum could be innervated by twigs of the sinuvertebral nerve entering the ligamentum flavum in association with blood vessels through the vascular channels (see Figs. 4.9 and 4.10). In spite of this, no nerves could be demonstrated in the ligamentum flavum by any of the methods employed in this study.

It is not surprising that no proprioceptive endings were demonstrated in this study, since they would be difficult to record from a highly elastic ligament. The fact that no substance P positive profiles were found in the ligamentum flavum is in keeping with the findings of Korkala et al (39), who found no substance P positive profiles (in small pieces of ligamentum flavum), despite their demonstration of substance P positive profiles in the posterior longitudinal ligament. The description of free nerve fibers and endings on the "outermost" posterior surface of the ligamenta flava by Pedersen et al (56) and Hirsch et al (57) may well have been in what is identified as the accessory capsule in this text or in posteromedial fibrous structures at higher lumbar levels.

Since blood vessels have been demonstrated in the posterolateral region of the ligamentum flavum in this study, one must presume the presence of paravascular vasomotor nerve fibers. These paravascular fibers could possibly mediate pain (see Chapter 5) from the ligamentum flavum.

Significance of Zygapophyseal Joint Innervation and the Relevance of the Innervation and Vascularization to Low Back Pain

There has been much discussion in the literature regarding the causes of low back pain, e.g., discogenic pain (58, 59) versus zygapophyseal joint pain (60), but in numerous cases of low back pain diagnostic uncertainty still remains because the structure causing pain often cannot be seen by even the latest diagnostic imaging procedures (61). In some cases, the injection of local anesthetic into the zygapophyseal joint cavity results in relief from low back pain (62, 63), presumably due to anesthetizing nerve receptors in the synovial folds or in the joint capsule. Therefore, it would appear that the synovial folds or the joint capsule are likely sources of such pain, although innervation of the zygapophyseal joint synovial folds has been denied historically (26; B. D. Wyke, personal communication, 1983).

Nerve fibers and/or fasciculi were found in the synovial folds of relatively young patients (25-32 years of age) with no evidence of zygapophyseal joint osteoarthritis, as well as in the synovial folds of older patients who had some degree of osteoarthritis. Thus, the nerve fibers found in the synovial folds are a normal anatomical finding and are not associated with degenerative joint disease.

It is acknowledged that it is not possible to categorically prove the function of the small nerve fibers which are unrelated to blood vessels in the synovial folds in vivo, and thus their function must be speculative. However, pain is generally accepted as being due to various types of physical stimuli to nerve fibers, or nerve receptors, such as mechanical, chemical, thermal, and electrical stimuli (64). Therefore, it seems reasonable to speculate that (a) mechanical "nipping" of synovial folds (65) or (b) traumatic synovitis with chemical irritation of nerve endings (66-68) due to the release of noxious chemical stimuli in the synovial folds could result in pain. The mechanism of the generation of pain producing nerve impulses from an inflamed area are not known, but a role may be played by pressure distortion of an axon and by some pain-producing substances, such as histamine, substance P, prostaglandins and polypeptides (e.g., bradykinin), which may be released due to cell damage, and potassium ions, released due to cell rupture, which must be present in the area of damaged tissue to stimulate nerve endings (69).

Tissue damage may cause ischemia with the genesis of ischemic pain due to an abnormal accumulation of metabolic products in the tissues such as lactic acid, potassium ions, histamine, and plasma kinins (70). However, it is possible that chemical agents such as bradykinin and proteolytic enzymes, which may be released in the tissues because of cell damage, rather than lactic acid, stimulate the free-nerve-ending pain receptors (71).

The presence of substance P immunofluorescent nerves does not differentiate between paravascular nerves and nonparavascular nerves. Thus, it cannot be said that the substance P immunofluorescent nerves are not associated with blood vessels; moreover, it is thought that paravascular nerve fibers may transmit pain of ischemic origin. In addition, nociceptors may well exist which do not contain substance P (P. J. Snow, personal communication, 1987).

Because the synovial folds have small (0.2 μm diameter) myelinated paravascular fibers and small (0.6–13 μm diameter) myelinated fibers which are remote from blood vessels, it is suggested that these fibers may be nociceptive in function. The immunohistochemical data clearly support such a proposal.

References

1. Giles LGF, Taylor JR: Histological preparation of large vertebral specimens. *Stain Technol* 58:45-49, 1983.
2. Giles LGF, Taylor JR: The effect of postural scoliosis on lumbar apophyseal joints. *Scand J Rheumatol* 13:209-220, 1984.
3. Miller MR, Ralston HJ, Kasahara M: The pattern of cutaneous innervation of the human hand. *Am J Anat* 102:183-197, 1958.
4. Munger BL: Patterns of organization of peripheral sensory receptors. In Loewenstein WR (ed): *Principles of Receptor Physiology*. New York, Springer-Verlag, 1971, pp 523-556.
5. Giles LGF, Taylor JR, Cockson A: Human zygapophyseal joint synovial folds. *Acta Anat* 126:110-114, 1986.
6. Courtney JT: *Studies on the structure and function of pericardial innervation*. Degree of Bachelor of Medical Science thesis, Department of Anatomy and Human Biology, University of Western Australia, Perth, 1978.
7. Disbrey BD, Rack JH: *Histological Laboratory Methods*. Edinburgh, E. & S. Livingstone, 1970, p 207.
8. Baker JR: *Principles of Biological Microtechnique. A Study of Fixation and Dyeing*. London, Methuen, 1958, p 114.
9. Stone J: Cited as a personal communication by J. Courtney: Studies on the structure and function of pericardial innervation. Bachelor of Medical Science

thesis, Department of Anatomy and Human Biology, University of Western Australia, Nedlands, 1978.

10. Drury RAB, Wallington EA: *Carleton's Histological Technique.* ed 5. Oxford, Oxford University Press, 1980, p 110.

11. Herdman PR, Taylor JJ: Suppression of connective tissue impregnation in a silver technique for demonstrating nerve fibers. *Stain Technol* 50:37-42, 1975.

12. Cox G: Neuropathological techniques. In Bancroft JD, Stevens A (ed): *Theory and Practice of Histological Techniques.* ed 2. Edinburgh, Churchill Livingstone, 1982, pp 332-363.

13. Lee AB: *The Microtomist's Vade-Mecum. A Handbook of the Methods of Microscopic Anatomy.* ed 7. London, U. & A. Churchill, 1913, p 212.

14. Green JD: The histology of the hypophysial stalk and medial eminence in man with special reference to blood vessels, nerve fibers and a peculiar neurovascular zone in this region. *Anat Rec* 100:273-295, 1948.

15. Hagen E, Knoche H, Sinclair DC, Weddell G: The role of specialized nerve terminals in cutaneous sensibility. *Proc R Soc Lond* 141:279-287, 1953.

16. Gough NG: The staining of nerves in serial sections. *J Anat* 106:437-448, 1970.

17. Schofield G: The Nervous System. In Drury RAB, Wallington EA (eds): *Carleton's Histological Technique,* ed 5. Oxford, Oxford University Press, 1980, p 384.

18. Clark G: *Staining Procedures.* ed 3. Baltimore, Williams & Wilkins, 1973, pp 102-103.

19. Polacek P: Die Nervenversorgung des Huft- und Kniegelenkes und ihre Besonderheiten. *Anat Anz Bd* 1125:243-256, 1963.

20. Polacek P, Peregrin J: Contribution to the relationship between the structure and the function of the sensory nerve endings. *Scripta Medica* 11:256-274, 1968.

21. Polacek P: Receptors of the joints: their structures, viability and classification. *Acta Fac Med Univ Brun* 23:9-107, 1966.

22. Burgess PR, Clark JF: Characteristics of knee joint receptors in the cat. *J Physiol (Lond)* 203:317-335, 1969.

23. Ferrell WR: The adequacy of stretch receptors in the cat knee joint for signalling joint angle throughout a full range of movement. *J Physiol (Lond)* 299:85-99, 1980.

24. Gandevia SC: Illusory movements produced by electrical stimulation of low-threshold muscle afferents from the hand. *Brain* 108:965-981, 1985.

25. Skoglund S: Joint receptors and Kinesthesis. In Iggo A (ed): *Handbook of Sensory Physiology: II. Somatosensory System.* New York, Springer-Verlag, 1973, pp 111-135.

26. Hadley LA: *Anatomico–Roentgenographic Studies of the Spine.* Springfield, IL, Charles C. Thomas, 1976, pp 186, 189.

27. Meek GA: *Practical Electron Microscopy for Biologists.* London, Wiley-Interscience, 1973, p 461.

28. Kushida H: A study of cellular swelling and shrinkage during fixation, dehydration and embedding in various standard media. *J Electron Microsc* 11:135, 1962.

29. Glauert AM: Fixation, dehydration and embedding of biological specimens. *Practical Methods in Electron Microscopy.* Amsterdam, North-Holland, 1975, pp 1-4.

30. Karnovsky MJ: A formaldehyde–glutaraldehyde fixative of high osmolality for use in electron microscopy. *J Cell Biol* 27:441, 1965.

31. Bullock GR, Christian RA, Peters RF, White AM: Rapid mitochondrial enlargement in muscle as a response to triamcinolone acetonide and its relationship to the ribosomal defect. *Biochem Pharmacol* 20:943-953, 1971.

32. Bullock GR: The current status of fixation for electron microscopy: a review. *J Microsc* 133:1-15, 1983.

33. Vaughn JE, Skoff RP: Neuroglia in experimentally altered central nervous system. In Bourne GH (ed): *The Structure and Function of Nervous Tissue.* New York, Academic Press, 1972, vol 5, pp 39-70.

34. Adams CWM, Davison AN, Gregson NA: Enzyme inactivity of myelin: histochemical and biochemical evidence. *J Neurochem* 10:383-395, 1963.

35. Angevine JB: The nervous tissue. In Bloom W, Fawcett DW (ed): *A Textbook of Histology.* ed 10. Philadelphia. W.B. Saunders, 1975, pp 333- 385.

36. Schumacher HR: Ultrastructure of the synovial membrane. *Ann Clin Lab Sci* 5:489-498, 1975.

37. Ralston HJ, Miller MR, Rasahara M: Nerve endings in human fasciae, tendons, ligaments, periosteum and joint synovial membrane. *Anat Rec* 136:137-139, 1960.

38. Hamashima Y: Immunofluorescence Techniques. In Barron JP (ed): *The Use of the Olympus Fluorescence Microscope.* Tokyo, Olympus, 1982, p 33.

39. Korkala O, Gronblad M, Liesi P, Karaharju E: Immunohistochemical demonstration of nociceptors in the ligamentous structures of the lumbar spine. *Spine* 10:156-157, 1985.

40. Liesi P, Gronblad M, Korkala O, Karaharju E, Rasanen M: Substance P: neuropeptide involved in low back pain. *Lancet* 1:1328-1329, 1983.

41. Gronblad M, Liesi P, Korkala O, Karaharju E, Polak J: Innervation of human bone periosteum by peptidergic nerves. *Anat Rec* 209:297-299, 1984.

42. Gronblad M, Korkala O, Liesi P, Karaharju E: Innervation of synovial membrane and meniscus. *Acta Orthop Scand* 56:484-486, 1985.

43. Gronblad M, Liesi P, Munck AM: Peptidergic nerves in human tooth pulp. *Scand J Dent Res* 92:319-324, 1984.

44. Henry JL: Relation of substance P to pain transmission: neurophysiological evidence. In Porter R, O'Connor M (eds): *Substance P in the Nervous System* (Ciba Foundation Symposium). London, Pitman, 1982, pp 206-224.

45. Richmond FJR, Bakker DA: Anatomical organization and sensory receptor content of soft tissues surrounding upper cervical vertebrae in the cat. *J Neurophysiol* 48:49-61, 1982.

46. Wyke BD: The neurology of joints. *Annals of the Royal College of Surgeons of England* 41:25, 1967.

47. Samuel EP: The innervation of the articular capsule of the knee joint. *J Anat* 83:80, 1949.

48. Mayhew TM, Sharma AK: Sampling schemes for estimating nerve fiber size: I. Method for nerve trunks and mixed fascicularity. *J Anat* 139:45-58, 1984.

49. Wyke BD: *Principles of General Neurology.* Amsterdam, Elsevier, 1969, pp 48-49.

50. Landon DN, Hall S: The myelinated nerve fibre. In Landon DN (ed): *The Peripheral Nerve.* London, Chapman and Hall, 1976, pp 1-105.

51. Landon DN: The structure of the nerve fibre. In Culp WJ, Ochoa J (eds): *Abnormal Nerves and Muscles as Impulse Generators.* Oxford, Oxford University Press, 1982, pp 27-53.

52. Barr ML, Kiernan JA: *The Human Nervous System. An Anatomical Viewpoint.* ed 4. Philadelphia, Harper and Row, 1983, p 43.

53. Guyton AC: *Textbook of Medical Physiology.* ed 5. Philadelphia, W.B. Saunders, 1976, pp 647-648.

54. Ballantyne JP: The peripheral nervous system. In Kyle J, Hardy J (ed): *Scientific Foundations of Surgery.* ed 3. London, William Heinemann Medical Books, 1981, p 236.

55. Bogduk N: The innervation of the lumbar spine *Spine* 8:286-293, 1983.

56. Pedersen HE, Blunck CFJ, Gardner E: The anatomy of lumbo-sacral posterior rami and meningeal branches of spinal nerves (sinu-vertebral nerves) with an experi-

mental study of their function. *J Bone Joint Surg* 38A:377-391, 1956.

57. Hirsch C, Ingelmark BE, Miller M: The anatomical basis for low back pain. *Acta Orthop Scand* 33:1-17, 1963.
58. Cyriax J: *Textbook of Orthopaedic Medicine. Vol. 1. Diagnosis of Soft Tissue Lesions.* London, Bailliere, Tindall and Cassell, 1969, pp 399-401.
59. Hall-Cragg ECB: *Anatomy as a Basis for Clinical Medicine.* Baltimore, Urban and Schwarzenberg, 1985, pp 52-65.
60. Bogduk N: The lumbar zygapophyseal joints. In *Proceedings of Low Back Pain Symposium.* Sydney, Manipulative Therapists Association of Australia, 1979, pp 32-40.
61. Nachemson AL: Recent advances in the treatment of low back pain. *Int Orthop* 9:1-10, 1985.
62. Kirkaldy-Willis WH: A comprehensive outline of treatment. In Kirkaldy-Willis WH (ed): *Managing Low Back Pain.* New York, Churchill Livingstone, 1983, pp 147-160.
63. Aprill C: Lumbar facet joint arthrography and injection in the evaluation of painful disorders of the low back (abstract). Presented at the meeting of the International Society for the Study of the Lumbar Spine, Dallas, 1986.
64. Keele CA, Neil E: *Samson Wright's Applied Physiology.* ed 10. London, Oxford University Press, 1961, p 322.
65. Kirkaldy-Willis WH: The relationship of structural pathology to the nerve root. *Spine* 9:49-52, 1984.
66. Guyton AC: *Textbook of Medical Physiology.* ed 3. Philadelphia, W.B. Saunders, 1966, p 694.
67. Lim RKS: Pain. *Ann Rev Physiol* 32:269-288, 1970.
68. Keele CA, Armstrong D: Mediators of pain. In Lim RKS (ed): *Pharmacology of Pain.* Oxford, Pergamon Press, 1968.
69. Wall PD: Physiological mechanisms involved in the production and relief of pain. In Bonica JJ, Procacci P, Pagni CA (eds): *Recent Advances in Pain: Pathophysiology and Clinical Aspects.* Springfield, IL, Charles C. Thomas, 1974, pp 36-63.
70. Arcangeli P, Galletti R: Endogenous pain producing substances. In Bonica JJ, Procacci P, Pagni CA (eds): *Recent Advances in Pain: Pathophysiology and Clinical Aspects.* Springfield, IL, Charles C. Thomas, 1974, pp 82-104.
71. Guyton AC: *Textbook of Medical Physiology.* ed 7. Philadelphia, W.B. Saunders, 1986, p 348.

CHAPTER 9

Pathologic Changes Affecting the Motion Segment

Intervertebral Disc

Just as the physiology of the zygapophyseal joints cannot be divorced from consideration of other elements of the mobile segment, so pathologic changes in the intervertebral disc may be expected to affect the function of the zygapophyseal joints (1, 2).

The age of onset and the rate of progression of intervertebral disc degeneration vary greatly in different individuals, and the role of excessive or chronic stress on the spine can initiate or accelerate disc degeneration (3). Degradative changes appear in the disc by the second decade and thereafter show variable but relentless progression (4). Considerable disc degeneration has been found in most spines of 40 years of age (5). In an investigation of aging and degeneration in lumbar intervertebral discs, Pritzker (6) found that (*a*) with aging, two new cell types appear, that is, giant chondrons in discs over 30 years of age and minichondrons in association with microfracture of the cartilage end-plate; (*b*) there was focal histologic changes in the cartilage end-plate which appeared to precede histologic changes in the nucleus pulposus and anulus fibrosis; and (*c*) there were generalized thinning, ossification, and disruption of the end-plates—this was seen only in collapsed discs and was indicative of advanced pathologic processes.

The major morphologic features of the aging disc, that is, a shrinking in the volume of the nucleus pulposus and a less distinct nucleus pulposus, have been repeatedly asserted (3, 7–12).

Progressive desiccation of the nucleus pulposus, or injury allowing the escape of nuclear material is said to allow adjacent vertebrae to approximate each other, leading to bulging of the anulus fibrosus, with lifting of the adjacent periosteum leading to osteophyte formation on the edges of the articulating surfaces of vertebral bodies (13).

However, in a survey of normal age changes in the human lumbosacral spine, Twomey (14) and Twomey and Taylor (15) suggest that loss of disc thickness is not an inevitable accompaniment of disc aging.

It is as the intervertebral joint degenerates, with loss of disc thickness and subsequent subluxation of the zygapophyseal joints (16), that osteoarthritic degenerative joint disease of the zygapophyseal joints develops (16, 17). Arthritic zygapophyseal joints possibly produce referred pain in the lower extremities (17).

With advancing age, the hallmarks of spondylosis appear in cases of spinal curvature, first on the concave side of the curvature, with the convex side being relatively spared. On the concave side, disproportionate loading together with reduced movement can be invoked as responsible for the changes, at least in part (4).

Since this text is mainly concerned with low back pain with or without leg pain of zygapophyseal joint origin, intervertebral disc degenerative changes, which have been discussed in detail elsewhere (2, 18–20) are not discussed further here.

Osteoarthritic Pathologic Changes Affecting the Lumbosacral Zygapophyseal Joints

Zygapophyseal joint hyaline articular cartilage changes associated with aging are different from those occurring in osteo-arthritis, i.e.,"degenerative joint disease"; aging results in thinning but not in the diffuse evidence of degradation and repair which is characteristic of osteoarthritis (21). With advancing years, the water content of hyaline articular cartilage is reduced, whereas in osteoarthritis, it is normal or increased (22). In adults the hyaline articular cartilage often develops areas of disintegration and erosion (23).

Osteoarthritis is said to be "primary" when no etiologic factors can be discerned and "secondary" when there is an identifiable cause (23) such as previous injury to a joint (24, 25). There are many and diverse opinions concerning the cause and development of osteoarthritis (26). According to Bland (27), four theories of the pathogenesis of osteoarthritis are (a) the initial event occurs in cartilage, because of a change in the microenvironment of the chondrocytes (most investigators hold this view); (b) the initial event occurs in subchondral bone with mechanical factors being the primary cause; (c) micro-osteonecrosis occurs in the subchondral bone as a result of vascular disease; and (d) a proteolytic enzyme from type A synovial cells (phagocytes), which is normally neutralized by an inhibitor from type B synovial cells, digests the protein core of chondroitin sulphate if the inhibitor is absent (28).

Osteoarthritis is regarded as exclusively a disease of synovial joints (29). The physical and chemical alterations may reflect repeated trauma of any degree (30) and can be brought about by an increase in the functional demands on essentially healthy tissues (31). For example, I have shown that hyaline articular cartilage changes can be found where zygapophyseal joint cartilage surfaces press against each other (32). Early evidence of pressure between the opposing cartilage surfaces at the anteromedial surfaces of zygapophyseal joint cartilages was indicated by tinctorial changes where the intra-articular synovial folds are pinched between the hyaline articular cartilages (Figs. 9.1–9.3). Hyaline articular cartilage and bone changes are illustrated in this area where the joint surfaces are in contact, but other areas are relatively normal.

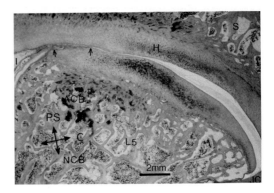

Figure 9.1. Horizontal light photomicrograph of the right lumbosacral zygapophyseal joint cartilages, from a 54-year-old male, showing an intra-articular synovial fold inclusion (I), with its fibrotic tip (*arrows*) projecting between the hyaline articular cartilages (H). L5 = inferior articular process of the L5 vertebra; S = superior articular process of the sacrum; JC = posterolateral fibrous joint capsule; ACB = abnormal cancellous bone; NCB = normal cancellous bone. The remaining part of the joint cartilage, where the cartilages are not adjacent to each other, is relatively normal, apart from some proliferation of the chondrocytes in the middle region of the joint. C = coronal plane; PS = parasagittal plane. (Ehrlich's hematoxylin stain with light green counterstain) (Reproduced with permission from Giles LGF: Pressure related changes in human lumbosacral zygapophyseal joint articular cartilage. *J Rheumatol* 13: 1093-1095, 1986.)

In these joints from middle-aged and elderly embalmed cadavers (aged 36–92 years; mean-67 years) the hyaline articular cartilage bearing on each side of the fibrous portion of the intra-articular synovial fold inclusion may show age changes which vary from (a) tinctorial changes within the matrix as seen in dark-field microscopy in 3 out of the 10 specimens, to (b) a loss of the normal chondrocyte population, with or without fibrillation of the hyaline articular cartilage. It is not the purpose of this text to describe these changes in detail, but the synovial fold tip fibrotic changes are due to pinching of the parts of the synovial fold between the cartilage surfaces. Therefore, the hyaline articular cartilage changes and subchondral bone changes in the same region of the joint suggest that these changes are pressure related.

The thickened subchondral bone on each side of the joint may show an intense stain-

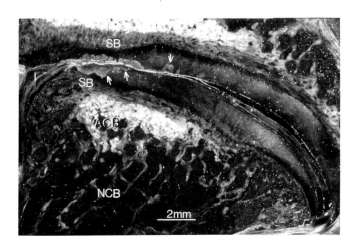

Figure 9.2. Dark-field light photomicrograph of the same histologic section shown in Figure 9.1. Note the areas of different staining which indicate matrix changes on each side of the intra-articular synovial fold inclusion, as well as where the joint surfaces have been in contact (*arrows*). Note the paucity of chondrocytes in the region of the matrix changes. The remaining parts of the cartilages appear to be relatively normal. I = intra-articular synovial fold inclusion; ACB = abnormal cancellous bone; NCB = normal cancellous bone; SB = subchondral bone. (Reproduced with permission from Giles LGF: Pressure related changes in human lumbosacral zygapophyseal joint articular cartilage. *J Rheumatol* 13:1093-1095, 1986.)

ing pattern in this age group, where the cartilages press against the fibrotic tip of the intra-articular synovial fold inclusion and against each other. Figures 9.2 and 9.3 show the same joint as in Figure 9.1, with the fibrous tip of its intra-articular synovial fold inclusion between the adjacent hyaline articular cartilages, as seen by dark-field microscopy. There is a distinct area of abnormal cartilage on either side of the fibrotic part of the intra-articular synovial fold inclusion, as well as slightly beyond this inclusion to the point at which the cartilages no longer press against each other, but there is no obvious fibrillation.

In some cases, one or both hyaline articular cartilage surfaces appear to become "molded" to accommodate the fibrous portions of intra-articular synovial fold inclusions. An example is shown in Figure 9.4, which shows the fibrotic tip of an intra-articular synovial fold (9 mm long) projecting more than half-way between the 16-mm-wide facet surfaces of the right lumbosacral zygapophyseal joint in the horizontal plane.

Osteoarthritis is a common progressive disorder characterized pathologically by degeneration of articular cartilage and pro-liferation of subchondral bone; osteoarthritis may begin with degenerative changes in the articular cartilage and other joint structures and occurs to some extent in most individuals with advancing age, but it may occur prematurely in joints subjected to abnormal wear and tear as a result of faulty joint mechanics (33–35) or mechanical overuse of joints (36) leading to "joint failure" (37).

Kellgren and Lawrence (38) and Lawrence et al (39) found no evidence that the "complaint rate" due to osteoarthritis was different in males and females, and Ingelmark (16, 40), Kellgren and Lawrence (38), and Lewin (41) found no difference between sexes in their studies on skeletal spinal columns. According to Lewin (41) and Dick (22), osteoarthritis is equally common in males and females.

According to Mears (42), fibrillation appears to be the initial abnormality in a joint destined to develop primary osteoarthritis, but the immediate cause of fibrillation remains unclear. In a quantitative histologic analysis of articular cartilage and subchondral bone from osteoarthritic human hips, Reimann and Christensen (43)

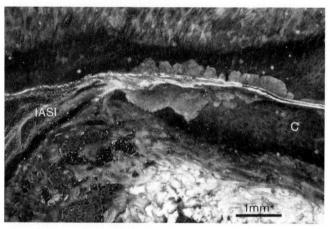

Figure 9.3. This high-powered dark-field photomicrograph of part of Figure 9.1 clearly shows the areas of matrix changes within the hyaline articular cartilages. C = chondrocytes; IASI = highly vascular fat-filled intra-articular synovial fold inclusion.

found consistently more marked cartilage and bony changes in the weight-bearing areas.

According to Radin and Rose (37), one of the mechanisms of initiation of osteo-

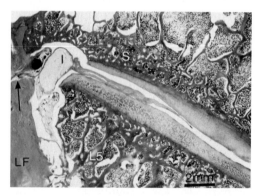

Figure 9.4. Horizontal light photomicrograph of the right lumbosacral zygapophyseal joint from a 75-year-old male. Note the long fibrotic portion of an intra-articular synovial fold inclusion (I) which projects from the inferomedial joint recess and extends more than half-way along the length of the joint. L5 = inferior articular process of the fifth lumbar vertebra; S = superior articular process of the sacrum. Part of the vascular channel (*arrow*), passing through the ligamentum flavum (LF) (see Figs. 4.9 and 4.10) is shown entering the inferomedial joint recess adjacent to the synovial fold. Early fibrillation of some areas of the cartilage surface is noted, as well as a loss of the normal cartilage thickness and chondrocyte population in some regions of the joint. (Ehrlich's hematoxylin stain with light green counterstain.)

arthritis may be increased "stiffness" in the underlying subchondral bone. However, Fazzalari et al (44), using human femoral heads, found no evidence for the hypothesis that increased numbers of subchondral microfractures play a role in maintaining osteoarthritic joint structure. They suggest that it is possible that microfractures act synergistically to maintain joint normality and that a reduction in the number of microfractures may lead to deterioration of a joint.

Regardless of the mechanisms of mechanical injury, according to Mitchell (45) the first changes are seen in the surface chondrocytes, and it has been postulated that stress on these chondrocytes releases lysosomal enzymes, which then cause degradation of cartilage matrix and a vicious cycle is thus established (Fig. 9.5).

Joint laxity is possibly one factor in the pathogenesis of osteoarthritis (46), and if any defects in the cartilage surface occur (e.g., clefts), which bring into direct contact with synovial fluid those parts of cartilage which are high in fixed-charge density, the collagen network will become locally exposed to considerably increased stresses and will therefore become more prone to failure (47). Increased hydration in degenerate cartilage is due to damage of the collagen network (48).

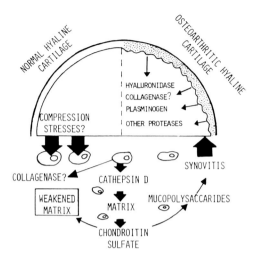

Figure 9.5. The possible mechanisms by which stress causes osteoarthritic changes in hyaline articular cartilage. (Modified from Mitchell NS: Current concepts of degeneration and repair in articular cartilage. In: *The Hip: Proceedings of the First Open Scientific Meeting of the Hip Society*: St. Louis, C.V. Mosby, 1973, p 27.)

Early osteoarthritis is not seen radiologically, but radiologic degenerative changes evidenced by eburnation, osteophytosis, and subarticular cysts in the zygapophyseal joints of the lumbar spine usually appear in approximately 20% of patients over the age of 35 years (22, 49). High intra-articular pressures have been implicated in the development of subarticular bone cysts which have been shown to communicate with the joint cavity. These are pseudocysts lined by dense fibrous connective tissue and reactive bone, and they contain mixed connective tissue elements and fluid (22). An example of a subarticular cyst is shown in Figure 9.6.

Autopsy studies by Sutro (50) did not show "very advanced" arthritic changes in the lumbar facets of elderly cadavers in his series.

According to Bland (27), the term "osteoarthritis" should be used since the process being described is a very anabolic, synthetic, and actually reparative process; therefore, the terms "osteoarthrosis," "degenerative joint disease," and "hypertrophic arthritis" are not satisfactory.

The findings of Giles and Taylor (51) that an extensive vascular supply extended ap-

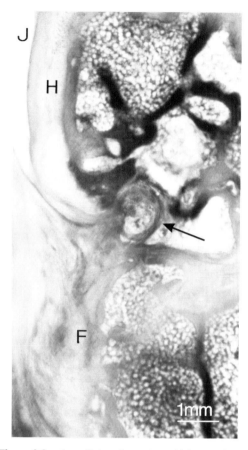

Figure 9.6. A sagittal section cut at a thickness of 150 μm from a block of tissue embedded in low-viscosity nitrocellulose and celloidin. Right L4–5 zygapophyseal joint of a 92-year-old female. Note the subarticular cyst (*arrow*). F = fibrocartilage; H = hyaline articular cartilage; J = joint space. (Ehrlich's hematoxylin stain with light green counterstain.)

proximately half-way into the surface of a lumbosacral zygapophyseal joint cartilage which exhibited minor osteoarthritis may well be indicative of an attempt at cartilage repair which is not limited to the periphery of the joint (Figs. 9.7 and 9.8)

According to Trueta (33), when a blood vessel penetrates into cartilage, the cartilage changes to become fibrous or bony. This may be an attempt to repair a joint at the site of biomechanical stress.

A major problem in studying osteoarthritis in human tissues is the extreme difficulty of defining the stage of disease represented in a given tissue sample (52). Neither the

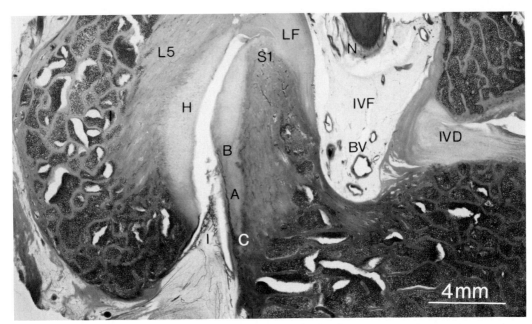

Figure 9.7. A sagittally cut histologic section from the medial one-third of the right zygapophyseal joint of a 56-year-old male cadaver. Note the blood vessel extending from the subchondral bone of the superior articular process of the sacrum into the hyaline articular cartilage surface which shows minor osteoarthritis. Note that this sagittal section reveals the anatomy of the inferomedial intra-articular synovial fold inclusion which projects into the wide opening of the inferior joint recess. The intra-articular synovial fold inclusion is a highly vascular adipose structure with a synovial lining membrane. BV = blood vessels; C = capillary—parts A and B; H = hyaline articular cartilage; I = intra-articular synovial fold inclusion; IVD = intervertebral disc at the lumbosacral joint; IVF = intervertebral "foramen"; LF = ligamentum flavum; L5 = inferior articular process of the fifth lumbar vertebra; N = nerve (spinal) ganglion; S1 = superior articular process of the first sacral segment. (Ehrlich's hematoxylin stain with light green counterstain) (Modified from Giles LGF, Taylor JR: Osteoarthrosis in human cadaveric lumbosacral zygapophyseal joints. *J Manipulative Physiol Ther* 8(4):239-243, 1985. Copyright National College of Chiropractic, Chicago.)

Figure 9.8. Magnification of the blood vessel shown in Figure 9.7. C = capillary—parts A and B; H = hyaline articular cartilage; I = intra-articular synovial fold inclusion. (Ehrlich's hematoxylin stain with light green counterstain) (Modified from Giles LGF, Taylor JR: Osteoarthrosis in human cadaveric lumbosacral zygapophyseal joints. *J Manipulative Physiol Ther* 8(4):239-243, 1985. Copyright National College of Chiropractic, Chicago.)

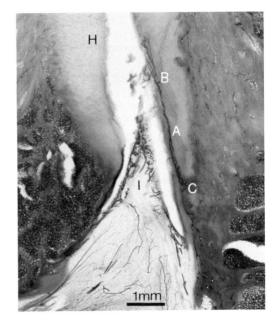

basic underlying causes of osteoarthritis nor the detailed temporal changes which occur in the tissues comprising the joints have been completely elucidated (53), and multiple etiologic factors cause cartilage cell injury (54). Furthermore, differences may exist between the asymptomatic lesions of aging cartilage and osteoarthritic cartilage changes (55).

Sometimes osteoarthritis of lumbar zygapophyseal joints occurs in association with degenerative disc disease, and this may be due to the increased stresses in the zygapophyseal joints resulting from disc degeneration (56). However, the two conditions may occur independently (13, 57, 58). Osteoarthritis of the zygapophyseal joints is regarded as a phenomenon of aging and inadequate repair of the effect of wear and tear of the joints (59).

According to McRae (13), osteoarthritis is seen radiographically most frequently at the lumbosacral joints because the zygapophyseal joints bear more weight there than at other levels.

According to Thompson and Oegema (60), histologic grading does not correlate uniformly with metabolic activity in the earlier stages of cartilage destruction, suggesting that repair of articular cartilage may occur in some osteoarthritic joints or at least in specific areas of some joints. Using femoral heads and humeral heads from cadavers aged 25–93 years, Lane et al (61) found that the number of blood vessels and the modeling activity in the calcified zone varied with age and the patterns of joint loading. More vessels and more active modeling occurred in joint areas subjected to greater loading, with the thickness of the calcified zone cartilage being approximately 10–15% thicker in the less stressed areas in all ages (62).

Lumbosacral Zygapophyseal Joint Tropism and Its Effect on Hyaline Articular Cartilage

Osteoarthritis has been linked to articular tropism (57, 63–65), that is, asymmetry in the horizontal plane of paired left and right zygapophyseal joints. Tropism may occur at all levels of the lumbar spine, but its oc-

currence is most frequent at the lumbosacral joint (63, 66–69). As previously noted, lumbar zygapophyseal joints are biplanar, with a coronally orientated anteromedial part and a sagittally orientated posterolateral part (15, 65). A difference of 5° or more between the horizontal planes of the left and right zygapophyseal joints represents tropism (70). Tropism may be found in 21–37% of the population (1, 5, 57, 66, 70).

A routine anteroposterior view of a patient's lumbosacral spine can show evidence of tropism between paired zygapophyseal joints (Fig. 9.9), but it cannot give the degree of tropism.

Many clinical investigations into articular tropism as a cause of joint degeneration and low back pain have been undertaken (57, 63, 68, 71–75). According to Putti (63), tropism may have a twofold effect on the intervertebral foramen: (a) It may alter its shape, thereby reducing its capacity; and (b) by altering spinal mechanics, it may induce localized osteoarthritis which could irritate the nerve trunk. Tropism strongly suggests mechanical instability and susceptibility to ligamentous injury (5, 67). According to Goldthwait (76) and von Luckum (77), when articulations are asymmetrical, their movements are irregular and contribute to weakness of some of the parts of the mobile segment, particularly at the lumbosacral joint where there is a junction between a mobile part (L5) and an immobile part (the sacrum). Between points of pressure within unstable zygapophyseal joints, where hyaline articular cartilage is not present, "bumper"-fibrocartilage develops and wraps around the facet margins as a protective cushioning mechanism (78). This bumper is not composed of hyaline articular cartilage (79) and it is located beyond the margin of the facet surfaces (see Fig. 13.9).

Cyron and Hutton (64) undertook a quantitative experiment in which they subjected lumbar intervertebral joints to long periods of sustained cyclic compressive and shear forces in order to correlate any instability of the lumbar spine with articular tropism. Their results indicated that spines with asymmetrical facets produced instability,

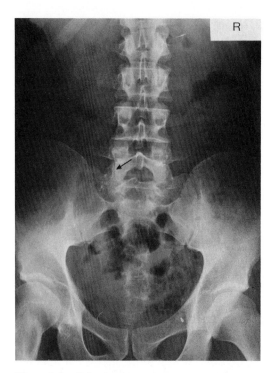

Figure 9.9. This anteroposterior erect posture pelvis and lumbar spine radiograph of a 35-year-old male with low back pain illustrates tropism at the L5–S1 level and, to a lesser extent, the L3–4 and L4–5 levels. The posterolateral portion of the left lumbosacral zygapophyseal joint plane is in the sagittal plane (*arrow*), whereas the right lumbosacral zygapophyseal joint plane is in the coronal plane. The right L3–4 and L4–5 zygapophyseal joint planes are slightly more sagittally oriented than are their left counterparts. Incidental findings are spina bifida occulta at S1 and bone remodeling of the left femur neck following surgery for fibrous dysplasia.

which manifested itself as rotation of the lumbar spine that put the ligaments of one zygapophyseal joint under extra strain, and greater interfacet forces in the more sagittally oriented facets, which may predispose these facets to osteoarthritis.

Since tropism of the lumbar zygapophyseal joints is of relevance to following chapters in this text, a histologic study I conducted is described in detail here. The study compared left and right paired lumbosacral zygapophyseal joint cartilage area and thickness in cadavers having equal leg lengths and either tropism of greater than 4° or no tropism (0–4°) (as a control group).

In order to ensure that cadavers used in the study had not had sacral base obliquity, since this may lead to unequal stresses at the lumbosacral joint (80, 81), 13 embalmed cadavers (aged 35–83 years; mean = 62.46 years) were surveyed for leg length equality, using orthoradiography to accurately measure leg lengths (82, 83). A pelvis–lumbar spine anteroposterior radiograph was also taken to look for pelvic anomalies which could cause pelvic obliquity. Cadavers were excluded from the study if they showed any structural asymmetry of the spine (other than tropism) or the pelvis, or any pathology except osteoarthritis.

Following this radiographic evaluation, the spines were further trimmed into rectangular blocks of tissue by means of a band-saw, to remove parts of the spinous and transverse processes and the vertebral bodies with their adjacent intervertebral disc, so as to facilitate histologic processing and mounting procedures (84, 85). Each block of spinal tissue included the zygapophyseal joints and the posterior one-third of the fifth lumbar and first sacral bodies, with their intervertebral disc, in order to maintain stability of the zygapophyseal joints.

Each trimmed block was placed in the center of the x-ray cassette with the x-ray beam perpendicular to it, then radiographed in the superior-to-inferior position at an x-ray tube-film distance of 128.5 cm. The overall angles of the joint planes on the left and right sides were measured by the method of Cyron and Hutton (64) (Fig. 9.10).

The lumbosacral spinal blocks were processed through the stages of postfixation, decalcification, dehydration, and embedding in low viscosity nitrocellulose and celloidin (85). Paired lumbosacral zygapophyseal joints were serially sectioned in the horizontal plane at a thickness of 100 μm by means of a Jung Tetrander (model K) microtome. One in seven of the serial sections was stained in Ehrlich's hematoxylin and light green stain, dehydrated, and mounted in DePex (85) for light microscopy.

The outlines of the articular cartilage were carefully traced in corresponding left and right middle serial sections (83) using a

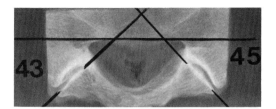

Figure 9.10. Superior-to-inferior radiograph of a trimmed lumbosacral block, showing the left and right zygapophyseal joints. A line is drawn across the back of the first sacral segment, and a line is drawn through the left and right zygapophyseal joints to bisect this line, enabling measurements of the plane of the left and right zygapophyseal joints to be made. (Reproduced with permission from Giles LGF, Taylor JR: The effect of postural scoliosis on lumbar apophyseal joints. *Scand J Rheumatol* 13:209-220, 1984.)

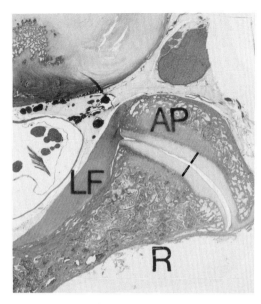

Figure 9.11. Anatomical structures traced and measured were the joint hyaline articular cartilage thickness across the center of the joint (*lines*) and the hyaline articular cartilage cross-sectional area. AP = superior articular process of the sacrum; LF = ligamentum flavum; R = right side of the specimen. (Ehrlich's hematoxylin stain with light green counterstain) (Modified from Giles LGF, and Taylor JR: The effect of postural scoliosis on lumbar apophyseal joints. *Scan J Rheumatol* 13:209-220, 1984.)

Leitz Aristophot overhead projector set at a projection magnification of 8, (Fig. 9.11).

From the tracings, a Reichert Kontron Manual Optical Analysis image analyzer system (MOP-3) was used to make accurate linear and area measurements at standardized positions within the zygapophyseal joints on each side so that mid-joint geometry could be established. The hyaline articular cartilage cross-sectional thickness, through the joint center, was found by moving the stylus of the image analyzer from the medial to the lateral margin of the subchondral surface of each facet. The digital reading was halved, then the stylus was moved from the medial margin half-way along the facet surface to find the center of the facet on the horizontal tracing. At this center point, a perpendicular line was drawn from the facet across any existing cartilage to bisect the cartilage. The stylus was then used to measure the length of these perpendicular lines, and the sum of these lines was used to record the cartilage thickness if cartilage was present. On each occasion, prior to using the MOP-3 system, it was checked for accuracy using the method suggested by the manufacturer (86).

Of the 13 cadavers radiographed, 8 had equal leg lengths. Four (aged 35–83 years; mean = 61 years) exhibited tropism of greater than 4°, and 4 (aged 46–73 years; mean = 59.5 years) exhibited no tropism (0–4°) and were used as a control group. The remaining 5 cadavers fell into the exclusion categories.

Figures 9.12–9.15 show the radiographs and histology obtained from a 73-year-old female with 26° of tropism.

Figure 9.12 shows a lateral view of the lumbosacral spine which shows only minor thinning of the lumbosacral disc with a small spur at the anterior margin of the sacral promontory.

Figure 9.13 shows left and right oblique views of the lower lumbar and lumbosacral joints.

Figure 9.14 shows a superior-to-inferior view of the lumbosacral zygapophyseal joints, and it can be seen that the left facets are in a more oblique plane than the right facets, which are mainly in the sagittal plane (except for the anteromedial [or coronal] part of the joint).

The corresponding histology for these paired lumbosacral joints is shown in

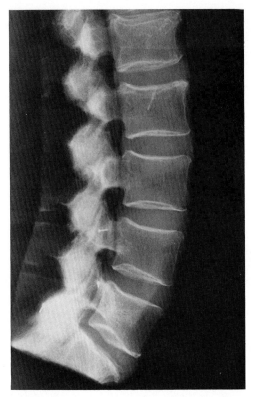

Figure 9.12. Radiograph of an excised lumbosacral spine: lateral view. (Reproduced with permission from Giles LGF: Lumbosacral zygapophyseal joint tropism and its effect on hyaline cartilage. *Clin Biomechan* 2:2-6, 1987. Copyright John Wright, Bristol.)

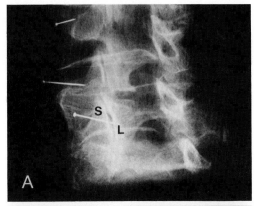

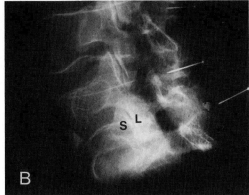

Figure 9.13. **A,** Left zygapophyseal joints. **B,** Right zygapophyseal joints. The radiographs show no great difference between the left and right lumbosacral facets with respect to joint space or subchondral sclerosis and eburnation. The pins were for clearly indicating the spinal levels during sectioning and radiography. L = inferior articular process of the fifth lumbar vertebra; S = superior articular process of the sacrum. (Reproduced with permission from Giles LGF: Lumbosacral zygapophyseal joint tropism and its effect on hyaline cartilage. *Clin Biomechan* 2:2-6, 1987. Copyright John Wright, Bristol.)

Figure 9.15, which shows a section from approximately the middle of each zygapophyseal joint.

The photomicrograph in Figure 9.15 clearly shows that in the more sagittal facing joint, virtually all the hyaline articular cartilage has been worn away. There is some os-

Figure 9.14. Superior-to-inferior radiographic view of paired zygapophyseal joints at the lumbosacral level. The *white dot* represents the left side of the lumbosacral specimen. There is tropism of 26° between the left and right joints. Small osteophytic spurs are seen at the posterior joint margins, particularly on the right side. Subchondral sclerosis and eburnation are also noted, particularly on the right side. S = sacrum; L5 = the lamina junction of the fifth lumbar vertebra. (Reproduced with permission from Giles LGF: Lumbosacral zygapophyseal joint tropism and its effect on hyaline cartilage. *Clin Biomechan* 1:2-6, 1987. Copyright John Wright, Bristol.)

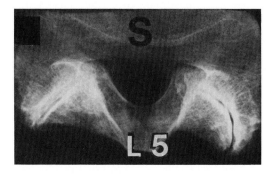

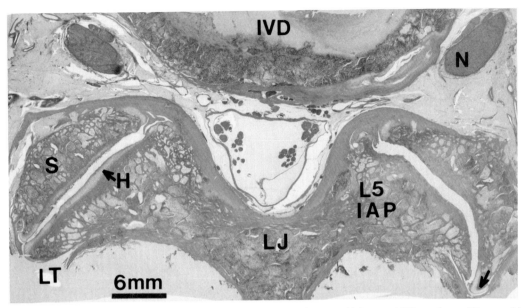

Figure 9.15.   Lumbosacral histologic section cut in the horizontal plane at a thickness of 100 μm, from a 73-year-old female with 26° of tropism. H = hyaline articular cartilage; IVD = intervertebral disc; LJ = lamina junction; LT = left side of the specimen; L5IAP = inferior articular process of the fifth lumbar vertebra; N = nerve root (spinal) ganglion; S = superior articular process of the sacrum. *Arrows* indicate bumper-fibrocartilage formation. Note the small fibrous intra-articular joint inclusions which project into the anteromedial region of each joint from the ligamentum flavum. (Ehrlich's hematoxylin stain with light green counterstain) (Reproduced with permission from Giles LGF: Lumbosacral zygapophyseal joint tropism and its effect on hyaline cartilage. *Clin Biomechan* 2:2-6, 1987. Copyright John Wright, Bristol.)

teoarthritic lipping of the right zygapophyseal facet margins in particular, and there is an increase in subchondral bone sclerosis. The left facets still have some hyaline articular cartilage, although this shows evidence of tinctorial changes, fibrillation, and thinning. Both left and right zygapophyseal joint facets show evidence of protective bumper-fibrocartilage formation beyond the facet margins where the articular processes are in close proximity to the joint capsules. Bumper-fibrocartilage is considered to be a completely anomalous "cushioning" structure which develops at points of pressure between bone and the tough capsule which opposes the sideways thrust of the joint (79). The considerable degenerative changes seen histologically are most likely due to instability caused by the tropism, since the lateral view radiograph (Fig. 9.12) shows a reasonably normal lumbosacral intervertebral disc.

Figure 9.16 shows paired lumbosacral zygapophyseal joints from a 35-year-old female. The joints have tropism of 11° but only minor osteoarthritic changes, as shown by fibrillation, are noted in the left joint at this age in this cadaver. The hyaline articular cartilage at the anteromedial region of the right joint shows early tinctorial changes when compared with the normal staining of most of the remaining hyaline articular cartilage in this joint.

The findings are typical of the four cadavers with tropism. The more sagittal-facing facets show greater degenerative changes than do the more coronal-facing facets.

Figure 9.17 shows the zygapophyseal joints from a 54-year-old male cadaver which did not exhibit tropism. On comparing the left and right joints there is virtually no difference in cartilage thickness, cartilage area, or cartilage staining, apart from a small area of fibrillation cleft formation in the cartilage of the right sacral facet.

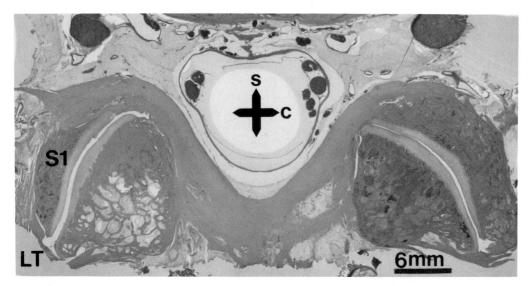

Figure 9.16.   Lumbosacral histologic section cut in the horizontal plane at a thickness of 100 μm. There is evidence of early fibrillation in the left hyaline articular cartilage, particularly of the superior articular process of the sacrum (S1) in this 35-year-old female specimen, with 11° of tropism. The right cartilages appear relatively normal, apart from minor tinctorial changes in the cartilage at the anteromedial portion of the joint. S = sagittal plane; C = coronal plane; LT = left side of specimen. (Ehrlich's hematoxylin stain with light green counterstain) (Reproduced with permission from Giles LGF: Lumbosacral zygapophyseal joint tropism and its effect on hyaline cartilage. *Clin Biomechan* 1:2-6, 1987. Copyright John Wright, Bristol.)

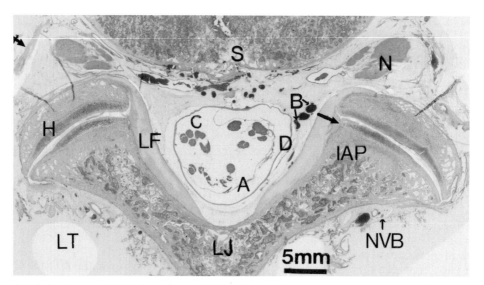

Figure 9.17.   Lumbosacral histologic section cut in the horizontal plane at a thickness of 100 μm, from a 54-year-old male. A = arachnoid membrane; B = Batson's venous plexus; C = cauda equina; D = dura mater; H = hyaline articular cartilage; IAP = inferior articular process of L5; LF = ligamentum flavum; LJ = lamina junction; LT = left side; N = nerve root (spinal) ganglion; S = sacrum. *Bisected arrow* shows part of a transforaminal ligament, an *arrow* shows a fibrous intra-articular inclusion projecting from the ligamentum flavum into the upper one-third of the right zygapophyseal joint. (Ehrlich's hematoxylin stain with light green counterstain) (Reproduced with permission from Giles LGF: Lumbosacral zygapophyseal joint tropism and its effect on hyaline cartilage. *Clin Biomechan* 2:2-6, 1987. Copyright John Wright, Bristol.)

Tables 9.1 and 9.2 list the mid-joint histologic measurements for each cadaver showing total hyaline articular cartilage cross-sectional area and cross-sectional thickness through the joint center.

Since only a small number of joints were compared in this study, a statistical analysis was not feasible. However, the histologic findings of this pilot study appear to confirm the hypothesis of Cyron and Hutton (64) that in tropism, there are greater interfacet forces in the more sagitally oriented facets. The more sagittal-facing facets had significantly less cross-sectional hyaline articular cartilage area and thickness at the joint center than did the coronal-facing facets. The changes of fibrillation, loss of hyaline articular cartilage, and greater subchondral sclerosis in the more sagittal-facing facets are typical of osteoarthritis.

The control group, with equal leg length, did not have a significant difference between left and right joint hyaline articular cartilage area and thickness, which probably indicates that biomechanical stresses are shared equally between the left and right zygapophyseal joints.

Tropism, Osteoarthritis, and Pain

In osteoarthritic joints, painful symptoms are due partly to joint wear (which involves degeneration of cartilage with loss of joint space, the formation of osteophytes and loose bodies, and fibrosis of the joint capsule); partly to episodes of synovial inflammation causing acute joint pain; and partly to degeneration, fraying, and inflammation of ligaments around the joints (87). Huskisson (88) concurs that osteoarthritis has an inflammatory component, and Bach-

Table 9.1.
Mid-Joint Geometrical Measurements for Each Cadaver Exhibiting Tropism of Greater Than 4°[a]

Age	Sex	Total Hyaline Articular Cartilage Cross-Sectional Area		Total Hyaline Articular Cartilage Cross-Sectional Thickness Through the Joint Center	
		Sagittal Joints	Coronal Joints	Sagittal Joints	Coronal Joints
		mm^2	mm^2	mm	mm
35	F	27.6	32.8	2.0	2.1
56	M	13.7	31.6	1.2	2.2
73	F	0	35.7	0	2.3
83	F	13.3	36.2	1.8	2.3
Total		54.6	136.3	5.0	8.9

[a]Reprinted with permission from Giles LGF: Lumbo-sacral zygapophyseal joint tropism and its effect on hyaline cartilage. *Clin Biomechan* 2:2-6, 1987. Copyright John Wright, Bristol.

Table 9.2.
Mid-Joint Geometrical Measurements for Each Cadaver with no Tropism[a]

Age	Sex	Total Hyaline Articular Cartilage Cross-Sectional Area		Total Hyaline Articular Cartilage Cross-Sectional Thickness Through the Joint Center	
		Left Joints	Right Joints	Left Joints	Right Joints
		mm^2	mm^2	mm	mm
46	M	32.0	29.7	1.8	1.9
45	M	50.9	54.7	3.2	3.2
65	M	34.4	40.1	2.6	2.9
73	M	21.0	21.5	1.8	1.8
Total		138.3	146.0	9.4	9.8

[a]Reprinted with permission from Giles LGF: Lumbo-sacral zygapophyseal joint tropism and its effect on hyaline cartilage. *Clin Biomechan* 2:2-6, 1987. Copyright John Wright, Bristol.

man and Noble (89) agree that synovitis secondary to degenerative changes is painful. However, according to Howell and Moskowitz (90) osteoarthritis is accompanied by a relative paucity of inflammatory response, although synovial proliferation can occur in osteoarthritis (91). According to Bland (27), venostasis occurs in the bone marrow, resulting in increased pressure and pain. Venous hypertension may produce pain by causing pressure on small nerves in bone (2, 92).

An additional factor in tropism which may result in low back pain is instability of the affected motion segment (64) causing strain on the innervated joint capsule (93) or pinching of the intra-articular synovial folds (94) which have small myelinated nerves (93).

"Dysfunction" Related to "Entrapment" of the Synovial Folds

Kos and Wolf (95) described vascular "menisci" in zygapophyseal joints and claimed that they are well innervated, although they did not present any histologic evidence of innervation. They advanced the theory that these may become entrapped between articular surfaces causing the syndrome of "vertebral block." The entrapment of "meniscoid inclusions" may mechanically interfere with movement (96), leading to pain and muscle spasm (94). Zukschwerdt et al (97), Bourdillon (98), Giles and Taylor (93, 99), and Giles and Harvey (100) have also implicated synovial fold inclusions in some cases of low back pain due to the impingement of the articular surfaces on synovial tissue. Kraft and Levinthal (101), Tondury (102), and Kirkaldy-Willis (103) believe impingement is accompanied by edema, synovitis, and then distention of the capsule. This causes nerve root irritation (104). According to Bogduk and Jull (105), meniscus entrapment as an explanation for the pathologic basis for acute locked back is inconsistent with the clinical features of acute back pain, because (a) fibrous inclusions "do not project into the joint space," and (b) there is the possibility of "cleavage" of the adipose type of inclusion when traction is applied to it. However, following the histologic examination of numerous zyg-

apophyseal joint synovial folds in serial sections, it is my opinion that by far the majority of synovial folds remain intact and do not undergo cleavage.

Ligamenta Flava

In young persons the ligamenta flava bulge little or not at all into the spinal canal, but with advancing age the ligamenta flava sometimes undergo liquefaction necrosis and edema in association with disc degeneration and spondylosis, and this can be a contributory factor in the sciatica of some patients who have normal-sized spinal canals (13). This ligament can undergo hyperplastic change with replacement of the normal yellow elastic tissue with white fibrous tissue containing calcareous deposits (106). It can become thickened, buckled inward, depressed by enlarged or overriding laminae, or incorporated into articular osteophytes at the site of its attachment to the zygapophyseal joint capsule (56). Ligamentum flavum thickening may result in a width ranging from 4 to 8 mm (107, 108).

According to Dockerty and Love (109), in the case of thickened ligamentum flavum, there is no true hypertrophy but rather thickening and fibrosis, and according to Farfan (110) ligamentum flavum thickening is a natural sequel of the shortening of an elastic structure.

According to Nachemson and Evans (111), increase in width of the ligamentum flavum is always secondary to severe disc degeneration. Thickening of the ligamentum flavum due to disc thinning with approximation of the pedicles and subluxation of the zygapophyseal facets can lead to compromise of the nerve root in the intervertebral foramen, even though the nerve root usually occupies about one-sixth to one-third of the intervertebral foramen (112).

Pathologic Changes Affecting Lumbar Spinous Processes

Interspinous Osteoarthritis (Baastrup's Disease, or "Kissing Spines")

Baastrup (113) described a clinical syndrome in which the lumbar spinous processes impinge upon each other—the so-called kissing spines.

An increase in the normal lumbar lordosis may produce approximation and contact of the "tips" of the spinous processes, which can result in trauma and injury to the interspinous tissues, with the formation of arthroses showing sclerosis and osteophytosis (5, 114).

Normal spinous processes are covered by periosteum, but, according to Bywaters and Evans (115), bursae develop between the kissing spinous processes as a result of a repeated shearing movement. However, according to Hadley (79), kissing spinous processes destroy the interspinous ligament, and bumper-fibrocartilage can develop when the spinous processes are subjected to intermittent pressure, and only an adventitious bursa may develop.

Figue 9.18 shows sclerosis of the cortex of the adjacent L3 and L4 spinous processes in an obese 72-year-old female. The inferior margin of the L3 spinous process has developed an osteophytic spur.

The histologic section shown in Figure 9.19, which was sectioned in the sagittal plane after the spinous processes had been decalcified and embedded in low-viscosity nitrocellulose and celloidin, shows parts of the L4–S1 spinous processes from an 80-year-old male cadaver. Between the spinous processes, the interspinous ligament has been destroyed as a result of intermittent pressure and shearing forces (Fig.9.19). At the L4–5 level, what appears to be bumper-fibrocartilage has developed, particularly on the inferior margin of the L4 spinous process. At the L5–S1 level, there is evidence of bony sclerosis and eburnation. Radiography of these joints, prior to decalcification, showed minimal sclerosis at the L4–5 level but some early eburnation at the L5–S1 level.

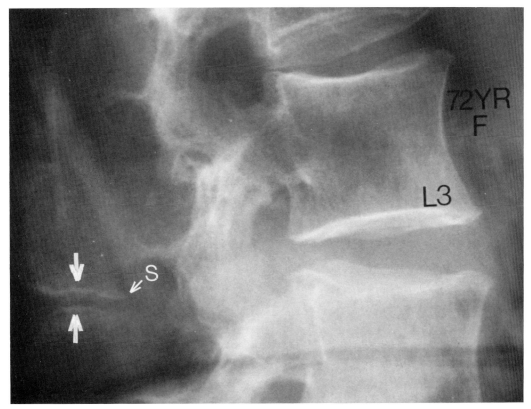

Figure 9.18. *White arrows* indicate the sclerotic changes of the L3 and L4 spinous processes. S = osteophytic spur.

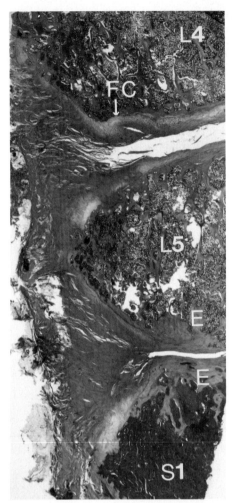

Figure 9.19. "Kissing spines." This histologic section, which was cut at a thickness of 100 μm in the sagittal plane, shows bumper-fibrocartilage (FC) on the spinous processes on each side of the L4–5 interspinous space. Only a few small remnants of the interspinous ligament remain between these spinous processes. On both sides of the L5–S1 space, the spinous processes show bony sclerosis and eburnation (E) where these processes underwent intermittent pressure and shearing forces. There is no residual interspinous ligament at the L5–S1 level.

According to Hadley (79), Schmorl and Junghanns (5), and Epstein (114), this impingement of adjacent spinous processes can cause chronic and sometimes severe pain, which may be aggravated by rotational movement or bending forward or backward.

References

1. Farfan HF: *Mechanical Disorders of the Low Back.* Philadelphia, Lea and Febiger, 1973, p 145.
2. Kirkaldy-Willis WH: The pathology and pathogenesis of low back pain. In Kirkaldy-Willis WH (ed): *Managing Low Back Pain.* New York, Churchill Livingstone, 1983, pp 23-43.
3. Donohue WL: Pathology of the intervertebral disc. *Am J Med Sci* 198:413-437, 1939.
4. Taylor TKF, Gosh P: Ageing and the intervertebral disc. Ageing in Australia. Australian Association of Gerontology. In JW Donald, AV Everett, PJ Wheeler (eds): *Proceedings of the Satellite Conference of the 11th Congress of the International Association of Gerontology.* Sydney, Pot Still Press, 1978, pp 113-115.
5. Schmorl G, Junghanns H: *The Human Spine in Health and Disease.* ed 2. New York, Grune and Stratton, 1971, p 211.
6. Pritzker KPH: Aging and degeneration in the lumbar intervertebral disc. Orthop Clin North Am 8:65-77, 1977.
7. Smith N: The intervertebral discs. *Br J Surg.* 18:358-375, 1930.
8. Saunders JB, Inman T: Pathology of the intervertebral disk. *Arch Surg* 40:389-416, 1940.
9. Peacock A: Observations on the postnatal structure of the intervertebral disc in man. *J Anat* 86:162-178, 1952.
10. Brown WD: The pathophysiology of disc disease. *Orthop Clin North Am* 2:359-370, 1970.
11. Taylor TKF, Akeson WH: Intervertebral disc prolapse: A review of morphologic and biochemic knowledge concerning the nature of prolapse. *Clin Orthop* 76:54-79, 1971.
12. Bijlsma F, Peeraboom JW: The aging pattern of human intervertebral disc. *Gerontology* 18:157-168, 1972.
13. McRae DL: Radiology of the lumbar spinal canal. In Weinstein PR, Ehni G, Wilson CB (eds): *Lumbar Spondylosis: Diagnosis, Management and Surgical Treatment.* Chicago, Year Book Medical Publishers, 1977, pp 92-114.
14. Twomey L: Age changes in the human lumbar vertebral column. Ph.D. thesis, Department of Anatomy and Human Biology, University of Western Australia, 1981.
15. Twomey L, Taylor JR: Age changes in the lumbar articular triad. *Australian Journal of Physiotherapy* 31:106-112, 1985.
16. Ingelmark BE: Function of and pathological changes in the spinal joints. *Acta Anat* 38:12-60, 1959.
17. Farfan HF: A reorientation in the surgical approach to degenerative lumbar intervertebral joint disease. *Orthop Clin North Am* 8:9-21, 1977.
18. Farfan HF: Biomechanics of the lumbar spine. In Kirkaldy-Willis (ed): *Managing Low Back Pain.* New York, Churchill Livingstone, 1983, pp 9-21.
19. Adams MA, Hutton WC: Gradual disc prolapse. *Spine* 10:524-531, 1985.
20. Howe JW, Yochum TR, Rowe LJ: Diagnostic imaging of spinal stenosis and intervertebral disc disease. In Yochum TR, Rowe LJ (eds): *Essentials of Skeletal Radiology,* Baltimore, Williams & Wilkins, 1987, Vol 1, pp 273-316.
21. Ferguson AB: The pathology of degenerative arthritis. In Cruess RL, Mitchell NS (eds): *Surgical Management of Degenerative Arthritis of the Lower Limbs.* Philadelphia, Lea and Febiger, 1975, pp 3-9.
22. Dick WC: *An Introduction to Clinical Rheumatology.* London, Churchill Livingstone, 1972, p 24.
23. Meachim G: Age changes in articular cartilage. *Clin Orthop* 64:33-44, 1969.

24. Boyle AC: *A Colour Atlas of Rheumatology. Wolfe Medical Atlases—10.* London, Wolfe Medical Books, 1976.
25. Huskisson EC, Hart FD: *Joint Disease: All the Anthropathies.* ed 3. Bristol, John Wright and Sons, 1978, p 89.
26. Tirgari M: Blood pattern changes in primary and secondary osteoarthritis of the dog: an experimental study using intraosseous venography. *Journal of American Veterinary Radiology* 19:83-91, 1978.
27. Bland JH: The reversibility of osteoarthritis: a review. *Am J Med* 74:16-26, 1983.
28. Glynn LE: Primary lesion in osteoarthritis. *Lancet* 1:574-575, 1977.
29. Shore LR: On osteoarthritis in the dorsal intervertebral joints. A study in morbid anatomy. *Br J Surg* 22:833-849, 1934.
30. Ehrlick GE: Osteoarthritis beginning with inflammation. Definitions and correlations. *JAMA* 232:157-159, 1975.
31. Editorial. Pathogenesis of osteoarthrosis. *Lancet* 2:1131-1133, 1973.
32. Giles LGF: Pressure related changes in human lumbo-sacral zygapophyseal joint articular cartilage. *J Rheumatol* 13:1093-1095, 1986.
33. Trueta J: Osteoarthritis of the hip. *Royal College of Surgeons of England Annals* 15:174-192, 1954.
34. Gartland JJ: *Fundamentals of Orthopedics*, ed 3. Philadelphia, W.B. Saunders, 1979.
35. Gracovetsky S, Farfan H: The optimum spine. *Spine* 11:543, 544, 1986.
36. Peyron JG: Osteoarthritis. The epidemiologic viewpoint. *Clin Orthop* 213:13-19, 1986.
37. Radin EL, Rose RM: Role of subchondral bone in the initiation and progression of cartilage damage. *Clin Orthop* 213:34-40, 1986.
38. Kellgren JH, Lawrence JS: Osteoarthrosis and disk degeneration in an urban population. *Ann Rheum Dis* 17:388, 1958.
39. Lawrence JS, Bremner JM, Bier F: Osteoarthrosis. Prevalence in the population and relationship between symptoms and x-ray changes. *Ann Rheum Dis* 25:1-24, 1966.
40. Ingelmark BE: De funktionellt anatomiska forhallandena i ruggraden med sarskild hansyn till dess smaleder. *Acta Uni Gothoburg* 62:1, 1956.
41. Lewin T: Osteoarthritis in lumbar synovial joints. *Acta Orthop Scand Suppl* 73:1-111, 1964.
42. Mears DC: *Materials and Orthopedic Surgery.* Baltimore, Williams & Wilkins, 1979, pp 162-181.
43. Reimann I, Christensen SB: A histological demonstration of nerves in subchondral bone. *Acta Orthop Scand* 48:345-352, 1977.
44. Fazzalari NL, Vernon-Roberts B, Darracott J: Osteoarthritis of the hip. Possible protective and causative roles of trabecular microfractures in the head of the femur. *Clin Orthop* 216:224-233, 1987.
45. Mitchell NS: Current concepts of degeneration and repair in articular cartilage. In: *The Hip: Proceedings of the First Open Scientific Meeting of the Hip Society.* St. Louis, C.V. Mosby 1973, pp 26-30.
46. Scott D, Bird H, Wright V: Joint laxity leading to osteoarthrosis. *Rheumatology and Rehabilitation* 18:167-169, 1979.
47. Maroudas A, Bayliss MT, Venn MF: Further studies on the composition of human femoral head cartilage. *Ann Rheum Dis* 39:514-523, 1980.
48. Maroudas A: Balance between swelling pressure and collagen tension in normal and degenerate cartilage. *Nature* 260:808, 1976.
49. Adams JC: *Outline of Orthopaedics.* ed 6. Edinburgh, E & S Livingstone, 1968, p 96.
50. Sutro CJ : Lumbar facets-spinal stenosis and inter-

mittent claudication: A mini review. *Bull Hosp Jt Dis Orthop Inst* 45:13-37, 1979.
51. Giles LGF, Taylor JR: Osteoarthrosis in human cadaveric lumbo-sacral zygapophyseal joints. *J Manipulative Physiol Ther* 8:239-243, 1985.
52. Moskowitz RW: Osteoarthritis. Studies with experimental models. *Arthritis Rheum* 20:104-108, 1977.
53. Shipiro F, Glimcher MJ: Induction of osteoarthrosis in the rabbit knee joint. *Clin Orthop* 147:287-295, 1980.
54. Howell DS: Biochemical studies of osteoarthritis. In McCarthy DJ (ed): *Arthritis and Allied Conditions.* ed 9. Philadelphia, Lea and Febiger, 1979, pp 1154-1159.
55. Vignon E, Arlot M, Menunier P, Vignon G: Quantitative histological changes in osteoarthritic hip cartilage. *Clin Orthop* 103:269-278, 1974.
56. Weinstein PR, Ehni G, Wilson CB: Clinical features of lumbar spondylosis and stenosis. In Weinstein PR, Ehni G, Wilson CB (eds): *Lumbar Spondylosis: Diagnosis, Management and Surgical Treatment.* Chicago, Year Book Medical Publishers, 1977, pp 115-133.
57. Badgley CE: The articular facets in relation to low back pain and sciatic radiation. *J Bone Joint Surg* 23:481-496, 1941.
58. Caplan PS, Freedman LMJ, Connelly TP: Degenerative joint disease of the lumbar spine in coal miners—a clinical and x-ray study. *Arthritis Rheum* 9:693-702, 1966.
59. Collins DH: Degenerative diseases. In Nassam R, Burrows JH (eds): *Modern Trends in Diseases of the Vertebral Column.* London, Butterworth, 1959.
60. Thompson RC, Oegema TR: Metabolic activity of articular cartilage in osteoarthritis. In Carone FA, Conn RB (eds): *1980 Year Book of Pathology and Clinical Pathology.* Chicago, Year Book Medical Publishers, 1980, pp 164-165.
61. Lane LB, Villacin A, Bullough PG: The vascularity and remodeling of subchondral bone and calcified cartilage in adult femoral and humeral heads. *J Bone Joint Surg* 59(B):272-278, 1977.
62. Lane LB, Bullough PG: Age-related changes in the thickness of the calcified zone and the number of tidemarks in adult human articular cartilage. *J Bone Joint Surg* 62(B):372-375, 1980.
63. Putti V: Pathogenesis of sciatic pain. *Lancet* 2:53-60, 1927.
64. Cyron BM, Hutton WC: Articular tropism and stability of the lumbar spine. *Spine* 5:168-172, 1980.
65. Giles LGF: Lumbo-sacral zygapophyseal joint tropism and its effect on hyaline cartilage. *Clin Biomech* 2:2-6, 1987.
66. Brailsford JF: Deformities of the lumbosacral region of the spine. *Br J Surg* 16:562-568, 1928-29.
67. Willis TA: Lumbosacral anomalies. *J Bone Joint Surg* 41(A):935-938, 1959.
68. Farfan HF, Sullivan JD: The relation of facet orientation to intervertebral disc failure. *Can J Surg* 10:179-185, 1967.
69. Guebert GM, Yochum TR, Rowe LJ: Congenital anomalies and normal skeletal variant. In Yochum TR, Rowe LJ (ed): *Essentials of Skeletal Radiology.* Baltimore, Williams & Wilkins, 1987, Vol 1, pp 95-167.
70. Cihak R: Variations of lumbosacral joints and their morphogenesis. *Acta Universitatis Carolinae Medica* 16:145-165, 1970.
71. Ferguson AB: The clinical and roentgenographic interpretation of lumbosacral anomalies. *Radiology* 22:548-558, 1934.
72. Ayers CE: Further case studies of lumbo-sacral pathology with consideration of the involvement of the intervertebral discs and the articular facets. *N Eng*

J Med 208:716, 1935.

73. Howard LG: Low back pain and the lumbosacral joint. *Med Clin North Am* 26:1551-1579, 1942.
74. Hirsch C: Etiology and pathogenesis of low back pain. *Isr J Med Sci* 2:362-370, 1966.
75. Downey EF, Nason SS, Majd M, McSweeney WJ: Asymmetrical facet joints. Another cause for the sclerotic pedicle. *Spine* 8:340-342, 1983.
76. Goldthwait JE: The lumbo-sacral articulation. An explanation of many cases of "lumbago," "sciatica" and paraplegia. *Boston Medical and Surgical Journal* 164:365, 1911.
77. von Luckum HL: The lumbosacral region. An anatomic study and some clinical observations. *JAMA* 82:1109, 1924.
78. Hadley LA: *Anatomico-Roentgenographic Studies of the Spine.* Springfield, IL, Charles C. Thomas, 1976, pp 186, 189, 190.
79. Hadley LA: *Anatomico-Roentgenographic Studies of the Spine.* Springfield, IL, Charles C. Thomas, 1964, p 179.
80. Giles LGF: Lumbosacral facetal "joint angles" associated with leg length inequality. *Rheumatology and Rehabilitation* 20:233-238, 1981.
81. Giles LGF, Taylor JR: Low-back pain associated with leg length inequality. *Spine* 6:510-521, 1981.
82. Green WT, Wyatt GM, Anderson M: Orthoroentgenography as a method of measuring the bones of the lower extremities. *J Bone Joint Surg* 28:60-65, 1946.
83. Giles LGF, Taylor JR: The effect of postural scoliosis on lumbar apophyseal joints. *Scand J Rheumatol* 13:209-220, 1984.
84. Giles LGF: *Leg length inequality with postural scoliosis: its effect on lumbar apophyseal jonts.* M.Sc. thesis, Department of Anatomy and Human Biology, University of Western Australia, Perth, 1982.
85. Giles LGF, Taylor JR: Histological preparation of large vertebral specimens. *Stain Technol* 58:45-49, 1983.
86. Reichert Kontron Messgerate GMBH. MOP4-AMO3 Quantitative Bildauswertung, March 1979.
87. Golding D: *General Management of Osteoarthritis, Joints and Their Disease.* London, British Medical Association, 1970, pp 95-102.
88. Huskisson EC: Routine drug treatment of rheumatoid arthritis and other rheumatic diseases. *Clin Rheum Dis* 5:697-706, 1979.
89. Bachman DC, Noble HB: Helping the patient with low back pain. *Modern Medicine of Australia* 1978, pp 15-18.
90. Howell DS, Moskowitz RW: Introduction: Symposium on osteoarthritis. A brief review of research and direction of future investigation. *Arthritis Rheum* 20:96-103, 1977.
91. Harris ED: Role of collagenases in joint destruction. In Sokoloff L (ed): *The Joints and Synovial Fluid.* New York, Academic Press, 1978, Vol 1, pp 243-272.
92. Arnoldi CC: Intraosseous hypertension. *Clin Orthop* 115:30-34, 1976.
93. Giles LGF, Taylor, JR: Human zygapophyseal joint capsule and synovial fold innervation. *Br J Rheumatol* 26:993-998, 1987.
94. Giles LGF, Taylor JR: Intra-articular synovial protrusions in the lower lumbar apophyseal joints. *Bull*

Hosp J Dis Orthop Inst 42:248-255, 1982.

95. Kos J, Wolf J: Les menisques intervertebraux et leur role possible dans les blocages vertebraux. *Annals de Medecine Physique* 15:203-217, 1972.
96. Lewit K: Beitrag zur reversiblen Gelenksblockierung. *Zeitschr Orthop* 105:150, 1968.
97. Zukschwerdt L, Emminger E, Biedermann F, Zettel H: *Wirbelgelenk und Bandscheibe.* Stuttgart, 1955.
98. Bourdillon JF: *Spinal Manipulation.* ed 2. London, William Heinemann Medical Books, 1973, pp 22-23.
99. Giles LGF, Taylor JR: Innervation of human lumbar zygapophyseal joint synovial folds. *Acta Orthop Scand* 58:43-46, 1987.
100. Giles LGF, Harvey AR: Immunohistochemical demonstration of nociceptors in the capsule and synovial folds of human zygapophyseal joints. *Br J Rheumatol* 26:362-364, 1987.
101. Kraft GL, Levinthal DH: Facet synovial impingement: a new concept in the etiology of lumbar vertebral derangement. *Surg Gynecol Obstet* 93:439-443, 1951.
102. Tondury G: Anatomie fonctionelle des petites articulations de rachis. *Ann Med Physique* 15:173-191, 1972.
103. Kirkaldy-Willis WH: The relationship of structural pathology to the nerve root. *Spine* 9:49-52, 1984.
104. Harmon PH: Congenital and acquired anatomic variations, including degenerative changes of the lower lumbar spine: role in production of painful back and lower extremity syndromes. *Clin Orthop* 44:171-186, 1966.
105. Bogduk N, Jull G: The theoretical pathology of acute locked back: a basis for manipulation. *Manual Medicine* 1:78-82, 1985.
106. Spurling RG, Mayfield FH, Rogers JB: Hypertrophy of the ligamenta flava as a cause of low back pain. *JAMA* 109:928, 1937.
107. Love JG, Walsh MN: Intraspinal protrusion of intervertebral discs. *Arch Surg* 40:454, 1940.
108. Pennal GF, Schatzker J: Stenosis of the lumbar spinal canal. *Clin Neurosurg* 6:86, 1971.
109. Dockerty MB, Love JG: Thickening and fibrosis (so-called hypertrophy) of the ligamentum flavum: a pathological study of fifty cases. *Proc Staff Meet Mayo Clin* 15:161-166, 1940.
110. Farfan HF: The biomechanical advantage of lordosis and hip extension for upright man as compared with other anthropoids. *Spine* 3:336-345, 1978.
111. Nachemson AL, Evans JH: Some mechanical properties of the third human lumbar interlaminar ligament (ligamentum flavum). *J Biomech* 1:211, 1968.
112. Hadley LA: Intervertebral joint subluxation, bony impingement and foramen encroachment with nerve root changes. *Am J Roentgenol* 65:377, 1951.
113. Baastrup CH: On the spinous processes of the lumbar vertebrae and the soft tissues between them, and on pathological changes in that region. *Acta Radiol (Stockh)* 14:52, 1933.
114. Epstein B: *The Spine: A Radiological Text and Atlas.* ed 4. Philadelphia, Lea and Febiger, 1976, p 417.
115. Bywaters EGL, Evans S: The lumbar interspinous bursae and Baastrup's syndrome. *Rheumatol Int* 2:87-96, 1982.

CHAPTER **10**

Low Back Pain Associated with Leg Length Inequality

Literature Review

Low back pain is frequently encountered in clinical practice. Its cause is usually obscure, but a possible association with leg length inequality, pelvic obliquity and postural scoliosis has been noted by Rush and Steiner (1), Stoddard (2), Nichols (3), Bourdillon (4), Giles (5), and Yates (6). Some of these authors attempt to correlate leg length inequality and low back pain by comparing the prevalence of leg length inequality in low back pain and control groups as shown in Tables 10.2 and 10.3. Maigne (7) and Fisk and Baigent (8) believe that leg length differences of 12.5 mm are not associated with an increased incidence of low back pain, but Maigne (7) does not give any data to support his view. According to Reid and Smith (9), a "mild" leg length inequality of up to 30 mm has not been convincingly linked to specific pathology, but they suggest that a therapeutic trial of correction may be warranted when pain is present. Clarke (10) suggests that the proportion of life during which an individual has symptoms of back pain increases with the degree of leg length inequality. Bourdillon (4) states that leg length inequality can also result in pelvic torsion with low back pain, and that this torsion may further increase the extent of sacral base obliquity. Pelvic torsion may be indicated by malaligned pubic crests on each side of the symphysis pubis. According to Dickson et al (11), nonstructural curves are associated with some rotation as evidenced in radiographs and by the fact that they can be detected on forward bending. In spite of the available literature regarding a possible association between leg length inequality

and low back pain, De Smet (12), who cites an incomplete bibliography on the topic, reports that "scoliosis due to leg length inequality is generally an infrequent and seldom significant problem."

However, because of the apparent association between leg length inequality and low back pain, the clinical and radiologic methods which have been used to measure leg "length" are reviewed. The accuracy of these methods is critically reviewed and the results of several investigators are summarized.

Methods of Measuring Leg Length Inequality

General Literature Review

Various methods of measuring leg lengths, or inequality in leg lengths, have been advocated in the literature. Some of these methods exclude the ankle–heel distance. Each method is briefly described here and a critical review of accuracy is given.

Clinical Methods

Leg "length" can be assessed by direct or indirect measurement.

Direct Measurement

In the supine position, a tape measure is used to measure the distance from each anterior superior iliac spine to the ipsilateral medial malleolus (3, 13–22) (Fig. 10.1). This is the most commonly used method in clinical practice (23, 24).

In population surveys, Taylor and Halliday (25) have used anthropometric measurements. Two anthropometers, fixed on a level platform, were used to measure tro-

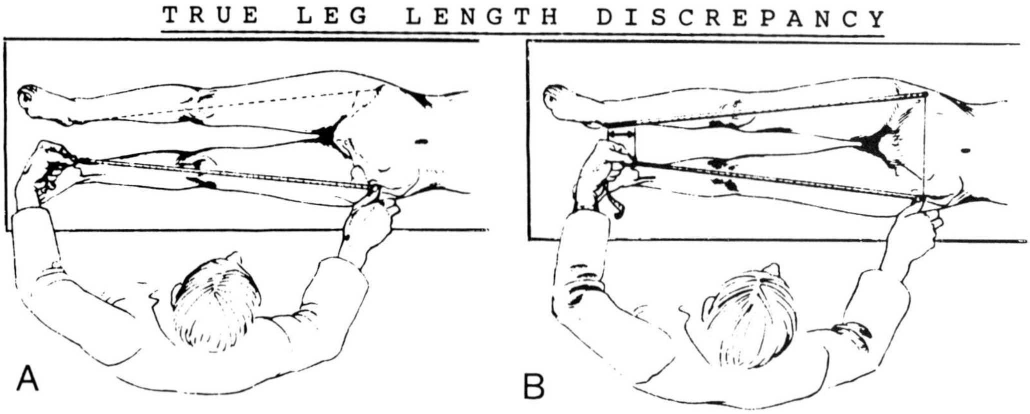

TRUE   LEG   LENGTH   DISCREPANCY

Figure 10.1.   Measurement of leg lengths using a tape measure. **A,** Measure from one fixed bony point to another to find true leg length. **B,** True leg length discrepancy. (Reproduced with permission from Hoppenfeld S: *Physical Examination of the Spine.* New York, Appleton-Century-Crofts, 1976.

chanteric height to the nearest millimeter on each side. The observer palpated the upper margin of both trochanters and marked these levels. These trochanteric heights were measured while the patient stood erect with the feet approximately 20 cm apart, the knees straight, and no lateral sway at the hips (26).

Indirect Measurement with the Patient in the Erect Posture with the Knees Straight

In one method of indirect measurement, the observer sits facing the patient with his or her hands on the trochanters, and his or her thumbs, pointing upwards, pressed against the notch on the lower border of the anterior superior iliac spines. The observer can then detect a difference in the level of the spines, and if shortening of one leg is present, it is measured by placing blocks of wood of known thickness under the foot of the short leg until the pelvis is level (27–29).

In another method, the observer sits behind the patient and (*a*) finds the posterior superior iliac spines from below with his or her thumbs and compares their relative heights (4, 30), and (*b*) finds the height of the left and right iliac crests by palpation compares these heights. When the distance from the iliac crest to the bottom of the feet is unequal, one observes a lateral tilt of the pelvis, and measurement of the leg length inequality is obtained by placing boards of known height under the shorter leg until the

pelvic obliquity is corrected (6, 20, 22, 23, 30–32). Instead of using boards of known height under the short leg, Schilgen (33, 34) devised an "ossometer" incorporating a system of blocks for measuring leg length inequality.

In a third method, the observer places a spirit level (which has sliding arms) on the iliac crests of the patient and checks for pelvic obliquity. Boards of known thickness are placed under the short leg until the bubble is centered (35).

Finally, the observer can use a plexiglass "Orthotractor," which incorporates a spirit level, to measure the level between the left and right anterior superior iliac spines (36).

Accuracy of Clinical Methods

Nichols and Bailey (14), Clarke (10) and Fisk and Baigent (8) performed remeasurement studies which indicated that clinical methods are inaccurate. This is suggested because there is difficulty in accurately locating bony points through soft tissues in obese or muscular subjects (37), and use is made of bony points on the pelvis, since the femur heads are not palpable, thus not making allowances for pelvic asymmetry (38).

Of the above authors, only Nichols and Bailey (14) conducted an "observer error" experiment in which four doctors (using the same tape measure) performed remeasurement studies on 50 randomly chosen patients. They concluded that differences of

12.5 mm or more may be diagnostically significant, whereas differences of less than 12.5 mm were not reliable, unless based on the average of at least four measurements. Clarke (10) and Fisk and Baigent (8) compared tape measurement studies with erect posture radiographs and found a difference of 5 mm or more between tape measurement and x-ray results.

Many other authors agree that tape measurement studies are inaccurate (22, 39–43). According to Gofton (37), it is doubtful if many would trust a measured difference of less than three-quarters of an inch (19 mm), and Henrard et al (41) found the same degree of inaccuracy , while Morscher and Figner (22) believe the degree of accuracy is about ± 5–10 mm.

Leg length estimations involving bilateral palpation of the anterior and superior iliac spines, and the iliac crests, in the erect posture, are unreliable because of pelvic torsion (4) and pelvic asymmetries (8, 10, 35, 44–46). On comparing the results of iliac crest palpation with x-ray measurements, Clarke (10) found that in only 16 out of 50 patients were two observers correct to within 5 mm of the x-ray results. The most accurate clinical method of estimating iliac crest height is the spirit level method devised by Hirschberg and Robertson (35). In their opinion, detection of differences of one-eighth of an inch (3 mm) in height of the iliac crests is possible, but they did not perform comparative or remeasurement studies to substantiate their claims.

Anthropometric Method

A remeasurement anthropometric study of trochanteric height estimation in 34 patients, with two separate observers, showed an "error" of 10 mm in 5% of these cases whose ages ranged from 6 years to maturity (26; J. R. Taylor, personal communication, 1979). A further remeasurement study involved comparison of anthropometric data with measurements made on erect posture A–P radiographs which showed no obvious pelvic rotation. Sixty-three adolescents were compared. Anthropometric trochanteric height difference was compared with the radiographic femoral head height difference in each case. Errors tended to cancel

each other out, and 65% of errors were within the range of ± 5 mm. Taking only those cases found anthropometrically to have 10-mm or more leg length difference, trochanteric height differences overestimated femoral head differences by 3.08 mm ± 3.07 mm (J. R. Taylor, personal communication, 1979).

According to Pope et al (47), the accuracy of anthropometric measurements of leg length inequality below 0.5 cm is subject to considerable measurement error.

Palpation and marking of corresponding levels of the left and right greater trochanters is difficult to perform accurately, particularly in obese subjects (J. R. Taylor, personal communication, 1979).

Radiographic Methods

Leg "length" can be assessed in the supine or erect posture position. Four main methods have been described in the literature, some of which do not take into account the ankle–heel distance.

Slit Scanography

Slit scanography (48, 49) is a method of taking radiographs with the patient in the supine position on the x-ray table. As the x-ray tube moves from one end of the x-ray table to the other, a narrow "slit" beam of x-rays traverses the part to be measured (Fig.10.2).

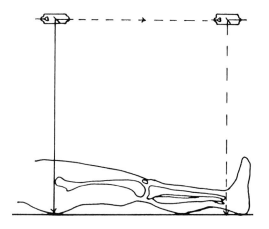

Figure 10.2. Slit scanography. The x-ray tube slowly moves horizontally over the lower extremities while emitting a constant narrow "slit" of x-radiation.

All the rays of the central beam pass through the part being radiographed at the same angle (50). The apparatus is so arranged that all the x-ray film is protected by lead, except the narrow strip which is being exposed. A perspex ruler is used to accurately measure leg lengths and differences in length from the x-ray films obtained.

Teleoradiography

Teleoradiography is a method in which the "total" length of both the lower extremities is radiographed in one exposure with the patient supine (51). In order to minimize magnification errors, a large tube–patient distance, such as 7 feet, should be used. This distance more nearly secures parallelism of the x-rays (50) (Fig. 10.3).

Orthoradiography (or Orthodiagraphy or Orthoskiagraphy)

A radiographic apparatus can be used to accurately record the form and size of structures inside the body, doing away with the distortion of the ordinary x-ray film (50). The orthoroentgenogram has been used for leg length measurements (52–54). This excludes the ankle–heel distance, but according to Laubach and McConville's (55) anthropometric measurements, the difference between the sphyrion height on the left and right sides is 0.2 mm (± 0.60 mm), hence the difference between the right and left hip joint–ankle joint distance can be taken to accurately reflect any total leg length inequality. Using radiographs from orthoradiography, corresponding points for measurement are chosen on the contralateral bone(s) of each leg.

Orthoradiography is considered to be an accurate method of measuring leg length (22). Although Nordentoft (56) found minor errors due to patient movement, these movement errors obviously would not apply to stabilized limbs.

With the subject supine and a 1-m steel calibrated ruler placed between the legs, A–P views are taken of the hip, knee, and upper ankle joints, respectively (Fig. 10.4A). By subtraction, the lengths of the femur and tibia can be measured accurately from the x-ray film (22) (Fig. 10.4B).

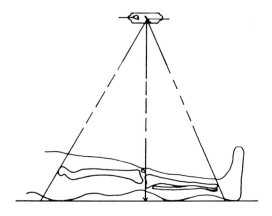

Figure 10.3. Teleoradiography. The "total" length of both lower extremities is x-rayed in one exposure.

Bell and Thompson (57) called this procedure modified spot "scanography," although the x-ray tube does not move during the exposure.

Orthoradiography as performed by Green et al (39) is used at a distance of 6 feet to measure the total length of each leg. These authors added the refinements of (*a*) using a long metal marker, which can be seen on the x-ray film opposite each joint, to ensure centering of the x-ray tube to the joint; and (*b*) restraining straps to keep the extremities still.

Goldstein and Driesinger (58) advocate the use of a similar method but with the added refinement of a brass cylinder, 26 inches long by 4½ inches in diameter, attached to the collimator, thus making it unnecessary to use lead to protect the unexposed parts of the film. They found the tube-film distance of 40 inches to be as accurate as greater distances and much easier for centering the x-ray tube.

Kunkle and Carpenter (59) incorporated elevation of the head of the x-ray table by 20–25° so that the patient's body weight pressed the feet against the foot rest of the table, and emphasized the importance of both feet exerting the same amount of pressure, using plywood boards, of known thickness, beneath the short leg when necessary. White (60) modified the foot rest of the x-ray table by replacing part of it with a thick glass window to enable him to observe equal

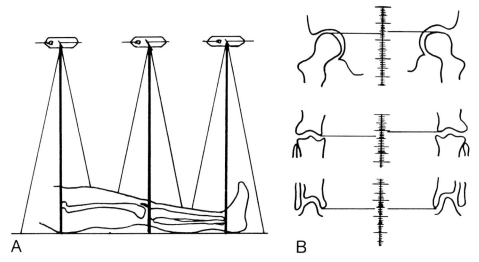

Figure 10.4. **A**, Orthoradiography. Perpendicular x-rays at the ends of the bones record the true length of the respective bones. **B**, Schematic representation of an x-ray showing the method of measuring leg length discrepancies (excluding the foot–heel height) from an x-ray film on which a calibrated metal rule was placed. (Modified from Cailliet R: *Scoliosis Diagnosis and Management.* Philadelphia, F.A. Davis, 1975 p 52.)

"pallor" of the sole of each foot which was compressed when supine patients pulled themselves down against the glass foot plate.

With the table vertical, and using an appropriate tube-stand, x-ray films may be taken in the erect posture (52).

Erect Posture Radiography

This method usually involves an A–P radiograph of the pelvis and lumbar spine in order to obtain information regarding leg length inequality and its effect on the pelvis and lumbar spine. It is used to measure any difference in total lengths of the legs, when the patient stands with his or her knees straight and buttocks against a vertical x-ray table or bucky.

Rush (61) devised a "roentgenographic spinal fixation and stabilization device" which was later used to measure lower limb lengths in 1,000 soldiers who complained of low back pain and 100 control asymptomatic soldiers (1).

Precautions were taken in order to ensure that the lower edge of the film and the platform on which the soldiers stood were parallel, and that the soldier's knees were straight. Any difference in leg length was determined by comparing the vertical height of each femoral head from the lower margin of the radiograph.

Judovich et al (62) stood patients behind a rigid fluoroscopic screen which had a water level attached to its frame. The screen was set so that the water level bubble was centered. A wire which was permanently attached to the front of the screen was lined across the iliac crests, and if leg lengths were equal, the wire was seen at corresponding levels on each iliac crest. If one iliac crest was low, lifts were placed under the appropriate heel until the pelvic obliquity was eliminated.

Gofton and Trueman (63, 64) used radiographs taken with the patient standing on a level platform with the feet placed parallel to each other at 7½ inches apart. The horizontal x-ray beam was centered to the hip joints, using a tube–film distance of 6 feet. A radiopaque plumb-line hung between the patient and the film. From the vertical image of this plumb-line on the film, a line was drawn at right angles to each femoral head, and the vertical difference between these lines was measured. A similar method was used by Clarke (10), Henrard et al (41), and Willman (65).

Wiltse (66) measured leg length inequality by simply getting the patient to stand "level" in stockinged feet, with both knees in the same degree of extension, in front of a level cassette, while the pelvic x-ray was taken. He then measured the femur head heights from the lower edge of the x-ray film.

Ottander (67) devised a simple water-level gauge device to establish a horizontal reference line. This device, a long radiotranslucent plastic cylinder with a 2-cm diameter, is half filled with a contrast medium, then stuck to the front of the bucky (behind the patient) by means of two small magnets. The total leg length inequality is measured on the film as the vertical distance between the top of each femur head and the reference contrast line. Mastrander (68) used a similar technique. Bolton (69) suggested a "U" tube containing mercury, attached to the front of the bucky, as a radiographic "spirit" level from which horizontal measurements could be made in the erect posture.

Henrard et al (41) assessed their accuracy by repeating x-ray exposures having artificially introduced known discrepancies in leg length.

Chamberlain (70), Henrard et al (41), Merrill (71), and Ladermann (72) showed that the center of the patient's sagittal plane must be centered to the midline of the bucky, and that the patient's feet must be at the same distance apart as the femoral heads in order to prevent errors of distortion in lateral sway of the pelvis (Fig. 10.5).

With the x-ray tube at any level other than at the femoral head height, the divergent x-ray beam may artificially cause apparent differences in femoral head heights as recorded on the film (73), should minor rotation of the pelvis be present. However, when the x-ray tube is at the femur head height, negligible differences in femoral head heights are recorded on the film (73, 74) (Fig. 10.6).

Papaioannou et al (76) and Gibson et al (77) took erect posture A–P pelvis–lumbar spine radiographs of patients who stood in front of a sheet of methylmethacrylate with accurately aligned horizontal and vertical steel wires set into its surface. A tube-to-film distance of 1 m was used; however, the x-ray beam was centered at the level of the fifth lumbar vertebra, and not at the femur head level.

Friberg (78) took erect posture radiographs of patients which exposed only the regions of the hip joints, but details of an accurate vertical or horizontal reference line on the x-ray film were not mentioned. The accuracy of the method was assessed by repeating the x-ray exposure with and without a shoe raise.

Cagnoli (79) also took erect posture radiographs of patients which showed only the upper regions of the left and right femurs and part of the pelvis. Horizontal lines were shown on the radiograph. The difference in femoral heads was measured in millimeters using the horizontal lines.

Erect Posture Pelvis and Lumbar Spine Anteroposterior Radiography

For a biomechanical evaluation of the lumbar spine and pelvis it is necessary for both these anatomical regions to be visualized on one x-ray film.

My technique is partly based on the methods of Chamberlain (70) Gofton (37), Clark (10), Howe (80), Henrard et al (41), Merrill (71), Willman (65), and F. Bauer (personal communication, 1973), incorporating the best elements of each with minor innovations. It is described in detail to explain the precautions used to obtain a precise evaluation of equality, or inequality, of the right and left femoral head heights at the focus film distance of 100 cm. The technique is as follows.

1. A thick steel plate, with spirit levels welded on to it, is screwed onto the floor in front of the bucky so that it is exactly horizontal. A perspex footplate is screwed onto the steel plate so that its back edge is parallel to the vertical x-ray bucky. The footplate is also centered to the middle of the bucky by means of thin-diameter wire with a plumb-bob which hangs centrally in front of the x-ray grid and cassette but behind the patient) (Fig. 10.7).
2. The patient stands barefoot with the heels in the inner or outer cups (Fig.

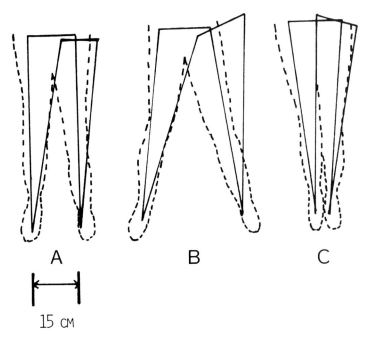

Figure 10.5. The effect on the femur head heights if lateral sway of the pelvis is present; **A**, when the patient's feet are below the femur heads, **B**, when the patient's feet are too far apart, and **C**, when the patient's feet are too close together. (Modified from the Henrard J-Cl, Bismuth V, de Molmont CH, Gaux J-C: Unequal length of the lower limbs: measurement by a simple radiological method. Application to epidemiological studies. *Revue de Rhumatisme* 41:773-779, 1974.)

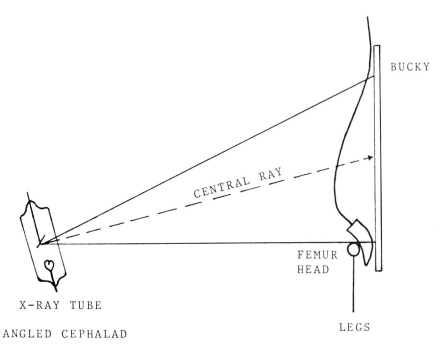

Figure 10.6. The x-ray tube is positioned at the level of the femoral heads for erect posture anteroposterior radiography. (Reproduced with permission from Giles LGF, Taylor JR: Low-back pain associated with leg length inequality. *Spine* 6:510-521, 1981. Copyright Harper and Row, Philadelphia.)

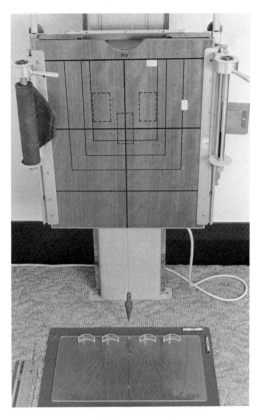

Figure 10.7. Perspex foot plate positioned in front of the bucky, Note the plumb-line "bob." (Reproduced with permission from Giles LGF, Taylor JT: Low-back pain associated with leg length inequality. *Spine* 6:510-521, 1981. Copyright Harper and Row, Philadelphia.)

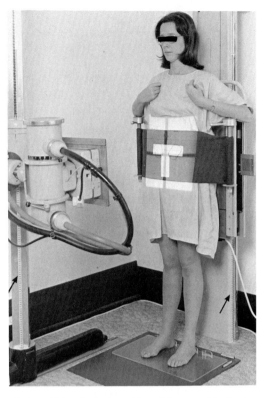

Figure 10.8. Patient positioned for a pelvis–lumbar spine anteroposterior radiograph. Arrows show the scale (in millimeters) on the x-ray tube stand and on the bucky stand. (Reproduced with permission from Giles LGF, Taylor JR: Low-back pain associated with leg length inequality. *Spine* 6:510-521, 1981. Copyright Harper and Row, Philadelphia.)

10.8) so that the heels are approximately below the femoral heads and the feet are kept parallel. (The paired inner and outer heel cups are 15 and 34 cm apart, respectively.)

3. The patient keeps the knees straight, and the superior aspect of each greater trochanter is palpated, then the x-ray beam is directed horizontally 2 cm higher, i.e., approximately to the femur head level. The bottom of the bucky is lowered 14 cm below this level so that the ischial tuberosities are located on the film.

4. The patient leans lightly against the bucky with the weight going "equally through both heels."

5. The x-ray tube is rotated slightly cephalad in order to center the central

ray to the center of the bucky. This allows the pelvis and lumbar spine to be included on the 35 × 43 cm film but docs not distort the accuracy of the femur head projection (Figs. 10.6 and 10.8).

6. The height of both the x-ray tube and bucky above the floor is read on scales on the tube stand and the bucky stand, respectively (Fig. 10.8), and these readings are recorded. This enables precise duplication of the film at a later date, if a check on the shoe-raise height is required for patients with a short leg.

7. The collimator is adjusted to allow only the lumbar spine and pelvis to be radiated.

8. In order to stabilize the patient (and to compress the abdominal tissues so as to

obtain good radiographic detail) a compression band is tightened equally on both sides of the patient. A cross, painted centrally on the front of the collimator, shows up as a black shadow on the compression band which has a white velcro "T" on it. During compression, the center of the "T" and the vertical line of the black cross are kept precisely in line to prevent introducing pelvic rotation (Fig. 10.8).

9. For radiation protection of the gonads, lead devices backed with velcro can be attached to parts of the velcro "T" (F. Bauer, personal communication, 1973), except in cases where this precaution may interfere with the examination of a particular patient.

10. The patient is instructed to breath in, then out, and then to keep absolutely still with the knees straight; at this point the exposure is made.

Measurement of Leg Length Inequality and Angle of Curvature of Postural Scoliosis

The A–P erect posture of radiographs of the pelvis and lumbar spine are used to determine leg length inequality.

Any difference in leg lengths is measured on the x-ray film by projecting a line at right angles from the plumb-line shadow to each femur head. Any vertical difference between these two lines represents leg length inequality which is measured using a perspex ruler marked in millimeters (Fig. 10.9).

This technique measures leg length differences accurately, except for very small magnification errors when pelvic rotation is present (10, 64, 70).

The angle of curvature of the lumbar spine is measured using a Cobb (81) method which has been shown to be reliable at all degrees of curvature (82) and is accepted as the standard method by the Scoliotic Research Society.

Measurement of Sacral Base Obliquity in Relation to Leg Length Inequality

The A–P erect posture radiographs of the pelvis and lumbar spine are used to determine whether the sacral base obliquity relates to the leg length inequality only, or

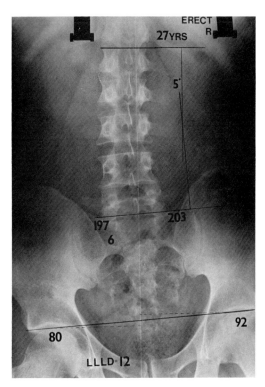

Figure 10.9. An erect posture radiograph of a 27-year-old male showing a left leg length deficiency (inequality) of 12 mm, sacral base obliquity, and postural scoliosis with a 5° angle of curvature. R = right side of the patient. Note the vertical plumb-line shadow which is used for measuring leg lengths and sacral base obliquity. (Reproduced with permission from Giles LGF, Taylor JR: Low-back pain associated with leg length inequality. *Spine* 6:510-521, 1981. Copyright Harper and Row, Philadelphia.)

whether a pelvic anomaly (such as hypoplasia of one side of the sacrum or of one ilium) is present above the femur heads. Real asymmetries in the distance from the roof of the acetabulum of the highest point on the iliac crest were found in 90% of the subjects examined by Ingelmark and Lindstrom (44). (A classification of sacral base obliquity in relation to leg lengths is shown in Figure A3.5.)

Any difference between the heights of the inferior margin of the superior sacral "notch" on the left and right sides of the sacrum is measured on the x-ray film by projecting a line at right angles from the plumb-line shadow to each inferior margin of the superior sacral "notch." Any vertical dif-

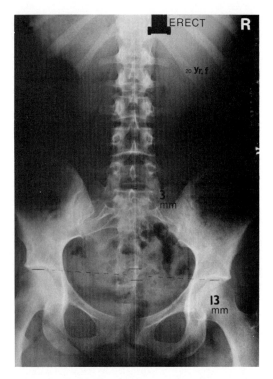

Figure 10.10. An erect posture anteroposterior radiograph of a 20-year-old female showing a right leg length deficiency of 13 mm, and a neglible (3 mm) sacral base obliquity on the same side, with a straight spine. (Reproduced with permission from Giles LGF: Letter to the editor. *Spine* 9(8):842, 1984. Copyright Harper and Row, Philadelphia.)

ference between these lines represents obliquity of the sacrum. If the sacral base obliquity is measured as being *half* the leg length inequality, on the same side, no pelvic asymmetry exists above the femur heads which would affect the relationship between leg length inequality and sacral base obliquity (Fig. 10.9).

It is essential to take into account sacral base obliquity because negligible sacral base obliquity can be found even in the presence of considerable leg length inequality. Figure 10.10 illustrates such an example in which a 20-year-old female had a right leg length deficiency of 13 mm but only a negligible sacral base obliquity of 3 mm and no scoliosis.

This example clearly shows why it is necessary to take a carefully standardized erect posture A–P radiograph of the pelvis

and lumbar spine. If pelvic–lumbar biomechanics are the reason for measuring leg length inequality, it is essential to take an erect posture A–P radiograph of the pelvis and lumbar spine. To radiograph only the region of the hip joints to determine leg length inequality, as advocated by Cagnoli (79) and Friberg (78), would be inexcusable, since the previously discussed pelvic osseous asymmetries would not be taken into account. Patients with leg length inequality who have a horizontal sacral base must not be provided with a shoe raise since a raise may cause strain in the lumbar spine joints and postural muscles as a result of introducing a postural scoliosis.

Accuracy of Radiographic Methods

Supine Radiographic Methods

Using radiographs in scanography, corresponding points for measurement are chosen on the contralateral bone(s) of each leg. It has been suggested that radiographic studies are more accurate, and Millwee (48) believes that slit scanography gives an exact measurement of bones, although Amstutz and Sakai (43) demonstrated a negligible error of 0.4 mm. According to Gofton and Trueman (64), slit scanography avoids the inaccuracies of centering and projection of other methods of orthoradiography.

In teleoradiography, divergence of the x-rays from the tube, even at a distance of 7 feet, produces an increasing degree of magnification and distortion with longer extremities (39).

Orthoroentgenograms show little deviation from the real length of bones, but comparison of x-ray results and direct measurement in one leg postmortem showed the femur to be 2 mm shorter on the x-ray film than on direct measurement (39). The tendency to cumulation of errors with "total" leg length (excluding the foot–ankle height) was estimated from summation of individual leg lengths by Nordentoft (56), who found leg movement and inaccuracy of positioning to be a major source of error. On rechecking the measurements of 25 patients having a short leg, he found a mean error of 0.52 mm (± 2.33 mm). Small projection errors remain, in spite of the sophisticated x-ray equipment required for orthoradiography (42).

Erect Posture Radiographic Methods

Judovich et al (62) did not give any objective assessment for the accuracy of their method. However, erect posture radiographic procedures which make use of iliac crest levels to evaluate leg length inequality must be considered to be unreliable in view of the pelvic asymmetries found by Ingelmark and Lindstrom (44) and pelvic torsion as described by Bourdillon (4).

Papaioannou et al (76) and Gibson et al (77) did not give any objective assessment for the accuracy of their method. However, erect posture radiographic procedures which use the x-ray beam centered at the fifth lumbar level cannot be accurate for estimating leg length inequality because of geometrical distortion errors; these errors become greater as the leg length inequality increases.

To accurately evaluate leg length inequality, erect posture radiography, with the patient's knees straight, should use (*a*) a plumb-line or a radio-opaque fluid level to produce a true vertical or horizontal axis as a reference line on the x-ray film, (*b*) a horizontal foot plate with each heel below the ipsilateral acetabulum so that lines joining heels and femoral heads form a parallelogram, and (*c*) an x-ray tube positioned at the femur head height. Gofton and Trueman (64), using a skeleton and the tube positioned at this height, showed that (*a*) with the femoral heads at the same level, pelvic rotation of 18° resulted in no error, and (*b*) with a difference of 18 mm in the level of the femoral heads, pelvic rotation of 18° resulted in a 1.5-mm error.

Accepting that radiologic methods are much more accurate in measuring an individual leg length inequality than clinical methods (84–86), particularly because of the difficulty of accurately palpating comparable osseous structures, and the fact that anomalies cannot be visualized without radiographs, clinical methods may be regarded as valid for (*a*) population studies, as long as the limitations of accuracy are clearly understood; (*b*) the ease with which they can be quickly performed to give some ap-proximate idea of leg length equality or inequality; and (*c*) the fact that they use noninvasive procedures. They are necessary as a screening procedure, but if there is reason to suspect leg length inequality, they cannot take the place of an adequately controlled erect posture radiographic study of the pelvis and lower extremities to determine the absolute leg length inequality (87). X-ray films must be taken under standardized conditions for accuracy (88) and it should be noted that Cleveland et al (89) found no significant difference by t-test between measurements of leg lengths obtained from standing and supine radiographs when these were carefully standardized.

Furthermore, it is important to repeat the A–P erect posture pelvis and lumbar spine radiograph with the patient standing on a raise equivalent to the leg length inequality, to determine what effect the raise has on the biomechanics of the pelvis and lumbar spine.

In an attempt to ascertain the accuracy of my radiographic method, the original and subsequent x-ray examination (using a measured perspex "raise" under the short leg) of each patient was compared, and a mean error of 1.12 mm (± 0.92 mm) was found. A comparison of the accuracy of some erect posture radiographic procedures is shown in Table 10.1.

Table 10.1.
Accuracy of Some Erect Posture Radiographic Procedures

Authors	Mean Error in Leg Length Inequality Determination	Standard Deviation
	mm	
Rush (61)[a]	2	—
Wilts (66)[a]	5	—
Gofton and Trueman (64)[b]	1.44	1.06
Henrard et al (41)[b]	—	2
Giles and Taylor (75)[b]	1.12	0.92
Friberg (78)[b]	0.6	<2

[a]These authors merely estimated their degree of accuracy.
[b]These authors performed remeasurement studies.

Prevalence of Leg Length Inequality

The incidence of leg length inequality in adults has usually been found to be greater in patients complaining of low back pain (with or without leg pain) than in asymptomatic control groups. The prevalence of leg length inequality has been reported as shown in Table 10.2 using clinical and anthropometric methods, and Table 10.3 using radiographic methods.

In general, there is a fair measure of agreement among the eight observers whose results are reviewed in Tables 10.2 and 10.3 that about 7% (range 4–8%) of the adult population with no history of low back pain have leg length inequality of 1 cm or more. In groups who have back pain severe or chronic enough to make them seek treatment, four author's out of five found a higher incidence of leg length inequality ranging from 13 to 22% (1–3, 75). Fisk and Baigent (8) disagree since they found a 6%

incidence of patients with low back pain and a leg length inequality of 12.5 mm or more.

In a study performed by this author, 2000 patients, aged 19–77 years, who presented with a complaint of low back pain with or without sciatica and 50 volunteer control cases aged 20–67 years (who complained of headaches and who had no history of low back pain) were subjected to erect posture radiography of (a) the pelvis and lumbar spine in the A–P position (b) left and right 45° oblique views of the lumbosacral spine, and (c) a lateral view of the lumbosacral spine. An A–P radiograph of the thoracic spine was taken if clinical examination indicated the presence of a structural scoliosis. Only patients presenting with no anomalies or pathology (other than thinning of the intervertebral discs with or without accompanying osteoarthritis of the zygapophyseal joints) and no malaligned

Table 10.2.
Incidence of Leg Length Inequality in Adults: Clinical and Anthropometric Measurements

				Incidence %	
Investigators	Low Back Pain	Control	Leg Length Difference	Low Back Pain	Control
			mm		
Nichols (3)[a]	180	1007	10+	22	7
Sicuranza et al (23)[a]		1000[c]	10+	16	
J. R. Taylor (personal communication, 1979)[b]		530[d]	10+	7	

[a]Clinical.
[b]Anthropometric.
[c]All admissions (females) were routinely screened irrespective of history of low back pain.
[d]Population group (young adult students) were routinely screened irrespective of history of low back pain.

Table 10.3.
Incidence of Leg Length Inequality in Adults: Radiographic Measurements

				Incidence %	
Investigators	Low Back Pain	Control	Leg Length Difference	Low Back Pain	Control
			mm		
Rush and Steiner (1)	1000	100	11+	15	4
Stoddard (2)	100	50	12.5+	17	8
Henrard et al (41)	—	50	10+	—	8
Fisk and Baigent (8)	206	—	12.5+	6	—
Giles and Taylor (75)	1309	50	10+	18	8

Table 10.4.
Leg Length Inequality in 1914 Consecutive Patients with Low Back Pain and 50 Controls

Subject	Total No. of Patients	No. with 1 cm or More Discrepancy	% with 1 cm or More Discrepancy
No history of low back pain	50	4	8.0
Chronic low back pain	1780	325[a]	18.3
Acute low back pain	134	29	21.6

[a]Six had previously broken a femur or tibia.

pubic crests (which may indicate sacroiliac joint subluxation or pelvic torsion) were used in this study. This was 1914 patients.

Of the 1914 patients, 354 had a leg length difference of 1 cm or more (Table 10.4). These 354 patients consisted of 325 chronic low back pain patients and 29 acute low back pain patients.

As shown in Table 10.4, 325 chronic low back pain patients had a leg length inequality of 1 cm or more. Of these 325 patients, 117 agreed to participate in this survey of the effectiveness of treatment. Eighty-nine of these patients had a 12-month follow-up examination, at which time the A–P pelvis and lumbar spine radiograph was repeated with the patient standing on an appropriate perspex block (equal to the leg length inequality). These patients fell into three arbitrarily chosen age groups of 19–30 years, 31–50 years, and older than 50 years.

A small group of 12 of the above patients (whose ages ranged from 21 to 59 years) were willing to undergo the second A–P pelvis and lumbar spine radiograph at the initial visit, so that the immediate response of postural scoliosis to the perspex raise could be assessed. Only this small sample of patients was subjected to two x-ray exposures at the initial visit, in order to minimize radiation dosage.

It is acknowledged that the number of 50 control cases in this study is too small to be statistically reliable as a true indication of the prevalence of leg length inequality in the "normal" community. However, the percentage of control cases with 1 cm or more leg length inequality was 8.0%, whereas the percentage of chronic low back pain patients with 1 cm or more leg length inequality was 18.3%. These results are in keeping with those of previously mentioned authors (Tables 10.2 and 10.3) and show that the prevalence of leg length inequality of 1 cm or more appears to be more common in patients suffering from low back pain than in the normal population.

References

1. Rush WA, Steiner HA: A study of lower extremity length inequality. *AJR* 56:616-623, 1946.
2. Stoddard A: *Manual of Osteopathic Technique.* London, Hutchinson Medical Publications, 1959, p 212.
3. Nichols PJR: Short-leg syndrome. *B Med J* 1:1863-1865, 1960.
4. Bourdillon JF: *Spinal Manipulation.* London, William Heinemann Medical Books Ltd, 1970.
5. Giles LGF: Leg length inequalities associated with low back pain. *Journal of the Canadian Chiropractic Association* 20:25-32, 1976.
6. Yates A: The lumbar spine and back pain. In Jayson M (ed): *Treatment of Back Pain.* London, Sector Publishing, 1967, pp 341-353.
7. Maigne R: *Orthopedic Medicine. A New Approach to Vertebral Manipulation.* Springfield, IL, Charles C. Thomas, 1972.
8. Fisk JW, Baigent ML: Clinical and radiologic assessment of leg length. *NZ Med J* 81:477-480, 1975.
9. Reid DC, Smith B: Leg length inequality: a review of etiology and management. *Physiotherapy Canada* 36:177-182, 1984.
10. Clarke GR: Unequal leg length: an accurate method of detection and some clinical results. *Rheumatology and Physical Medicine* 11:285-390, 1972.
11. Dickson RA, Lawton JO, Butt WP: The pathogenesis of idiopathic scoliosis. In Dickson RA, Bradford DS (eds): *Orthopaedics 2. Management of Spinal Deformities.* London, Butterworths, 1984, p 1-100.
12. De Smet AA: *Radiology of Spinal Curvature.* St. Louis, C. V. Mosby, 1985, p 228.
13. Hoppenfeld S: *Physical Examination of the Spine and Extremities.* New York, Appleton-Century-Crofts, 1976.
14. Nichols PJR, Bailey NTJ: The accuracy of measuring leg-length differences. *Br Med J* 2:1247-1248, 1955.
15. Mennell JMcM: *Back Pain. Diagnosis and Treatment using Manipulative Techniques.* ed 1. Boston, Little, Brown 1960, p 63.
16. Riley LH: Musculoskeletal system. In Judge RD, Suidema GD (eds): *Physical Diagnosis.* ed 2. Boston, Little, 1968, p 338.
17. Keim HA: Scoliosis. *Ciba Clinical Symposia* 24:12, 1972.
18. Keim HA: Low back pain. *Ciba Clinical Symposia* 25:4, 9, 1973.
19. Bradford DS, Moe JH, Winter RB: Scoliosis. In Roth-

man RH, Simeone FA (eds): *The Spine.* Philadelphia, W.B. Saunders, 1975, Vol 1, p 276, 279.

20. Cailliet R: *Scoliosis Diagnosis and Management.* Philadelphia, F.A. Davis, 1975, p 52.
21. D'Ambrosia RA: *Musculoskeletal Disorders, Regional Examination and Differential Diagnosis.* Toronto, J.B. Lippincott, 1977, pp 404-413.
22. Morscher E, Figner G: Measurement of leg length. In Hungerford DS (ed): *Leg Length Discrepancy. The Injured Knee* (Progress in Orthopedic Surgery) New York, Springer-Verlag, 1977, pp 21-27.
23. Sicuranza BJ, Richards J, Tisdall LH: The short leg syndrome in obstetrics and gynecology. *Am J Obstet Gynecol* 107:217-219, 1970.
24. Woerman AL, Binder-Macleod SA: Leg length discrepancy assessment: accuracy and precision in five clinical methods of evaluation. *Journal of Orthopedics and Sports Physical Therapy* 5:230-239, 1984.
25. Taylor JR, Halliday M: Limb length asymmetry and growth. *J Anat* 126:634-635, 1978.
26. Halliday M: *Limb length asymmetry and scoliosis.* Bachelor of Science honors thesis, Department of Anatomy and Human Biology, University of Western Australia, Perth, 1976.
27. Wiles P. Sweetman R: *Essentials of Orthopaedics.* London, J. and A. Churchill, 1965, pp 16-17.
28. Beard RG: Spinal curvature. In Douthwaite (ed): *French's Index of Differential Diagnosis.* ed 9. Bristol, John Wright and Sons, 1967, p 765.
29. Subotnick SI: The short leg syndrome. *J Am Podiatr Assoc* 66:720-723, 1976.
30. Cailliet R: *Low Back Pain Syndrome.* ed 2. Philadelphia, F.A. Davis, 1968.
31. Redler I: Clinical significance of minor inequalities in leg length. *New Orleans Medical Surgical Journal* 104:308-312, 1952.
32. Rickenbacher J, Landolt AM, Theiler K: *Applied Anatomy.* Berlin, Springer-Verlag, 1985, pp 30, 31.
33. Schilgen L: A new, simplified, technique to measure differences in leg-length, measurement-steps. *Z Orthop* 111:805-808, 1973.
34. Schilgen L: Beinlangendifferenzmessung mit dem "Ossometer." *Z Orthop* 113:818-820, 1975.
35. Hirschberg GG, Robertson KB: Device for determining differences in leg length. *Arch Phys Med Rehab* 53:45-46, 1972.
36. Okun SJ, Morgan JW, Burns MJ: Limb length discrepancy. A new method of measurement and its clinical significance. *J Am Podiatr Assoc* 72:595-599, 1982.
37. Gofton JP: Studies in osteoarthritis of the hip: Part IV. Biomechanics and clinical considerations. *Can Med Assoc J* 104:1007-1011, 1971.
38. Ober FR, Brewster AH: *Lovett's Lateral Curvature of the Spine and Round Shoulders.* ed 5. Philadelphia, P. Blakiston's Son, 1931.
39. Green WT, Wyatt GM, Anderson M: Orthoroentgenography as a method of measuring the bones of the lower extremities. *J Bone Joint Surg* 28:60-65, 1946.
40. Dunlap K, Kooda JC: Determination of differences in leg length by x-ray. *The Military Surgeon* 106:373-375, 1950.
41. Henrard J-CI, Bismuth V,de Molmont Ch, Gaux J-C: Unequal length of the lower limbs: measurement by a simple radiological method. Application to epidemiological studies. *Revue de Rhumatisme* 41:773-779, 1974.
42. Eichler J: Methodological errors in documenting leg length and leg length discrepancies. In Hungerford DS (ed): *Leg Length Discrepancy. The Injured Knee* (Progress in Orthopaedic Surgery, Vol. 1). New York, Springer-Verlag,1977, pp 29-39.
43. Amstutz HC, Sakai DN: Equalization of leg length (editorial comment) *Clin Orthop*136-2-5, 1978.

44. Ingelmark BE, Lindstrom T: Asymmetries of the lower extremities and pelvis and their relations to lumbar scoliosis. *Acta Morphol Scand* 5-6:227-234, 1963.
45. Stoddard A: *Manual of Osteopathic Technique.* London, Hutchinson Medical Publications, 1969.
46. D'Eschougues JR and associates: Inequality of length of lower limbs. A simplistic affirmation too often erroneous or inadequate. *Rheumatologie Review of Osteoarthricular Conditions* 27:227-230, 1975.
47. Pope MH, Bevins T,Wilder DG, Frymoyer JW: The relationship between anthropometric, postural, muscular, and mobility characteristics of males ages 18–55. *Spine* 10:644-648, 1985.
48. Millwee RH: Slit scanography. *Radiography* 28:483-486, 1937.
49. Pugh DG, Winkler NT: Scanography for limb-length measurement. An essay satisfactory method. *Radiology* 87:130-133, 1966.
50. *Dorland's Illustrated Medical Dictionary.* ed 25. Philadelphia, W.B. Saunders, 1974.
51. Hickey PM: Teleoroentgenography as an aid to orthopedic measurements. *AJR* 11:2232-2233, 1924.
52. Merrill OE: A method for the roentgen measurement of the long bones. *AJR* 48:405-406, 1942.
53. Ferill J: Orthoradiographic measurement of shortening of the lower extremity. *Med Radiogr Photogr* 29:32, 1980.
54. Mosely CF: Growth. In Lovell W,Winter RB (eds): *Pediatric Orthopedics.* Philadelphia, B. Lippincott, 1978, pp 28-29.
55. Laubach LL, McConville JT: Notes on anthropometric technique: anthropometric measurements—right and left sides. *Am J Phys Anthropol* 26:367-370, 1967.
56. Nordentoft EL: The accuracy of orthoroentgenographic measurements. *Acta Orthop Scand* 24:283-288, 1964.
57. Bell S, Thompson WAL: Modified spot scanography. *AJR* 63:615-616, 1950.
58. Goldstein LA, Driesinger F: Spot orthoroentgenography. *J Bone Joint Surgery* 32(A): 449–452, 1950.
59. Kunkle HM, Carpenter EB: A simple technique for x-ray measurement of limb-length discrepancies. *J Bone Joint Surg* 36(A):152-155, 1954.
60. White JW: A practical graphic method of recording leg length discrepancies. *South Med J* 33:946-949, 1940.
61. Rush WA: Roentgenographic spinal fixation and stabilization device. *American Journal of Roentgenology and Radiologic Therapy* 54:187-189, 1945.
62. Judovich B, Bates W, Yashin JC: *Pain Syndromes, Treatment by Paravertebral Nerve Block,* ed 3. Philadelphia, F.A. Davis, 1949, pp 46-49.
63. Gofton JP, Trueman GE: Unilateral idiopathic osteoarthritis of the hip. *Can Med Assoc J* 87:1129-1132, 1967.
64. Gofton JP, Trueman GE: Studies in osteoarthritis of the hip. Part II. Osteoarthritis of the hip and leg-length disparity. *Can Med Assoc J* 104:791-799, 1971.
65. Willman MK: Radiographic technical aspects of the postural study. *JAOA* 76:739-744, 1976.
66. Wiltse LL: *Lumbo-Sacral Strain and Instability.* American Academy of Orthopaedic Surgeons, Symposium on the Spine, St. Louis, C.V. Mosby, 1969, p 66.
67. Ottander H: Simple x-ray method for measuring leg length discrepancy. *X-ray Focus* 15:83-85, 1977.
68. Mastrander F: Leg length deficiency and tilt in fundament of the spine. *Tidsskr Nor Laegeforen* 7:435-436, 1980.
69. Bolton PS: A radiographic spirit level. *Journal of the Australian Chiropractors Association* 16:48-50, 1986.
70. Chamberlain WE: Measurements of differences in leg length. In Merrill V (ed): *Atlas of Roentgenographic Positioning,* St. Louis, C.V. Mosby, 1967, vol 1.
71. Merrill V: *Atlas of Roentgenographic Positions and Stan-*

dard *Radiologic Procedures,* ed 4. St. Louis, C.V. Mosby, vol 1, 1975.

72. Ladermann JP: About inequalities of the lower extremities. *Annals of the Swiss Chiropractors Association* 6:37-57, 1976.

73. Howe JW, Buehler MT, Palmateer DC, Hollen WV: Research on several parameters relating to full-spine radiography. *ACA Journal of Chiropractic* 4:S57-S64, 1970.

74. Giles LGF: Leg length inequality: its measurement, prevalence and effects on the lumbar spine. Master's degree preliminary thesis, Department of Anatomy and Human Biology, University of Western Australia, Perth, 1979.

75. Giles LGF, Taylor JR: Low-back pain associated with leg length inequality. *Spine* 6:510-521, 1981.

76. Papaioannou T, Stokes I, Kenwright J: Scoliosis associated with leg length inequality. *J Bone Joint Surg* 64(A):59-62, 1982.

77. Gibson PH, Papaioannou T, Kenwright J: The influence on spine and leg length discrepancy after femoral fracture. *J Bone Joint Surg* 65(B):584-587, 1983.

78. Friberg O: Clinical symptoms and biomechanics of lumbar spine and hip joint in leg length inequality. *Spine* 8:643-651, 1983.

79. Cagnoli H: Un procede rediographique simple de mesure de la difference de longueur des membres inferieurs. *Revue de Chirurgie orthopedique et reparatrice de l'Appareil moteur (Pans)* 58(8): 817-819, 1972.

80. Howe JW: Facts and fallacies, myths and misconceptions in spinography. *Journal of Clinical Chiropractic Archives* 2:34-45, 1972.

81. Cobb JR: Outline for the study of scoliosis. Instructional course lectures. *Am Acad Orthop Surg* 5:261-175, 1948.

82. Greenspan A, Pugh JW, Norman A, Norman RS: Scoliotic index: a comparative evaluation of methods for the measurement of scoliosis. *Bull Hosp Jt Dis Orthop* 39:117-125, 1978.

83. Giles LGF: Lumbar apophyseal joint arthrography. *J Manipulative Physiol Ther* 7:21-24, 1984.

84. Hughes JL, Hogue RE: Basic rehabilitation principles of persons with leg length discrepancy: an overview. In Hungerford DS (ed): *Leg length Discrepancy. The Injured Knee* (Progress in Orthopaedic Surgery, Vol. 1). New York, Springer-Verlag, 1977, pp 3-8.

85. Lawrence D: Chiropractic concepts of the short leg: a critical review. *J Manipulative Physiol Ther* 8:157-161, 1985.

86. Friberg O, Nurminen M, Korhonen K, Soininen E, Manttari T: Accuracy and precision of clinical estimation of leg length inequality and lumbar scoliosis: comparison of clinical and radiologic measurements. *International Disability Studies* 10:49-53, 1988.

87. McKenzie RA: *The Lumbar Spine. Mechanical Diagnosis Therapy.* Waikanae, New Zealand, Spinal Publishers, 1981, p 36.

88. Lewit K: Rontgenologische kriterien statischer storungen der wirbelsaule. *Manuelle Medizine* 20:26-35, 1982.

89. Cleveland RH, Kushner DC, Ogden MC, Herman TE, Kermond W, Correia JA: Determination of leg length discrepancy. A comparison of weight-bearing and supine imaging. *Investigative Radiology* 23:301-304, 1988.

CHAPTER 11

Lumbosacral Spine Posture

This chapter discusses some of the normal and abnormal biomechanical forces associated with the erect posture.

Normal Lumbosacral Biomechanical Forces

Because of humans' erect posture, the lumbosacral joint supports most of the incumbent weight of the trunk and upper extremities, and this joint is considered to be the most stressed spinal joint (1, 2). Also, the lumbosacral junction is in an area where high stresses occur (3) between the mobile presacral vertebrae and the relatively stable pelvic girdle (4, 5). According to Kenesi and Lesur (6), the shearing force is much greater at L5–S1 than at L4–5. As previously shown, the biomechanical stresses of the lumbosacral junction in a person with a normal sacral base angle of approximately 41° and equal leg lengths are summarized in Figure 11.1.

Some authors have emphasized that the weight-bearing stresses at the lumbosacral joint are associated with humans' erect posture and that this predisposes them to low back pain (11–13). It has been suggested by Cailliet (14) that an abnormal sacral base angle is responsible for low back pain, and Robinson and Grimm (15) believe that low back pain can be due to a variation in the degree of angulation at the base of the spine. According to von Lackum (16), backache may be caused by an increased sacral base angle and consequently increased joint strain. Changes in lumbar spine posture may influence the load borne by the zygapophyseal joints which have been estimated to bear 16–40% of the total compressive spine load in the erect posture (17–19). According to McRae (20) the lumbosacral zygapophyseal joints bear more weight than do zygapophyseal joints at higher levels. Because the human erect posture involves a permanent lordosis, the lower lumbar joints are always subject to a shearing force (21).

Lumbar Spine Postural and Structural Changes Associated with Leg Length Inequality

Literature Review

In the literature, there is very little reference to postural and structural changes of the lumbar spine associated with leg length inequality. Although Ingelmark (22) compared corresponding left and right zygapophyseal joints in a large series of spines from skeletons and autopsy material, he did not consider the question of any related leg length inequality.

It is generally accepted that leg length inequality is the most common cause of pelvic obliquity in the erect posture and that the usual response to pelvic obliquity is a postural scoliosis of the spine with the curve being convex toward the short leg side (23–28). It has been suggested that a short leg increases the compressive load across the zygapophyseal joints on the concave side of the postural scoliosis with signs of zygapophyseal osteoarthritis (29, 30).

Using discography, some authors have noted wedging of the intervertebral discs in scoliotics, with the nucleus pulposus asymmetrically placed closer to the convex side of the scoliosis (31).

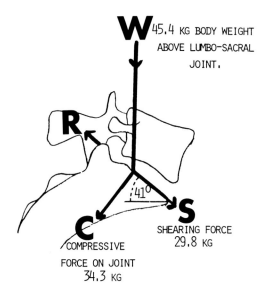

W 45.4 KG BODY WEIGHT
ABOVE LUMBO-SACRAL
JOINT.

R

41°

C   S
SHEARING FORCE
29.8 KG

COMPRESSIVE
FORCE ON JOINT
34.3 KG

Figure 11.1.   Biomechanical forces at the lumbosacral junction. W = 45.4 kg body weight above the lumbosacral joint; S = 29.8 kg shearing force; C = 34.3 kg compressive force on the joint; R = counter reactive force to the shearing force S. (Modified from Davis PR: Human lower lumbar vertebrae: some mechanical and osteological considerations. *J Anat* 95:337-334, 1961; Kapandji IA: *The Physiology of the Joints* (Vol. 3, *The Trunk and the Vertebral Column*). Edinburgh, Churchill Livingstone, 1974, p 78; Lafferty JF, Winter WG, Gambaro SA: Fatigue characteristics of posterior elements of vertebrae. *J Bone Joint Surg* 59A:154-158, 1977; LeVeau B: Williams and Lissner: *Biomechanics of Human Motion,* ed 2. Philadelphia, W.B. Saunders, 1977.)

Voluminous literature exists regarding idiopathic scoliosis and its gross structural changes (23, 27, 32) and Enneking and Harrington (33) undertook a comprehensive study to compare left and right zygapophyseal joints in idiopathic scoliosis. However, this type of scoliosis will not be discussed in this text. Wiles and Sweetman (34), James (27), Apley (35), Apley and Solomon (36), and De Smet (37) state that postural curves never become fixed and that there are no changes in the shape of the lumbar vertebrae.

Radiographic Assessment and Results of Postural Changes in the Lumbosacral Zygapophyseal Joints

I examined asymmetrical postural differences in the right and left lumbosacral zygapophyseal "joint angles" in 100 patients having a mean leg length difference of 13.0 mm and in 100 patients having no leg length difference (0-3 mm), who did not exhibit tropism of the lumbosacral zygapophyseal joints on the A-P radiographic view.

Oblique radiographs were taken in the erect posture with each patient standing on the horizontal steel plate in front of the x-ray bucky (Fig. 10.7). The patient was placed in the 45° posterior oblique radiographic position with relation to the bucky, this angle being achieved by means of a 45° firm foam rubber spacer placed behind the low back. This position was maintained by means of the compression band being applied across the patient's abdomen so as not to change the 45° angle. The horizontal x-ray beam was directed at the right lumbosacral joint, 2.5 cm medial to the anterior superior iliac spine, and a 100-cm film focus distance was used. The same procedure was used for the contralateral projection with the height of the x-ray tube remaining unchanged.

The right and left oblique radiographs obtained showed the vertical plumb-line shadow. This line was used as a reference point and a horizontal pencil line was drawn at right angles to it on each radiograph (Fig. 11.2). A line was drawn through the plane of each lumbosacral zygapophyseal joint to bisect the horizontal line and the zygapophyseal "joint angle" was measured on both sides.

Measurements of the left and right lumbosacral zygapophyseal "joint angles" showed that in 100 patients with a short leg there was always a smaller angle with the horizontal on the short leg side (Fig. 11.2). A comparison of the right and left lumbosacral zygapophyseal "joint angles" in these 100 patients and in 100 controls is given in Table 11.1

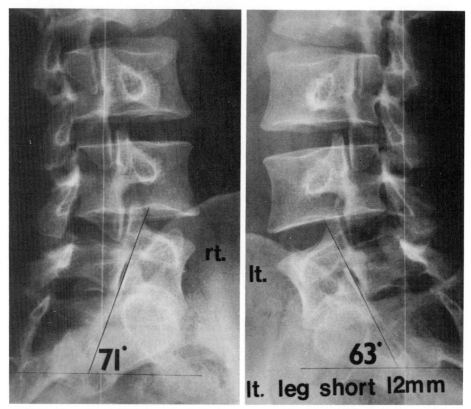

Figure 11.2. Measurement of each right and left lumbosacral zygapophyseal "joint angle" in a 27-year-old male with a left leg length deficiency of 12 mm. These oblique view radiographs are of the patient shown in Figure 10.9. (Reproduced with permission from Giles LGF: Lumbosacral facetal "joint angles" associated with leg length inequality. *Rheumatology and Rehabilitation* 20:233-238, 1981. Copyright Bailliere Tindall, London.)

Table 11.1.
Comparison of the Left and Right Lumbosacral Zygapophyseal "Joint Angles"[a]

Patients	Mean	SD
With a mean leg length difference of 13.0 mm[b]		
Lumbosacral zygapophyseal joint angle—short leg side	65.2°	7.0
Lumbosacral zygapophyseal joint angle—long leg side	73.8°	7.4
Difference between lumbosacral zygapophyseal joint angles on the long leg side and the short leg side	8.7°	4.5
With no leg length difference (0-3 mm)[b]		
Difference between lumbosacral zygapophyseal joint angles on the left and right sides	1.6°	1.5

[a]Modified from Giles LGF: Lumbosacral facetal "joint angles" associated with leg length inequality. *Rheumatology and Rehabilitation* 20:233-238, 1981.
[b]N = 100.

Student's t-test was used to compare the difference between the lumbosacral zygapophyseal "joint angles" in groups A (short leg group) and B (control group), and this difference was found to be very highly significant (p < 0.0005).

Sacral Base and Sacrovertebral Angles

Literature Review

Because of the inaccessibility of the lumbosacral joint, direct assessment of the sacral base angle and of the forces acting on this region is extremely difficult (7). Therefore, measurement of angles at the junction of L5 and S1 have been confined to measurements made in cadavers (39, 40), skeletal vertebral columns (7), erect posture radiographs (40, 41), and recumbent radiographs (42–44). However, with the patient in the recumbent position no information is obtained concerning carriage of the lumbar spine (45).

Values for the sacral base angle have previously been reported to range from 30° (8) to 80° (16). Using normal subjects, aged 17–58 years for erect posture lateral lumbosacral "spot" radiography, Hellems and Keats (41) found an overall mean of 41.1°, with a standard deviation of 7.7°.

Radiographic Assessment and Results

I investigated the sacral base and sacrovertebral angles in the erect posture to determine whether there is a difference in pelvic tilt (forward tilting of the sacrum in the median (sagittal) plane) in chronic low back pain patients having pelvic obliquity due to leg length inequality of 1 cm or more, and those with no pelvic obliquity. An asymptomatic volunteer group with no leg length inequality was used as a control.

The erect posture lateral lumbosacral spine radiographs were used for measurements of the sacral base and sacrovertebral angles in 40 patients complaining of chronic low back pain and having a leg length inequality of 1 cm or more and pelvic obliquity, in 40 patients complaining of chronic low back pain and having no leg length inequality or pelvic obliquity and a control group of 20 asymptomatic volunteers.

Lateral radiographs were taken in the erect posture with patients and controls standing on the horizontal steel plate in front of the vertical x-ray bucky. Each subject was carefully positioned in the center of the bucky and at right angles to it. The central ray of the x-ray tube was centered over the lumbosacral joint. This position was maintained by means of the compression band.

Because there is considerable confusion in the literature regarding the angles at the lumbosacral transition (41, 46), the sacral base and sacrovertebral angles described in this text are defined in Figure 11.3.

The sacral base and sacrovertebral angles were measured from the erect posture lateral view radiographs using the vertical plumb-line shadow as a reference point, as shown in Figure 11.4.

The measurement results of the sacral

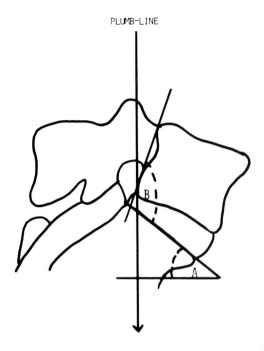

PLUMB-LINE

Figure 11.3.   **A**, Sacral base angle. The angle is made by the plane of inclination of the sacral base to the horizontal. (From Ferguson AB: *Roentgenogram Diagnosis of the Extremities and Spine*. New York, Hoeber, 1939.) **B**, Sacrovertebral angle. The angle is made by drawing a line along the posterior part of the L5 vertebral body to bisect the sacral base line. (From Morris J: *Human Anatomy*, ed 6. Philadelphia, P. Blackiston's Son, 1921, p 276.)

base and sacrovertebral angles are shown in Table 11.2.

It can be seen that there is no statistically significant difference between the sacral base and sacrovertebral angles, respectively, on comparing the results in the two groups of patients suffering from chronic low back pain. Therefore, in patients having chronic low back pain, leg length inequality of 1 cm or more, and pelvic obliquity, it appears that there is no statistically significant difference in the angle of pelvic tilt in the median plane. However, on comparing the chronic low back pain patients with the asymptomatic volunteers, there is a slightly greater degree of pelvic tilt in the asymptomatic group as shown by a marginally greater sacral base angle. Also, in asymptomatic volunteers, there appears to be a slight increase in the sacrovertebral angle con-

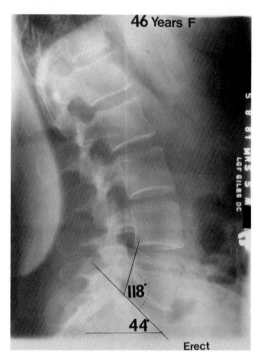

Figure 11.4. The vertical plumb-line shadow on the radiograph was used to measure the sacral base and sacrovertebral angles.

comitant with an increase in the sacral base angle.

The findings in asymptomatic patients give an average sacral base angle of 44.8° (± 6.8) which approximates the findings of 41.4° (± 7.7) found by Hellems and Keats (41).

Splithoff (43) hypothesized that patients with low back pain may automatically assume a "flattening" of the lumbar spine lordosis since this position may be more comfortable; they may also have a degree of muscle spasm causing some flattening of the lumbar spine. The results in this study appear to support this hypothesis in that the low back pain patients have a slightly smaller sacral base and sacrovertebral angle than do the asymptomatic control group.

Radiographic Assessment and Results of Structural Changes in Vertebral Bodies

Radiographs of 100 of the chronic low back pain patients, which included 50 with 1 cm or more of leg length inequality and postural scoliosis and 50 of comparable age groups with straight spines, were examined for any asymmetrical structural changes in the lumbar vertebrae.

Inferior end-plate contours of the vertebral bodies were measured for asymmetry according to a method similar to that used by Dietz and Christensen (49) (Fig. 11.5). A perspex ruler, calibrated in millimeters, was used for making the measurements.

The L5 vertebral body contour was not measured since this is known not always to be clearly shown on the A–P projection (49).

Concavities in the end-plates of lumbar vertebral bodies were asymmetrically situated nearer to the convex side of the scoliotic curvature in patients with a leg length inequality of greater than 9 mm (Fig. 11.6). This asymmetry was most frequently

Table 11.2.
Comparison of the Sacral Base and Sacrovertebral Angles

Patients	Sacral Base Angle		Sacrovertebral Angle	
	Mean	SD	Mean	SD
With chronic low back pain				
40 patients with leg length inequality of 1 cm or more (19–79 years)	39.8	8.1	115.8	5.7
40 patients with no leg length inequality (0–3 mm) (19–68 years)	38.5	7.1	115.0	6.4
With no low back pain history				
20 asymptomatic volunteers with no leg length inequality (0–3 mm) (19–67 years)	44.8	6.8	117.9	5.1

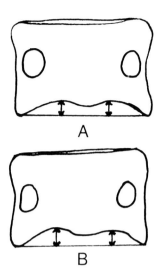

Figure 11.5. Measurement of end-plate contours (using a perspex ruler calibrated in millimeters). **A**, Symmetrical contour. **B**, Asymmetrical contour. (Reproduced with permission from Giles LGF, and Taylor JR: Lumbar spine structural changes associated with leg length inequality. *Spine* 7:159, 162, 1982, Copyright Harper and Row, Philadelphia.)

observed in the apical vertebra and was more evident on the lower surface than the upper surface of the vertebra. (Table 11.3).

Vertebral body height for each fifth lumbar vertebra was measured by means of a perspex ruler, using the end-plate margins at their left and right lateral aspects (Fig. 11.7).

"Wedging" of the fifth lumbar vertebra in the A–P view (Fig. 11.8) was sometimes noted. (Table 11.3).

"Traction" spurs and osteophytes, when present on the vertebral margins, were com-

Figure 11.6. **A**, Radiograph of a 27-year-old male with a left leg length deficiency of 31 mm. Note the asymmetry of the concavities in the end-plates—the concavities are nearer to the convex side of the postural scoliosis; the sagittal plane of part of the right L4–5 zygapophyseal joint, which indicates the presence of tropism, since there is no corresponding joint plane on the left side at this level; the subluxation (imbrication) of the right L4–5 zygapophyseal joint facets; and the bilateral sacralization of the presacral segment. **B**, The same patient standing on a 33-mm left shoe raise. Note that the end-plate concavities exist and are not due to radiographic distortion. The right L4–5 zygapophyseal joint subluxation is still present. (Reproduced with permission from Giles LGF, Taylor JR: Lumbar spine structural changes associated with leg length inequality. *Spine* 7:159-162, 1982. Copyright Harper and Row, Philadelphia.)

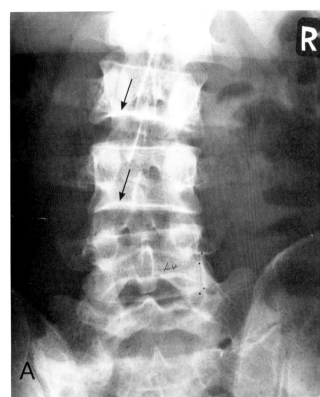

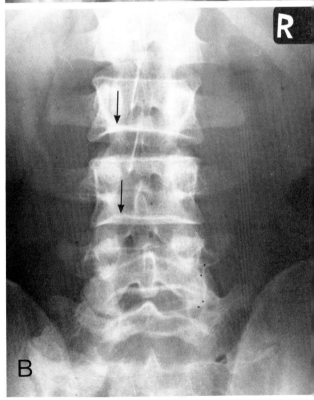

Table 11.3.
Structural Changes in Lumbar Vertebral Bodies [a]

Patients	Asymmetric Concavities in the End-Plates	Asymmetric Wedging of L5 Vertebral Body	Bilateral "Traction" Spurs and Osteophytes (40 years and older)
With a leg length difference of 1 cm or more and a postural scoliosis[b,c]	28%	10%	83%
With no leg length difference (0–3 mm) and straight spine[b,d]	2%	0	25%

[a]From Giles LGF, Taylor JR: Lumbar spine structural changes associated with leg length inequality. *Spine* 7:159-162, 1982. Copyright Harper and Row, Philadelphia.
[b]$N = 50$.
[c]18 were 40 years and older.
[d]13 were 40 years and older.

Figure 11.7. Measurement of vertebral body height. (Reproduced with permission from Giles LGF, Taylor JR: Lumbar spine structural changes associated with leg length inequality. *Spine.* 7:159-162, 1982. Copyright Harper and Row, Philadelphia.)

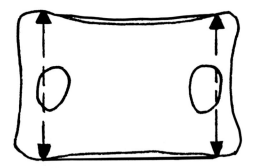

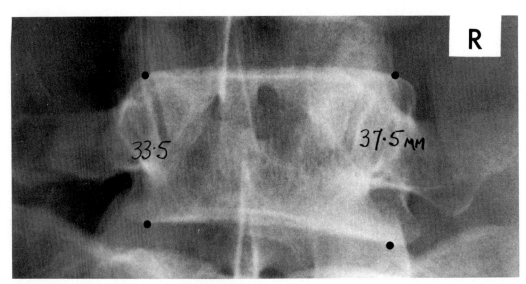

Figure 11.8. An example of an L5 wedged vertebral body in a 37-year-old male, with a right leg length deficiency of 26 mm. There is very little rotation of the L5 vertebral body as judged by the fact that the pedicles are almost clearly seen bilaterally, using the method of Nash and Moe (1969) (51) for determining vertebral rotation. (Reproduced with permission from Giles LGF, Taylor JR: Lumbar spine structural changes associated with leg length inequality. *Spine* 7:159-162, 1982. Copyright Harper and Row, Philadelphia.)

pared visually in the short leg and control groups. (Table 11.3). Lateral osteophytes were common, more frequent, and larger on the vertebral margins at the convex side of the curve in patients over 40 years (Fig. 11.9).

Late degenerative changes were seen in the apical vertebra and intervertebral disc which appeared to be "squeezed" between approximated vertebral bodies on the concavity of the scoliosis (Fig. 11.9).

The data in Table 11.3 show that the 50 adult patients who did not exhibit any postural lumbar scoliosis showed no discernible pattern of asymmetrical changes.

Response of Postural Scoliosis to Shoe-Raise Therapy in Three Age Groups

Comparison of Figures 11.10 and 11.11 illustrates the reduction in scoliosis with use

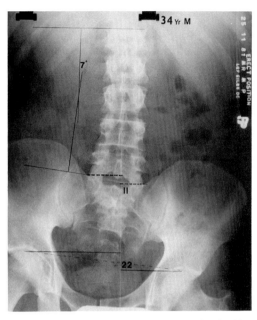

Figure 11.10. Radiograph of a 34-year-old male with a right leg length deficiency of 22 mm and a postural scoliosis of 7°.

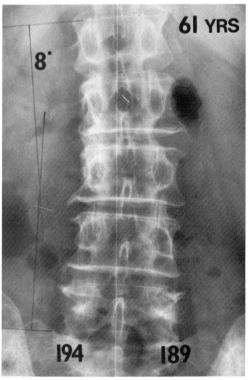

Figure 11.9. Radiograph of a 61-year-old female with a right leg length deficiency of 10 mm and a postural scoliosis of 8°. Chronic intermittent low back pain with no history of trauma. (Reproduced with permission from Giles LGF, Taylor JR: Lumbar spine structural changes associated with leg length inequality. *Spine* 7:159-162 1982. Copyright Harper and Row, Philadelphia.)

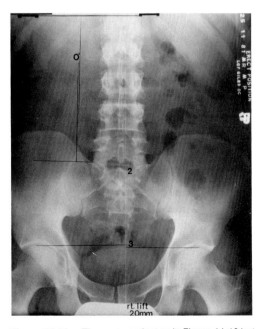

Figure 11.11. The same patient as in Figure 11.10 but standing on a right shoe raise of 20 mm.

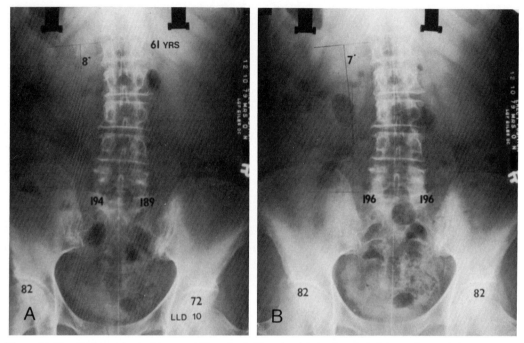

Figure 11.12.   Radiograph of a 61-year-old female. **A**, Note the right leg length deficiency (LLD) of 10 mm and the postural scoliosis of 8°. **B**, The patient is standing on a right shoe raise of 10 mm. Note that the postural scoliosis has become fixed.

of a shoe raise in a supple lumbar spine.

This reduction is less in older people (Fig. 11.12).

In the small group of 12 patients (21–59 years) who were x-rayed with and without a shoe raise at the initial visit, it appears that the immediate response to shoe raise, up to the age of 53 years, is the same as at 12 months. Over this age, there is a slower improvement in response, and the scoliosis is never entirely eliminated, as can be seen from Figure 11.13.

Postural and Structural Changes in the Lumbar Spine

In an electromyographic study, Taillard (53) found anomalies of pelvic and spinal posture, as well as abnormalities in the dynamics of postural muscles when there was a leg length difference of 1 cm or more. According to Kay (54), balance is maintained by a constant equilibrium of forces and any disturbance of these forces will create an imbalance of forces in the spinal column.

In the curving spine, the articulating surfaces of the zygapophyseal joints are probably no longer congruous, and consequently, increased friction may occur at some point of the gliding movement (55). According to Huskisson and Hart (56), abnormally shaped or positioned zygapophyseal joint surfaces appear to be a cause of osteoarthritis. van der Korst (57) also believes that osteoarthritis is primarily a disturbance of the anatomical integrity of the joint cartilage with fractures of the collagen network. Increased stress or low-level repetitive trauma may initiate a self-perpetuating cycle of events in articular cartilage, which eventually leads to progressive osteoarthritic changes (58, 59) that are initially asymptomatic (60).

The measured differences in the lumbosacral zygapophyseal "joint angles" on the two sides of the spinal curvature suggest the likelihood of asymmetrical stress involving the left and right lumbosacral zygapophyseal joints. However, the probable effects are difficult to assess in terms of mechanical shearing "stress," but there is evidence to support the view that leg length

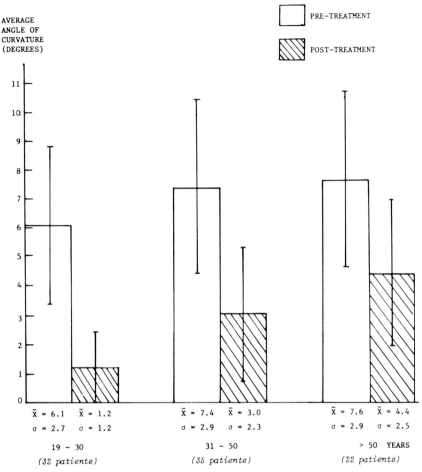

Figure 11.13.   Age-related response of postural scoliosis to treatment by shoe raise. (Modified from Giles LGF, Taylor JR: Low-back pain associated with leg length inequality. *Spine* 6:510-521, 1981. Copyright Harper and Row, Philadelphia.)

inequality is associated with asymmetrical bilateral stresses. Unfortunately, plane oblique radiographs of zygapophyseal joints are not reliable for comparison of arthritic changes on the right and left (61). However, comparison of the left and right lumbosacral zygapophyseal "joint angles" (Table 11.1) in 100 patients with a mean leg length difference of 13.0 mm and 100 patients with no leg length difference (0–3 mm) was very highly significant.

There is no detailed information on the effect of pelvic obliquity on the spine (40). Therefore, I undertook autopsy studies to compare the right and left zygapophyseal joints at the lumbosacral and apical zyg-

apophyseal joints with respect to degenerative changes in cases of postural scoliosis and controls (see Chapter 13).

The asymmetrical angulation of the lower lumbar zygapophyseal joints can be corrected in a supple postural lumbar scoliosis by the use of a shoe raise, thereby presumably equalizing the stresses on the left and right lumbosacral zygapophyseal joints.

It has been shown that a postural scoliosis does in fact become structural with the passage of time (Fig. 11.3); therefore, clinicians should be cognizant of the likely postural and structural changes involving the lumbar spine and their possible relationship with chronic low back pain.

Asymmetrical concavities in the inferior end-plates of some lumbar vertebrae have been noted (62). It has been shown (63) that the nucleus pulposus normally changes its position within the intervertebral disc during infancy in response to assumption of the erect posture and that its position influences the position and shape of the concavity which develops on the vertebral end-plate between 3 and 7 years. It has also been shown that in scoliosis the nucleus pulposus moves toward the convex side of the curve (31). The present study demonstrates that structural asymmetry of the vertebral end-plates may be common in compensatory scoliosis. This skeletal asymmetry is presumably associated with a fixed eccentric position of the nucleus pulposus during growth. When the nucleus is pushed toward the convex side of the scoliosis, the result may be that it affects Junghanns's motion segment (46). It is suggested by the early appearance of "traction" osteophytes that asymmetrical degeneration of the intervertebral discs occurs when they are stretched at the convexity of the scoliosis (62, 64). Where they are squeezed on the concavity of the scoliosis, a later degenerative change is seen (28, 65). The greater frequency of vertebral traction osteophytes on the convex side of the curve, as indicated in the present study, suggests that they are produced in response to tension in the anulus since such outgrowths are known to occur at the point of insertion of ligament into bone (66). Intervertebral joint traction "spurs" are probably the most useful indication of lumbar instability (67). Their earlier appearance on the convex side of the curve suggests greater tension here than on the concave side.

Farfan (40) has stated that if the anulus becomes sufficiently stretched and torn, a significant degree of distortion may be produced in the form of radial tears characteristic for the shape of the disc. Furthermore, forced torsion of the disc may cause it to bulge in one location, while it becomes depressed in another. Farfan et al (68) and Koreska (69) showed that torsional stresses of a magnitude encountered in daily activity may play a major role in initiating degeneration of lumbar intervertebral discs.

References

1. Willis TA: Anatomical variations and roentgenographic appearance of the low back in relation to sciatic pain. *J Bone Joint Surg* 23:410-416, 1941.
2. Ehni G: Historical writings on spondylotic caudal radiculopathy and its effects on the nervous system. In Weinstein PR, Ehni G, Wilson Scoliosis (CB (eds): *Lumbar Spondylosis: Diagnosis Management and Surgical Treatment*. Chicago, Year Book Medical Publishers, 1977, pp 1-12.
3. Levine DB: The painful low back. In McCarthy DJ (ed): *Arthritis and Allied Conditions*, ed 9. Philadelphia, Lea and Febiger, 1979, pp 1044-1079.
4. Cyron BM, Hutton WC: The fatigue strength of the lumbar neural arch in spondylolysis. *J Bone Joint Surg* 60B:234-238, 1978.
5. Carmichael SW, Burkart SL: Clinical anatomy of the lumbo-sacral complex. *Phys Ther* 59:965-968, 1979.
6. Kenesi C, Lesur E: Orientation of the articular processes at L4, L5, and S1. Possible role in pathology of the intervertebral disc. *Anat Clin* 7:43-47, 1985.
7. Davis PR: Human lower lumbar vertebrae: some mechanical and osteological considerations. *J Anat* 95:337-344, 1961.
8. Kapandji IA: The Physiology of the Joints (Vol. 3 in *The Trunk and the Vertebral Column*). Edinburgh, Churchill Livingstone, 1974, p 78.
9. Lafferty JF, Winter WG, Gambaro SA: Fatigue characteristics of posterior elements of vertebrae. *J Bone Joint Surg* 59A:154-158, 1977.
10. LeVeau B: *Williams and Lissner: Biomechanics of Human Motion*, ed 2. Philadelphia, W.B. Saunders, 1977.
11. Friberg S: Anatomical studies on lumbar disc degeneration. *Acta Orthop Scand* 17:224-230, 1948.
12. Rasch PJ, Burke RK: *Kinesiology and Applied Anatomy*. ed 3. Philadelphia, Lea and Febiger, 1967.
13. Gross D: Multifactorial diagnosis and therapy for low back pain. In Bonica JJ, Liebeskind JC, Albe-Feffard DG (eds): *Advances in Pain Research Therapy*. New York, Raven Press, 1979, vol 3, pp 671-683.
14. Cailliet R: Rehabilitation management of the patient with low back pain. In Buerger AA, Tobis JS (eds): *Approaches to the Validation of Manipulation Therapy*. Springfield, IL, Charles C Thomas, 1977, pp 84-100.
15. Robinson WH, Grimm HW: Sacro-vertebral angle, its measurement and the clinical significance. *Arch Surg* 11:911, 1925.
16. von Lackum HL: The lumbosacral region. An anatomic study and some clinical observations. *JAMA* 82:1109, 1924.
17. Hakim NS, King AI: Static and dynamic articular facet loads. In *Proceedings, 20th Stapp Car Crash Conference*, 1976, p 609-637.
18. Hutton WC, Adams MA: The forces acting on the neural arch and their relevance to low back pain. In: *Engineering Aspects of the Spine*. London, Mechanical Engineering Publications, 1980, pp 49-55.
19. Farfan HF: Biomechanics of the lumbar spine. In Kirkaldy-Willis (ed): *Managing Low Back Pain*. New York, Churchill Livingstone, 1983, pp 9-21.
20. McRae DL: Radiology of the lumbar spinal canal. In Weinstein PR, Ehni G, Wilson CB (eds): *Lumbar Spondylosis: Diagnosis, Management and Surgical Treatment*. Chicago, Year Book Medical Publishers, 1977, pp 92-114.
21. Farfan HF: The biomechanical advantage of lordosis and hip extension for upright man as compared with other anthropoids. *Spine* 3:336-345, 1978.
22. Ingelmark BE: Function of and pathological changes in the spinal joints. *Acta Anat* 38:12-60, 1959.

23. Keim HA: Scoliosis. *Ciba Clinical Symposia* 24:2-32, 1972.
24. Bradford DS, Moe JH, Winter RB: Scoliosis. In Rothman RH, Simeone FA (eds): *The Spine.* Philadelphia, W.B. Saunders, 1975, vol 1, p 276, 279.
25. Cailliet R: *Scoliosis Diagnosis and Management.* Philadelphia, F.A. Davis, 1975, p 44.
26. Riseborough EJ, Herndon JH: *Scoliosis and Other Deformities of the Axial Skeleton.* Boston, Little, Brown, 1975, p 263.
27. James JIP: *Scoliosis,* ed 2. Edinburgh, Churchill Livingstone, 1976, p 33.
28. Morscher E: Etiology and pathophysiology of leg length discrepancies. In Hungerford DS (ed): *Leg Length Discrepancy. The Injured Knee.* (Progress in Orthopaedic Surgery, Vol. 1). New York, Springer-Verlag, 1977, pp 9-20.
29. Kendall H, Kendall F, Boynton D: *Posture and Pain.* New York, Kreiser, 1977.
30. Turek SL: *Orthopedics—Principles and Their Application.* ed 3. Philadelphia, J.B. Lippincott, 1977, p 1384.
31. O'Brien JP, Dwyer AP, Hodgson AR: Discography in paralytic scoliosis. *Acta Orthop Scand* 46:216-220, 1975.
32. Roaf F: *Scoliosis.* London, E.&S. Livingstone, 1966.
33. Enneking WF, Harrington P: Pathological changes in scoliosis. *J Bone Joint Surg* 51(A):165-184, 1969.
34. Wiles P, Sweetman R: *Essentials of Orthopaedics,* London, J. and A. Churchill, 1965, pp 16-17.
35. Apley A: *System of Orthopaedics and Fractures,* ed 5. London, Butterworth Scientific, 1977.
36. Apley A, Solomon L: *Apley's System of Orthopaedics and Fractures.* ed 6. London, Butterworth Scientific, 1982, pp 216-247.
37. DeSmet AA: *Radiology of Spinal Curvature.* St. Louis, C.V. Mosby, 1985, p 228.
38. Giles LGF: Lumbosacral facetal "joint angles" associated with leg length inequality. *Rheumatology and Rehabilitation.* 20:233-238, 1981.
39. Mitchell GAG: The lumbosacral junction. *J Bone Joint Surg* 26:233-254. 1934.
40. Farfan HF: *Mechanical Disorders of the Low Back.* Philadelphia, Lea and Febiger, 1973, pp 21, 31, 145.
41. Hellems HK, Keats TE: Measurement of the normal lumbosacral angle. *Radiology* 113:642-645, 1971.
42. Ferguson AB: The clinical and roentgenographic interpretation of lumbo-sacral anomalies. *Radiology* 22:548-558, 1934.
43. Splithoff CA: Lumbosacral junction. Roentgenographic comparison of patients with and without backaches. *JAMA* 152:1610-1613, 1952.
44. Chaffin DB, Moulis EF: An empirical investigation of low back strains and vertebrae geometry. *J Biomech* 2:89-96, 1969.
45. Hasner E, Schalimtzek M, Snorrason E: Roentgenological examination of the function of the lumbar spine. *Acta Radiol* 37:141-149, 1952.
46. Schmorl G, Junghanns H: *The Human Spine in Health and Disease,* ed 2. New York, Grune and Stratton, 1971, p 420.
47. Ferguson AB: *Roentgenogram Diagnosis of the Extremities and Spine.* New York, Hoeber, 1939.
48. Morris J: *Human Anatomy.* ed 6. Philadelphia, P. Blakiston's Son, 1921, p 276.
49. Dietz GW, Christensen EE: Normal "cupid's bow" contour of the lower lumbar vertebrae. *Radiology* 121:577-579, 1976.
50. Giles LGF, Taylor JR: Intra-articular synovial protrusions in the lower lumbar apophyseal joints. *Bull Hosp Jt Dis Orthop Inst* 42:248-255, 1982.
51. Nash CL, Moe JH: A study of vertebral rotation. *J Bone Joint Surg* 51A:223-229, 1969.
52. Giles LGF, Taylor JR: Low-back pain associated with leg length inequality. *Spine* 6:510-521, 1981.
53. Taillard W: Colonne lambaire et inegalite des membres inferieures. *Acta Orthop Belg* 35:601-613, 1969.
54. Kay SP: A new conception and approach to the problem of scoliosis. *Clin Orthop* 81:21, 1971.
55. Cailliet R: *Low Back Pain Syndrome.* ed 2. Philadelphia, F.A. Davis, 1968, pp 30, 52.
56. Huskisson EC, Hart FD: *Joint Disease: All the Arthropathies.* ed 3. Bristol, John Wright and Sons, 1978.
57. van der Korst JK: Osteoarthrosis— the doctor's dilemma. *Rheumatology and Rehabilitation* 18:1-9, 1979.
58. Radin EL, Simon SR, Rose RM, Paul IL: *Practical Biomechanics for the Orthopedic Surgeon.* New York, John Wiley & Sons, 1979.
59. Weiss C: Normal and osteoarthritic articular cartilage. *Orthop Clin North Am* 10:175-189, 1979.
60. Muir H: Cartilage structure and metabolism and basic changes in degenerative joint disease. *Aust NZ J Med* (Supp 1) 8:1-5, 1978.
61. Reichman S: Radiography of the lumbar intervertebral joints. *Acta Radiol* 14:161-171, 1973.
62. Taylor JR, Giles LGF: Lower limb length inequality and compensatory scoliosis. *J Anat* 126:634-635, 1978.
63. Taylor JR: Growth of human intervertebral discs and vertebral bodies. *J Anat* 120:49-68, 1975.
64. Farkas A: Physiologic scoliosis. *J Bone Joint Surg* 23:607-627, 1940.
65. Fahrni WH: *Backache Relieved.* Springfield, IL, Charles C. Thomas, 1966, p 19.
66. Allbrook D: Movements of the lumbar spinal column. *J Bone Joint Surg* 39B:339-345, 1957.
67. Macnab I: The traction spur. *J Bone Joint Surg* 53(A):663-670, 1971.
68. Farfan HF, Sossette J, Robertson G, Wells R: The effects of torsion in the production of disc degeneration. *J Bone Joint Surg* 52(A):468-497, 1970.
69. Koreska J: Biomechanics of the lumbar spine and its clinical significance. *Orthop Clin North Am* 8:121-133, 1977.

CHAPTER 12

Clinical Assessment of Low Back Pain and the Result of Treatment

Clinical assessment of low back pain, pre- and posttreatment, incorporating the use of a subjective questionnaire and measurements of pain-related ranges of movement is now described.

Subjective Questionnaire

Alteration of pain was judged by the use of a simple subjective questionnaire which was filled in by each patient at the initial visit, but prior to consulting the author (Fig. 12.1). Following treatment (see Treatment Methods section), patients were requested to complete a second questionnaire at 12 and 24 months posttreatment (Fig. 12.2).

The pre- and posttreatment questionnaires indicated the character of the pain. A method of "scoring" the responses to the character of pain recorded on the questionnaires was used (Fig. 12.3).

Measurement of Ranges of Movement

Functional improvement for 50 randomly chosen patients between the initial and final visits was judged by (*a*) the degree of *passive straight leg raising* measured by a Leighton Flexometer (1) (Fig. 12.4), a highly reliable and valid measurement (2); (*b*) the extent of *spine and hip flexion*, using a perspex calibrated device to measure the distance from the middle fingers to the floor (on forward bending with straight knees) (Fig. 12.5); and (*c*) the range of *lumbar spine lateral bending* from the normal erect posture as measured by a Leighton Flexometer (1). At the time of the posttreatment measurements of spine and hip flexion, an appropriate perspex block was placed under the short leg, equal to the leg length inequality. It should be noted that the ranges of movement may be restricted by pain.

Treatment Methods

Shoe raise with or without lumbosacral manipulation was applied. Lumbosacral manipulation was performed specifically with patients lying on their side with the short leg side uppermost and both knees partly bent.

Lumbosacral manipulation is a common method of treatment in all chronic low back pain patients when no neurologic or radiologic evidence of spinal pathology, other than osteoarthritis, is present.

This study compared the responses of 88 chronic low back pain patients who had greater than 9 mm leg length inequality with two treatment methods:

1. Patients received lumbosacral manipulation and a shoe raise appropriate to the leg length inequality;
2. Patients were given shoe-raise therapy only, but if the low back pain was to persist for 1 month, such patients were to be manipulated. It is acknowledged that, to some extent, this prejudges the issue under examination. However, clinicians have a moral and ethical duty to do whatever they can to assist their patients. The period of 1 month was chosen since patients receiving lumbosacral manipulation and a shoe raise were usually asymptomatic within 7 to 10 days.

The two groups were randomly selected but the numbers are unequal since initially all patients were manipulated.

A) PLEASE TICK THE CLOSEST CORRECT ANSWER:

  (1) I have **NO** low back pain   ....

  (2) The low back pain is:

            Slight   ....
            Moderate   ....
            Severe   ....
            Unbearable   ....

B) FEMALE PATIENTS ONLY

  For x-ray purposes – Are you pregnant?   YES/NO

              On what date did your last menstrual

              period begin? ....

                        SIGNED: ....
                        DATE: ....

Figure 12.1.   Initial low back pain research questionnaire.

Dear,

It would greatly assist my research programme into the effectiveness of
treatment for <u>LOW BACK</u> pain, if you would please fill in this follow-up
confidential questionnaire and return it to me in the enclosed stamped
envelope.

1) Since treatment, has your <u>LOW BACK</u> pain been –

              UNBEARABLE   ....

              SEVERE   ....

              SLIGHT   ....

              OR, HAS IT
              DISAPPEARED
              COMPLETELY   ....

	<u>DURING 12 MONTHS BEFORE TREATMENT</u>	<u>DURING 12 MONTHS AFTER TREATMENT</u>
2) Can you state –		
(A) The number of attacks of low back pain.	....	....
(B) The number of days of work lost due to low back pain (if applicable).	....	....

Yours sincerely,

<u>L.G.F. Giles.</u>

Figure 12.2.   Follow-up (12 month/24 month) low back pain research questionnaire.

Character of Pain	Score
None	0
Slight	1
Moderate	2
Severe	3
Unbearable	4

Figure 12.3. Method of "scoring" responses to the character of pain. (From Giles LGF, Taylor JR: Low-back pain associated with leg length inequality. Spine 6:510-521, 1981. Copyright Harper and Row, Philadelphia.)

Clinical Results

Clinical Tests Measuring Pain-Related Limitations of Movement

On straight leg raising, pain was felt by 18 out of 50 patients, and the average angle of straight leg raising before pain prevented further movement (on the side of most pain) was 56°. No patients experienced pain on straight leg raising after treatment. The average ranges of spine and hip flexion and left

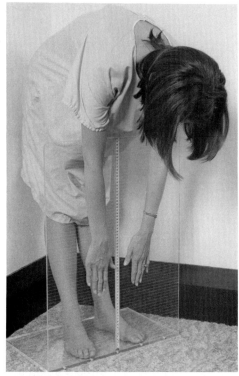

Figure 12.5. Apparatus for measuring spine and hip flexion. (Reproduced with permission from Giles LGF, Taylor JR: Low-back pain associated with leg length inequality. Spine 6:510-521, 1981. Copyright Harper and Row, Philadelphia.)

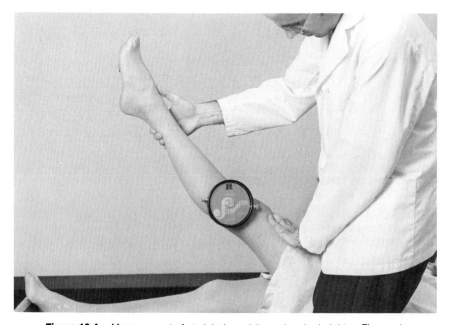

Figure 12.4. Measurement of straight leg raising using the Leighton Flexometer.

Table 12.1.
Ranges of Movement[a]

Patients	Average Spine and Hip Flexion (Middle Fingers to Floor Distance)	Lateral Flexion of Lumbar Spine (Using Leighton Flexometer)	
		Average Total Range in Degrees	Average Difference between Left and Right Lateral Flexion in Degrees
19–30 Years (N = 16)	cm		
Pretreatment	14	42	6.5
Posttreatment[b]	6	48	3.1
31–50 Years (N = 18)			
Pretreatment	7	42	5.3
Posttreatment[b]	6	45	1.6
>50 Years (N = 16)			
Pretreatment	16	36	5.9
Posttreatment[b]	14	38	3.9

[a]Used with permission from Giles LGF, Taylor JR: Low-back pain associated with leg length inequality. *Spine* 6:510–521, 1981. Copyright Harper and Row, Philadelphia.
[b]With appropriate perspex raise.

and right lateral bending, which gave an approximate estimate of pain-related limitation of movement, are shown in Table 12.1. Differences between left and right lateral bending of the lumbar spine are also shown.

"Scored" Results of the Subjective Questionnaire

The data (Fig. 12.6) indicate that patients thought the treatment was beneficial. However, since there was no untreated group, one cannot attach great significance to the results. The available data show no difference between the two groups.

For ethical reasons, there was no untreated control group. However 94% of the patients had recently received treatments (usually multiple) from other health professionals (Fig. 12.7), which must be presumed to have failed to achieve long-lasting relief.

When patients filled in the questionnaires 12 and 24 months posttreatment they generally stated that there was a very significant decrease in the frequency and number of attacks of low back pain. Also, less working days were lost as a result of low back pain. The number is small, but the questionnaire results which are given in Table 12.2 for a 2-year follow-up period show these

results expressed according to adjectives used by the patients.

Of the 88 patients who received the 24-month final questionnaire, only 52 could recollect details enabling them to answer Part 1 of the questionnaire.

Difficulties Experienced in this Clinical Trial

In a clinical trial it is not possible to have as carefully controlled conditions as in an animal experiment. Some of the following difficulties were experienced.

A large number of patients were unwilling to take part in the x-ray reassessment program because they were concerned about the "invasive" nature of radiography, particularly since they felt better. This resulted in the small number of patients in each follow-up group. No "untreated" control group was used for the reasons previously mentioned, that is, most patients had recently been treated by other practitioners and it was considered unethical not to attempt to alleviate the pain experienced by the patients. Patient groups and the types of treatment administered can be compared. However, no two patients are identical, for example, in their response to pain. It is acknowledged that while one measure of the effectiveness of treatment is the reduction of

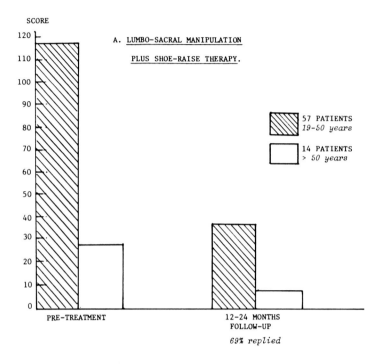

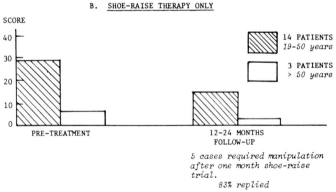

Figure 12.6. "Scored" subjective questionnaire replies from patients with 1 cm or more leg length inequality. The data indicate that patients thought the treatment was beneficial. (Modified from Giles LGF, Taylor JR: Low-back pain associated with leg length inequality. *Spine* 6:510-521, 1981. Copyright Harper and Row, Philadelphia.)

pain, measurements of pain are notoriously difficult and a totally objective measure of pain intensity has yet to be devised. I performed as both the assessor and the therapist; however, (*a*) the clinical assessment was made using calibrated pain-related measuring devices and radiographic measurement; (*b*) two standardized forms of therapy were used, and (*c*) a questionnaire was used to subjectively assess the response of patients.

These difficulties were responsible for the multiplicity of the approach used in this clinical trial in an attempt to seek evidence of a correlation between leg length inequality and low back pain.

Low Back Pain Associated with Leg Length Inequality

Over the past 50 years there has been a great deal of controversy as to whether leg length inequality results in low back pain (5–8) and

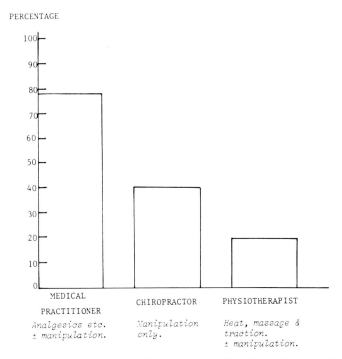

Figure 12.7.   Other health practitioners consulted recently by 50 patients with chronic low back pain.

Table 12.2.
Number of Attacks of Low Back Pain and Working Days Lost[a]

Number of Attacks	During 12 Months Before Treatment	During 12 Months After Treatment
Constant	20	1
Several/often/frequent/quite a few	20	3
5-6 attacks	3	2
3-4 attacks	4	5
1-2 attacks	5	11
No attacks	—	13
Marked decrease or improvement	—	17
Number of Working Days Lost		
29-42 days	3	—
21-28 days	2	—
Several/quite a few	2	1
3-4 days	2	1
1-2 days	3	2
No days	40	48

[a]Used with permission from Giles LGF, Taylor JR: Low-back pain associated with leg length inequality. *Spine* 6:510-521, 1981. Copyright Harper and Row, Philadelphia.

whether treatment should be undertaken to eliminate pelvic obliquity in patients presenting with low back pain, either because of the relatively high incidence of leg length inequality in low back pain patients or because of a good response to shoe-raise therapy (4, 9–12). Although the number of patients followed up in this study is small, the study supports the view that patients thought the treatment was beneficial. In the group of 17 patients who were given a shoe raise only, 5 required manipulation to relieve their low back pain after a 1-month trial period, which may indicate that manipulation plus shoes raise results in quicker remission of symptoms.

Although the 12- and 24-month questionnaires showed a recurrence of low back pain in a few patients, some patients who had experienced chronic low back pain for 20 years or more stated that they no longer experienced low back pain, as long as they wore their shoe raise. This finding is supported by Gofton (17) who found that patients with long-standing low back pain had major or total relief over a long period of follow-up, as a result of using an appropriate shoe raise. I found the number of attacks of low back pain and the number of working days lost appeared to be reduced.

The greater prevalence of "short leg" in low back pain patients compared with "normal" controls is presented as evidence of the importance of leg length inequality as an etiological factor in the production of low back pain.

It is suggested that clinical screening for leg length inequality should be conducted at the age of 13–14 years (well before the femoral epiphyses have united and the legs have reached their final length at approximately 19 years of age). In cases suspected of having a leg length inequality of 1–2 cm a shoe raise may be required to level the sacral base. Follow-up examinations should be conducted in case there is a significant change in leg length inequality before growth ceases. In cases where the leg length inequality is greater than 1–2 cm, the opinion of an orthopedic surgeon should be sought to determine whether predictions of growth in the lower extremities (13) suggest that a surgical procedure is necessary to equalize leg lengths (14–17).

In order to investigate the effect of leg length inequality and pelvic obliquity on the zygapophyseal joints of the lumbosacral spine, a histologic survey was undertaken, and the materials and methods used are described in Chapter 13.

References

1. Giles LGF, Taylor JR: Low-back pain associated with leg length inequality. *Spine* 6:510-521, 1981.
2. Leighton JR: The Leighton Flexometer and flexibility test. 20:86-93, 1966.
3. Hoehler FK, Tobis JS: Low back pain and its treatment by spinal manipulation: measures of flexibility and asymmetry. *Rheumatology and Rehabilitation* 21:21-26, 1982.
4. Hoppenfeld S: Back pain. *Pediatr Clin North Am* 24:881-887, 1977.
5. Hazleman B, Bulgen D: Low back pain. *Med 13. Rheumatic Disorders* Part 2:649-654, 1979.
6. Browne PSH: *Basic Facts in Orthopaedics*. Oxford, Blackwell Scientific Publications, 1981, pp 11-13.
7. Klenerman L: The orthopedic viewpoint. *Clin Obstet Gynecol* 8:27-32, 1981.
8. Stoddard A: *Manual of Osteopathic Technique*. London, Hutchinson Medical Publications, 1959, p 212.
9. Cyriax J: *Textbook of Orthopaedic Medicine*. ed 5. London, Bailliere, Tindall and Cassell, 1969, Vol 1, p 442.
10. Sicuranza BJ, Richards J, Tisdall LH: The short leg syndrome in obstetrics and gynecology. *Am J Obstet Gynecol* 107:217-219, 1970.
11. Yates A: The lumbar spine and backpain. In Jayson M (ed): *Treatment of Back Pain*. London, Sector Publishing, 1976, pp 341-353.
12. Anderson M, Green WT, Messner MB: Growth and predictions of growth in the lower extremities. *J Bone Joint Surg* 45A:1-14, 1963.
13. Anderson M, Green WT: Lengths of the femur and the tibia. *Am J Dis Child* 75:279-290, 1948.
14. Anderson WV: Lengthening of the lower limbs: its place in the problem of limb length discrepancy. In Graham WD (ed): *Modern Trends in Orthopaedics*. London, Butterworth, 1967, Vol 5, pp 1-22.
15. Poirier H: Epiphyseal stapling and leg equalization. *J Bone Joint Surg* 50B:61-69, 1968.
16. D'aubignet RM, Dubousset J: Surgical correlation of large length discrepancies in the lower extremities of children and adults. *J Bone Joint Surg* 53A(3):411-430, 1971.
17. Gofton JP: Persistent low back pain and leg length disparity. *J Rheumatol* 12:747-750, 1985.

CHAPTER 13

Histologic Survey of Lumbar Zygapophyseal Joints in Cadavers with Leg Length Inequality and in Controls

Design of Histologic Survey

In a preliminary investigation of any possible zygapophyseal joint degenerative changes which may be associated with leg length inequality, lumbar spines were obtained over a 5-year period from two groups of cadavers—cadavers which had been bequeathed to the department of anatomy and human biology at the University of Western Australia and cadavers from the mortuary of one of the University's teaching hospitals. The cadavers were aged 36–80 years (mean-68 years). The lumbar spines were unselected in that the first 10 cadavers with equal leg lengths and the first 7 with leg length inequality were collected, except when certain other anomalies were present. Because of the time factor involved and the difficulty experienced in obtaining cadaveric material, it was not possible to obtain 10 short leg specimens. Some cadavers were rejected because of evidence of injury, surgery, pathology (other than osteoarthritis), or structural asymmetries such as tropism of the zygapophyseal joints or asymmetries which could have mimicked leg length inequality. These included prosthetic implants (femoral heads), idiopathic scoliosis, structural asymmetry in the pelvis, or fixed deformities of long bones of the legs, e.g., lower limb joints and femoral neck/shaft angles (coxa valga and coxa vara).

From 75 cadavers x-rayed, 7 with a leg length inequality of greater than 9 mm and 10 controls with no leg length inequality (0–3 mm) and virtually no scoliosis (0–2°) were obtained.

Cadavers from the department of anatomy were embalmed, within 12–24 hours of death, by infusion of embalming fluid (glycerine 14 fluid ounces, phenol 30 fluid ounces, and formalin 80 fluid ounces, made up to 4 gallons with a resultant pH of 5). Lumbar spines from the mortuary were obtained within 12–24 hours and were fixed in embalming fluid.

An A–P radiograph of the pelvis and lumbar spine was taken on a 35 × 43 cm film at the film focus distance of 128.5 cm (40 inches) using a stationary grid to minimize "scatter" radiation and thereby clarify film detail. The leg lengths of the cadavers were measured by orthoradiography (see Fig. 10.4).

The cadaver was placed supine on the table so that a calibrated 1-m steel ruler, firmly attached to the center of the x-ray table, was situated between and parallel to the legs. Separate A–P views were taken of hips, knees, and ankle joints in succession, by centering the horizontally mobile x-ray tube over each of these joints in turn. The ruler extended from the upper sacral region to beyond the cadaver's feet, permitting accurate orthoradiographic measurements to be made of "leg lengths," from the femoral head to the tip of the medial malleolus, excluding the ankle–heel distance (Fig. 13.1).

The Cobb (2) method is the most widely used method of measuring scoliotic curvatures and has been shown to be reliable at all degrees of curvature (3). It is accepted as the standard method by the Scoliotic Research Society. A modification of this method was used to measure any angle of curvature of the lumbar spine in both controls and short leg cadavers. A line drawn through the inferior margin of the left and

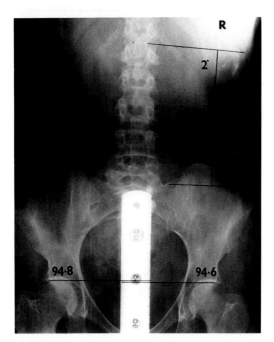

Figure 13.1. Anteroposterior radiograph of the pelvis and lumbar spine of a cadaver. The application of the modified Cobb method for measurement of the curvature of the lumbar spine is indicated. (Reproduced with permission from Giles LGF, Taylor JR: The effect of postural scoliosis on lumbar apophyseal joints. *Scand J Rheumatol* 13:209-220, 1984.)

loss of diagnostic detail of the osseous structures was noted in the pelvic–lumbar spine radiographs (Fig. 13.1). Also, because it was not possible to x-ray the heavy cadavers in the lateral and oblique positions, the complete excised lumbar spines with the first sacral segment were re-x-rayed using the posteroanterior, lateral (Fig. 13.2), and left and right oblique positions (Fig. 13.3), once the muscles had been trimmed off. This permitted exclusion of the pathologic changes in the vertebral structures and the intervertebral discs.

Following this further radiographic evaluation, spines retained for this study were trimmed by means of a band-saw to remove part of the spinous and transverse processes. Blocks including the paired left and right zygapophyseal joints at the apex of the lumbar curve and at the lumbosacral joint were then cut as shown in Figure 13.4

By retaining the posterior one-third of the intervertebral disc and the adjacent bony structures (Fig. 13.5), the zygapophyseal joints were kept rigid to maintain existing alignment of zygapophyseal joint structures.

right superior sacral "notches" was used as the inferior baseline in this study, and a line drawn across the top of the uppermost vertebral body in the curve was used as the superior line (Fig. 13.1).

The data relating to the cadavers used in this study are as follows: In the control group the mean age was 58.3 years, while the average leg length inequality was 1.8 mm and the average scoliosis was 1.5°. In the short leg group the mean age was 70.6 years, while the average leg length inequality was 11.5 mm and the average scoliosis was 5.0°. Vertical and anteroposterior dimensions of the L5 body, as measured on radiographs, showed the linear dimensions in the controls, on average, to be only 2% less than the short leg group.

From these cadavers, the lumbosacral spines were removed by means of a band-saw and stored in embalming fluid.

Because of the distension and high fluid content of the embalmed cadavers, some

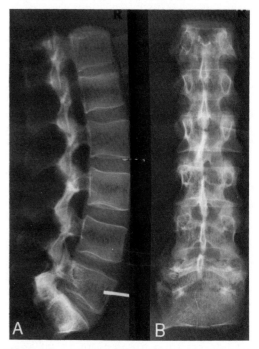

Figure 13.2. Radiographs of excised lumbar spines. A = lateral view; B = posteroanterior view.

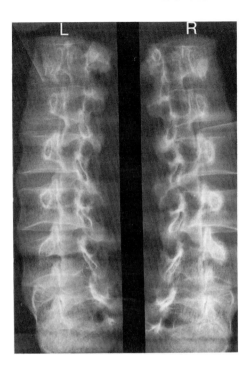

Figure 13.3. Left and right oblique views showing the left (L) and right (R) zygapophyseal joints, respectively.

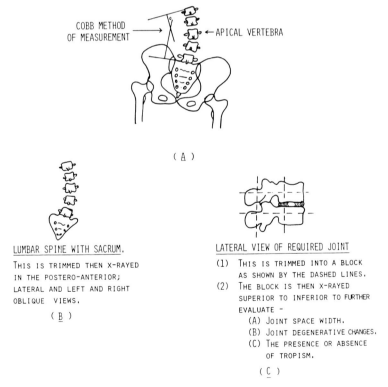

Figure 13.4. **A**, Cobb's method for measuring the angle of curvature of the lumbar spine. **B**, An excised lumbosacral spine. **C**, Trimming of spinal blocks. (Reproduced with permission from Giles LGF, Taylor JR: The effect of postural scoliosis on lumbar apophyseal joints. *Scand J Rheumatol* 13:209-220, 1984.)

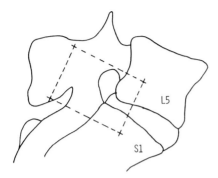

Figure 13.5. The structures within the rectangle represent a lumbosacral block of tissue retained for further radiography and histologic processing. (Reproduced with permission from Giles LGF, Taylor JR: Histological preparation of large vertebral specimens. *Stain Technol* 58(1):45-49, 1983. Copyright Williams & Wilkins, Baltimore.)

In order to ascertain whether paired zygapophyseal joints exhibited tropism, superior-to-inferior radiograph views were used so that the angle of the left and right joints could be measured using the method suggested by Cyron and Hutton (5) (Fig. 13.6).

Spines whose "blocks" exhibited tropism of greater than 4° were not used.

The blocks were processed for histologic evaluation by the method of Giles and Taylor (4) (see Appendix 2), and serial sections were cut at a thickness of 100 μm.

The serial sections were numbered by using interleaved pieces of paper, then stored in 70% ethanol prior to staining.

In a measurement study it is obviously of vital importance to compare corresponding regions of bilaterally symmetrical structures.

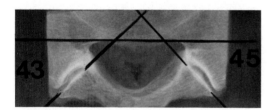

Figure 13.6. Superior-to-inferior radiographic view of a trimmed lumbosacral block showing left and right zygapophyseal joints (see Fig. 9.10). (Reproduced with permission from Giles LGF, Taylor JR: The effect of postural scoliosis on lumbar apophyseal joints. *Scand J Rheumatol* 13:209-220, 1984.)

Since it is not possible to cut all sections in a precisely horizontal plane, particularly in a scoliotic spine, the following method of ensuring comparability was developed. The problem of comparing corresponding histologic microtome sections in left and right joints is overcome by counting from the first histologic section obtained which shows part of the superior region of the zygapophyseal joint to the least histologic section which shows part of the inferior region of the zygapophyseal joint on one side of the lumbar spine. Then the same procedure is used to obtain the numerically corresponding histologic sections for the opposite joint. This makes it possible for the mid-joint section for each joint to be accurately located (Fig. 13.7).

Plane of Sections

It is acknowledged that in postural scoliosis, which becomes fixed after the age of approximately 53 years (6), there are small differences between the left and right sides of the spine in the amount of overlap (facet imbrication/telescoping) between opposing zygapophyseal joint articular facet surfaces (in paired zygapophyseal joints). Therefore, it was proposed to compare corresponding sections from areas of minimal overlap at the center of the "contact areas" of paired joint surfaces. Also, it was noted that peripheral areas of zygapophyseal joint cartilage showed more degenerative changes, so for this particular study, only the center of the mid-joint sections was used in order to compare areas of minimal change. Thus, three 100-μm-thick horizontal sections from the middle of each pair of left and right joints were compared for the 17 specimens (17 blocks at the lumbosacral zygapophyseal joints and 17 blocks at the zygapophyseal joints at the apex of the postural curve).

The main object was to compare left and right sides, which are of necessity sectioned in the same plane in serial sections on an intact vertebral arch. By comparing the corresponding three middle sections of each joint, a legitimate comparison of left and right joints was possible. The sections were processed and mounted for histologic ex-

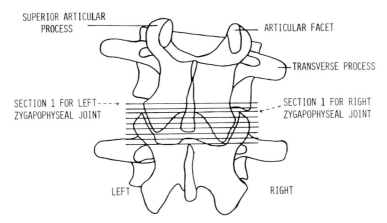

Figure 13.7. Lateral "tilt" of one vertebra upon another, and the method used for numbering corresponding histologic microtome sections in left and right zygapophyseal joints. (Reproduced with permission from Giles LGF, Taylor JR: The effect of postural scoliosis on lumbar apophyseal joints. *Scand J Rheumatol* 13:209-220, 1984.)

amination by the method of Giles and Taylor (4).

The corresponding left and right middle serial sections were carefully traced using an overhead projector, set at a projection magnification of 8. It is emphasized that great care was taken to make comparable measurements on the left and right sides of these tracings. Taking into account the aforementioned possible sources of error, the method of joint analysis is shown in Figure 13.8, which clearly shows the cartilage–subchondral bone plate junction, which was used as a reliable reference for measurement.

From the tracings, the Reichert Kontron

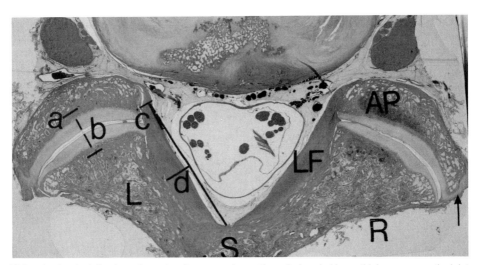

Figure 13.8. Anatomical structures traced and measured were the *subchondral bone thickness* across the joint center (from each bone cartilage junction to the corresponding line "a"); the *joint hyaline articular cartilage thickness* across the center of the joint, and the *cross-sectional area* (b); the *ligamentum flavum thickness* at the anterior cartilage bone junction (c); and the ligamentum flavum thickness (d) mid-way between "c" and the lamina junction (s). In addition, measurements were made of the area of bumper-fibrocartilage (*arrow*) extending beyond the hyaline articular cartilage on the facet surface, but in continuity with it, around the articular process. AP = superior articular process; L = lamina; LF = ligamentum flavum; R = right side of the specimen; S = remains of spinous process/lamina junction. (Ehrlich's hematoxylin stain with light green counterstain) (Modified from Giles LGF, Taylor JR: The effect of postural scoliosis on lumbar apophyseal joints. *Scand J Rheumatol* 13:209-220, 1984.)

Manual Optical Analysis image analyzer system (MOP-3) was used to make accurate linear and area measurements (*a*) at the standardized positions within the zygapophyseal joints on each side so that mid-joint geometry could be established (see Chapter 9, section entitled Lumbosacral Zygapophyseal Joint Tropism and Its Effect on Hyaline Articular Cartilage for discussion of joint cartilage measurements in tropism), and (*b*) of the bumper-fibrocartilage area when this was present. The area of bumper-fibrocartilage was found by drawing a line in continuity with the hyaline articular cartilage–subchondral bone junction to cross the hyaline articular cartilage-bumper-fibrocartilage junction, then measuring the area of bumper-fibrocartilage (see Figs. 13.8 and 13.9).

A high-magnification photomicrograph of a horizontal section from the middle of the left lumbosacral zygapophyseal joint of a 74-year-old male cadaver, with a right leg length deficiency of 21 mm and a right convex postural scoliosis of 6.5°, is shown in Figure 13.9 to clearly demonstrate the bumper-fibrocartilage.

The various data from the measurements made were grouped as shown in Tables 13.1–13.4. Student's t test on 16° of freedom was used to analyze the data obtained from the paired mid-joint histologic sections.

Preliminary Results of the Histologic Survey

Lumbosacral Zygapophyseal Joints

Control Group

Table 13.1 summarizes the results for the control group. There was no significant asymmetry between the left and right zygapophyseal joints for any of the measurements made.

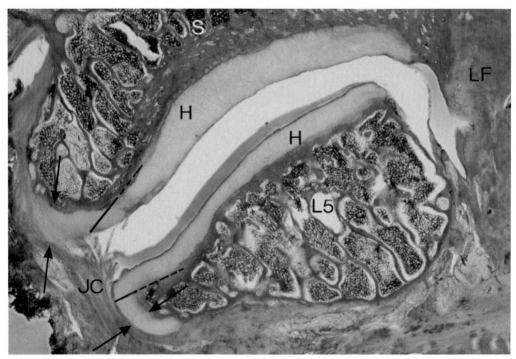

Figure 13.9. Note the large areas of bumper-fibrocartilage (*arrows*) beyond the lateral margins of the facet surfaces of the sacral superior articular process (S) and the fifth lumbar inferior articular process (L5) in a 74-year-old male cadaver with a leg length deficiency of greater than 9 mm. These large bumper-fibrocartilages appear to have developed between points of pressure between the bone and the tough fibrous joint capsule (JC) as a result of joint instability in postural scoliosis. The lines show the approximate junction between the hyaline articular cartilage (H) and the bumper-fibrocartilage. LF = ligamentum flavum. (Ehrlich's hematoxylin stain with light green counterstain.)

Table 13.1.
Histologic Findings: L5–S1 in the Control Group [a]

Finding	Left		Right	
	Mean	SD	Mean	SD
	mm	*mm*	*mm*	*mm*
Subchondral bone thickness across the joint center	1.72	0.49	1.76	0.67
Joint hyaline articular cartilage				
Thickness across the center of the joint	2.33	0.54	2.25	0.57
Cross-sectional area	30.73[b]	8.95[b]	29.37[b]	8.86[b]
Ligamentum flavum thickness at the anterior hyaline articular cartilage bone junction	2.20	1.06	2.18	0.64
Ligamentum flavum thickness midway between the anterior cartilage bone junction and the lamina junction	3.66	1.28	3.70	1.13

[a]From Giles LGF, Taylor JR: The effect of postural scoliosis on lumbar apophyseal joints. *Scand J Rheumatol* 13:209–220, 1984.
[b]mm².

Short Leg Group

Table 13.2 summarizes the results for the short leg group. The lumbosacral zygapophyseal joints on the *convex* side of the scoliotic curvature show a tendency toward thinner hyaline articular cartilage ("b" in Fig. 13.8) and thicker subchondral bone ("a" Fig. 13.8) compared with the concave side, and also to joints in the controls. These differences between concave and convex sides are probably significant (at the 10% level). See Figures 13.10 and 13.11.

No statistical difference's were found regarding the joint hyaline articular cartilage cross-sectional area, although it is greater on the concave side of the scoliotic curvature; the ligamentum flavum thickness "c" (Fig. 13.8) at the anterior hyaline articular cartilage bone junction; or the ligamentum flavum thickness "d" (Fig. 13.8)

Table 13.2.
Histologic Findings: L5–S1 in the Short Leg Group [a]

Finding	Concave		Convex	
	Mean	SD	Mean	SD
	mm	*mm*	*mm*	*mm*
Subchondral bone thickness across the joint center	1.47	0.56	1.94	0.81
Joint hyaline articular cartilage				
Thickness across the center of the joint	2.36	0.99	1.89	0.91
Cross-sectional area	29.04[b]	14.65[b]	26.03[b]	13.05[b]
Ligamentum flavum thickness at the anterior hyaline articular cartilage bone junction	2.04	0.88	1.96	0.70
Ligamentum flavum thickness midway between the anterior cartilage bone junction and the lamina junction	3.35	1.07	2.84	1.07

[a]From Giles LGF, Taylor JR: The effect of postural scoliosis on apophyseal joints. *Scand J Rheumatol* 13:209–220, 1984.
[b]mm².

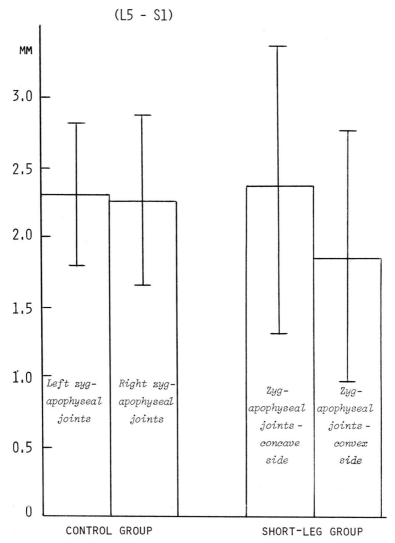

Figure 13.10. Joint hyaline articular cartilage thickness across the center of the joint (L5–S1). (Reproduced with permission from Giles LGF, Taylor JR: The effect of postural scoliosis on lumbar apophyseal joints. *Scand J Rheumatol* 13:209–220, 1984.)

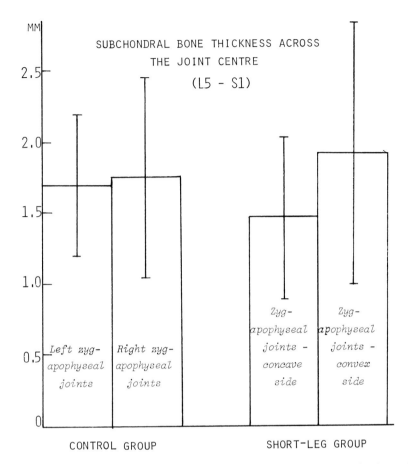

Figure 13.11.   Subchondral bone thickness across the center of the joint (L5–S1). (Reproduced with permission from Giles LGF, Taylor JR: The effect of postural scoliosis on lumbar apophyseal joints. *Scand J Rheumatol* 13:209-220, 1984.)

mid-way between "c" and the lamina junction.

There appeared to be more bumper-fibrocartilage area in the short leg group at the lumbosacral mid-joint level (Fig. 13.12).

Upper Lumbar Zygapophyseal Joints (Corresponding to the Apical Joints of the Scoliotic Curve)

Control Group

Table 13.3 summarizes the results for the control group. There was no significant asymmetry between the left and right zyg-apophyseal joints regarding any of the measurements made.

Short Leg Group

Table 13.4 summarizes the results for the short leg group. There was a difference at the 5% level between the joints on the concave and convex sides of the curvature regarding the joint hyaline articular cartilage cross-sectional area at the apex of the scoliotic curvature (which was greater on the concave side of the curvature)—see Figure 13.13.

At the apical joint, the hyaline articular cartilage had a tendency towards being thicker on the concave side of the scoliotic curvature, while the subchondral bone had a tendency to be thicker on the convex side

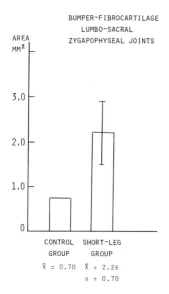

1 OUT OF 7 CONTROL SPECIMENS HAD BUMPER-FIBROCARTILAGE.
4 OUT OF 7 SHORT-LEG SPECIMENS HAD BUMPER-FIBROCARTILAGE.
BUMPER-FIBROCARTILAGE APPEARS UNRELATED TO THE CONVEX OR
CONCAVE SIDE BUT IT APPEARS TO BE RELATED TO THE DEGREE
OF POSTURAL SCOLIOSIS ($>4^0$).

Figure 13.12. The mid-joint bumper-fibrocartilage area at the lumbosacral joints, which appeared in only one control but in four short leg specimens.

of the scoliotic curvature, but at this joint level these differences are not statistically significant. No statistically significant difference was found regarding the ligamentum flavum thickness "c" at the anterior hyaline articular cartilage bone junction, the ligamentum flavum thickness "d" midway between "c" and the lamina junction, or the area of bumper-fibrocartilage in the short leg or control groups.

Thus the principal findings of the measurement study are that in lumbar spines of short leg cases, there is a tendency (*a*) for zygapophyseal joint hyaline articular cartilage to be thinner, and the subchondral bone to be thicker, on the convex side of the curve both at the apical level and the lumbosacral joint level (Fig. 13.14), and (*b*) for there to be a difference in the area of bumper-fibrocartilage in the short leg group at the L5–S1 joints (Fig. 13.12).

Zygapophyseal Joint Geometric Analysis

Over the 5-year period of this research, a great number of cadavers (75) had to be radiographed in order to obtain the seven short leg specimens because of the exclusion categories and the fact that only 8–18% of the population has a leg length inequality of 1 cm or more, depending on whether they are low back pain sufferers or not (6).

Table 13.3.
Histologic Findings: Upper Lumbar Level in the Control Group[a]

Finding	Left		Right	
	Mean	SD	Mean	SD
	mm	*mm*	*mm*	*mm*
Subchondral bone thickness across the joint center	1.25	0.37	1.26	0.39
Joint hyaline articular cartilage				
Thickness across the center of the joint	2.39	0.62	2.24	0.75
Cross-sectional area	26.84[b]	9.43[b]	24.46[b]	10.73[b]
Ligamentum flavum thickness at the anterior hyaline articular cartilage bone junction	2.36	0.56	2.50	0.54
Ligamentum flavum thickness midway between the anterior cartilage bone junction and the lamina junction	2.93	0.93	2.90	0.97

[a]From Giles LGF, Taylor JR: The effect of postural scoliosis on lumbar apophyseal joints. *Scand J Rheumatol* 13:209-220, 1984.
[b]mm².

Table 13.4.
Histologic Findings: Apex in the Short Leg Group[a]

Finding	Concave		Convex	
	Mean	SD	Mean	SD
	mm	*mm*	*mm*	*mm*
Subchondral bone thickness across the joint center	1.38	0.52	1.54	0.36
Joint hyaline articular cartilage				
Thickness across the center of the joint	2.78	0.41	2.42	0.36
Cross-sectional area	28.88[b]	5.27[b]	24.66[b]	4.82[b]
Ligamentum flavum thickness at the anterior hyaline articular cartilage bone junction	2.31	1.02	2.25	0.78
Ligamentum flavum thickness midway between the anterior cartilage bone junction and the lamina junction	2.72	0.54	2.88	0.82

[a]From Giles LGF, Taylor JR: The effect of postural scoliosis on lumbar apophyseal joints. *Scand J Rheumatol* 13:209-220, 1984.
[b]mm^2.

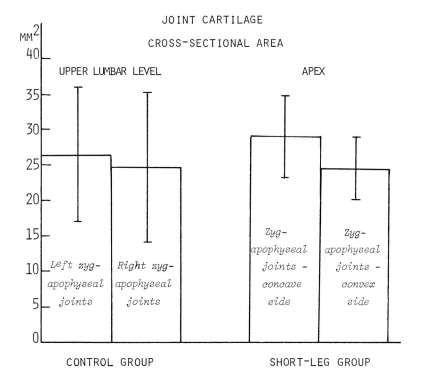

Figure 13.13.   Joint hyaline articular cartilage cross-sectional area. (Reproduced with permission from Giles LGF, Taylor JR: The effect of postural scoliosis on lumbar apophyseal joints. *Scand J Rheumatol* 13:209-220, 1984.)

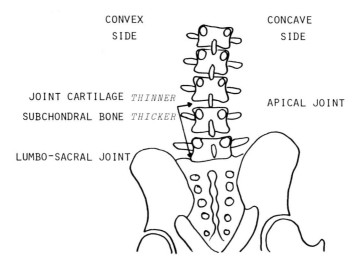

Figure 13.14. Diagram summarizing mid-joint hyaline articular cartilage and subchondral bone thickness at the center of the zygapophyseal joint facets.

In this study there were two sets of controls: the control population, which was on average 12 years younger than the short leg group (i.e. 58.3 years: 70.6 years), and the zygapophyseal joints on one side, which acted as controls for the contralateral joints.

The possible influence of leg length inequality on the lumbar spine is controversial. Some clinical and epidemiologic evidence suggests that differences greater than 1 cm give a greater likelihood of low back pain (6, 7), but others claim that leg length inequality of this order does not lead to structural changes in the spine (8, 9) and that any degenerative changes observed in the spine cannot be attributed to leg length inequality (10). Giles and Taylor (11) demonstrated some structural changes in vertebral bodies and intervertebral discs associated with leg length inequality, and Giles (12) showed differences in the angle to the vertical plane of the right and left lumbosacral zygapophyseal joints in postural scoliosis. This suggested the possibility that (a) the facets are probably no longer congruous, and consequently increased friction may occur at some point of the gliding movement; and (b) asymmetrical biomechanical stress involving the left and right lumbosacral zygapophyseal joints is likely in cases of pelvic obliquity.

The controversy about zygapophyseal joint pathology in relation to leg length inequality is not easily resolved radiographically since osteoarthritis is advanced before it appears on radiographs. On the other hand, although a postmortem investigation can effectively study structural changes in zygapophyseal joints, it cannot relate leg length inequality directly to low back pain. A new method of processing large osteoligamentous blocks with good preservation of tissue and minimal contraction artifact was developed for the present study of zygapophyseal joints (13).

The present study shows that the asymmetrical stresses arising from leg length inequality are associated with structural asymmetry in the lumbar zygapophyseal joints, both in hyaline articular cartilage and subchondral bone thickness. The control group mid-joint combined hyaline articular cartilage thickness was measured as 2.3 mm with no significant variation at different lumbar zygapophyseal joint levels. Allowing for the measured shrinkage of 8.6% (13) (Appendix 2) during processing, this gives an average thickness of 2.5 mm, considerably less than the 4 mm reported by Fick (14) and Delmas et al (15). Fick (14) did not record the ages or the number of subjects from which his data were obtained, and the method of Delmas et al (15) of es-

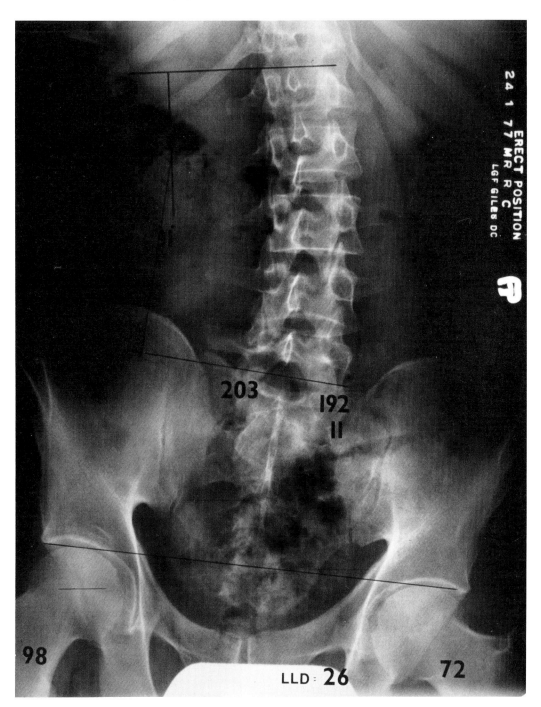

Figure 13.15.   Radiograph of a 37-year-old male with a right leg length deficiency of 20 mm and a postural scoliosis of 11°. The following can be noted: The L3–4 facets on the concave side of the postural scoliosis are apparently more closely apposed than on the convex side; the L4–5 facets appear to be more closely apposed on the convex side; the L4-5 facet surfaces are subluxated (imbricated) and the concavity in the inferior surface of the L4 vertebral body is asymmetrical—the concavity is nearer to the convex side of the postural scoliosis.

timating hyaline articular cartilage thickness by sticking a pin in it would appear to be highly inaccurate. In the short leg cases in the current study, the joint hyaline articular cartilage showed a tendency towards being thicker at the apical zygapophyseal joint on the concave side of the curvature, compared with both the contralateral joint and upper lumbar controls, and the cartilage showed a tendency towards being thinner at the lumbosacral joint on the convex side of the curvature than in the contralateral joint and in controls. At both levels, the hyaline articular cartilage was relatively thinner in the joints on the convex side of the curvature.

Subchondral bone thickness at lumbosacral joints showed asymmetry in an inverse manner to hyaline articular cartilage thickness, being relatively thicker on the convex side of the scoliotic curvature. This could represent early changes leading to osteoarthritis in the lumbosacral zygapophyseal joint at the convex side. However, at the apical joints, subchondral bone showed a tendency towards being thicker on both sides in the short leg group compared with controls, the greater "thickening" being on the convex side.

These asymmetries are difficult to interpret, but they would appear to be a response to the asymmetrical posture and stress associated with leg length inequality. The problem of interpreting the histologic findings is highlighted by the erect posture anteroposterior radiograph shown in Figure 13.15. This radiograph of a 37-year-old male with a right leg length deficiency of 26 mm shows that at the L3–4 zygapophyseal joints, the facets on the concave side are apparently more closely apposed than those on the convex side. However, at the L4–5 level, the facets appear to be more closely apposed on the convex side of the scoliosis.

The lumbar articular facets are said to carry 16–40% of the total compressive spine load (16–17). The presence of a lateral curvature would tend to increase this load since increased postural muscle activity would be required. Lange (18) found a close association between "scoliosis" and osteoarthritis of the zygapophyseal joints of the lumbar spine.

The question of relative stress on concave and convex sides of a scoliotic spine is complex. It has been claimed that short leg increases the compressive load on the concave side of the curvature (19). This would be true of the static loading, without postural muscle support, since the vertical load of body weight acts down across the concavity of the curve. On the other hand, higher levels of postural muscle tone on the convex side of the curve would be required to balance body weight around the fulcrum in the zygapophyseal joint on the convex side of the curved column of each level. The tendency towards greater subchondral bone thickness in the joints on the convex side of the curve would support this view, since this suggests they are responding to higher stresses in these joints. The tendency to thinning of the lumbosacral hyaline articular cartilage in the joint on the convex side of the curve also suggests greater "wear and tear" on this side, although articular cartilage is sometimes said to be thicker where it is most subject to pressure (20). At the apical joints, while there may be subchondral bone thickening in both joints, the joint at the convex side of the curve shows a tendency towards greater thickening, and relative to the contralateral joint, the hyaline articular cartilage also has a tendency to be thinner here. This may be taken to suggest increased stress in both apical zygapophyseal joints, particularly in the joint at the convex side of the curve. These interpretations of the findings of this study receive some support from the observations of Taillard (21) that the anomalies of spinal posture resulting from leg length inequality are associated with increased activity in the spinal postural muscles, which is easily corrected in recent leg length inequality of less than 3 cm.

Bumper-Fibrocartilage

Aberrations of posture in scoliosis may play a role in the genesis of low back pain by disturbing the even distribution of stresses over the respective structures, thereby overloading some of them, causing strain, collapse, and pain (22). The bumper-fibrocartilage suggests sideways "thrusting" of the lateral margins of the joints against the fibrous joint capsule, which may cause pain as a result of stretching of the innervated fibrous joint capsule and irritation of the innervated synovial lining membrane. Leg length inequality and postural scoliosis of the lumbar spine may cause perpetuating muscle strain with myofascial pain arising from trigger points in the quadratus lumborum muscle and/or its associated fascia (23).

As previously mentioned, the lumbosacral joint is the site of tremendous shearing strain, and anything which unlevels the pelvis or shifts the weight, e.g., leg length inequality, increases the shearing strain (24). Equal distribution of the force of body mass to the spine, pelvis, and lower extremities must be maintained by the body, otherwise unstable posture will result (25).

Rush and Steiner (26) and Nichols (27) believe that there is a clinical association between leg length inequality and lumbar spine pain, and according to Golding (28), the importance of a short leg in throwing abnormal postural strain on the spine, with consequent backache, must be emphasized, and the lumbar pain may not be resolved until leg lengths are equalized (29). Giles and Taylor (6) also found that provision of a shoe raise to such individuals who complained of chronic low back pain often led to long-term relief of symptoms.

References

1. Giles LGF, Taylor JR: The effect of postural scoliosis on lumbar apophyseal joints. *Scand J Rheumatol* 13:209-220, 1984.
2. Cobb JR: Outline for the study of scoliosis. Instructional course lectures. *Am Acad Orthop Surg* 5:261-275, 1948.
3. Greenspan A, Pugh JW, Norman A, Norman RS: Scoliotic Index: A comparative evaluation of methods for the measurement of scoliosis. *Bull Hosp Jt Dis Orthop Inst* 39:117-125, 1978.
4. Giles LGF, Taylor JR: Histological preparation of large vertebral specimens. *Stain Technol* 58:45-49, 1983.
5. Cyron BM, Hutton WC: Articular tropism and stability of the lumbar spine. *Spine* 5:168-172, 1980.
6. Giles LGF,Taylor JR: Low-back pain associated with leg length inequality. *Spine* 6:510-521, 1981.
7. Rush WA, Steiner HA: A study of lower extremity length inequality. *AJR* 56:616-632, 1946.
8. Fisk JW, Baigent ML: Clinical and radiological assessment of leg length. *NZ Med J* 81:477-480, 1975.
9. Amstutz HC, Sakai DN: Equalization of leg length (editorial comment). *Clin Orthop* 136:2-5, 1978.
10. Saunders WA, Gleeson JA, Timlin DM, Preston TD, Brewerton DA: Degenerative joint disease in the hip and spine. *Rheumatology and Rehabilitation* 18:137-141, 1979.
11. Giles LGF,Taylor JR: Intra-articular synovial protrusions in the lower lumbar apophyseal joints. *Bull Hosp Jt Dis Orthop Inst* 42:248-255, 1982.
12. Giles LGF:Lumbosacral facetal "joint angles" associated with leg length inequality. *Rheumatology and Rehabilitation* 20:233-238, 1981.
13. Giles LGF: Leg length inequality with postural scoliosis: its effect on lumbar apophyseal joints. M.Sc. thesis, Department of Anatomy and Human Biology, University of Western Australia, Perth, 1982.
14. Fick R: *Handbuch der Anatomie und Mechanik der Gelenke.* Jena, Verlag G. Fischer, 1904, pp 77-89.
15. Delmas A, Ndjaga-MbaM,Vannareth T: Le cartilage articulaire de *Comptes Rendus de l'Association des Anatomistes* L4-5 et L5-S1. 147:230-234, 1970.
16. Hakim NS, King AI: Static and dynamic articular facet loads. In *Proceedings 20th Stapp Car Crash Conference,* 1976, pp 609-637.
17. Hutton WC, Adams MA: The forces acting on the neural arch and their relevance to low back pain. In: *Engineering Aspects of the Spine.* London, Mechanical Engineering Publications, 1980, pp 49-55.
18. Lange M: Veranderungen an den kleinen Wirbelgelenken, eine bisher wenig beobachtete Ursache von Ruckenschmerzen. *Munch Med Wschr* 80:1134, 1933.
19. Kendall H, Kendall F, Boynton D: *Posture and Pain.* New York, Kreiser Publishing, 1977.
20. Davies DV: The biology of joints. In Copeman WSC (ed): *Textbook of the Rheumatic Diseases,* ed 4. Edinburgh, London, 1969, pp 40-86.
21. Taillard W: Colonne lambaire et inegalite des membres interieures. *Acta Orthop Belg* 35:610-613, 1969.
22. During J, Goudfrooij H, Keessen W, Beeker ThW, Crowe A: Toward standards for posture. Postural characteristics of the lower back system in normal and pathologic conditions. *Spine* 10:83-87, 1985.
23. Simons DG: Myofascial pain syndromes due to trigger points: (1) Principles, diagnosis, and perpetuating factors. (2) Treatment of single-muscle syndromes. *Manual Medicine* 1:67-77, 1985.
24. von Lackum HL: The lumbosacral region. *JAMA* 82:1109-1114, 1924.
25. Triano JJ: Objective electromyographic evidence for use and effects of lift therapy. *J Manipulative Physiol Ther* 6:13-16, 1983.
26. Rush WA, Steiner HA: A study of lower extremity length inequality. *AJR* 56:616-623, 1946.
27. Nichols PJR: Short-leg syndrome. *Br Med J* 1:1863-1865, 1960.
28. Golding D: *General Management of Osteoarthritis: Joints and Their Disease.* London, British Medical Association, 1970, pp 95-102.
29. Mennell JMcM: *Back Pain: Diagnosis and Treatment Using Manipulative Techniques,* ed 1. Boston, Little, Brown, 1960, p 63.

CHAPTER 14

Summary of Anatomical Findings and Their Possible Role in the Treatment of Low Back Pain with or without Leg Pain

The main conclusions arising from the anatomical studies can be summarized as follows:

1. Each lower lumbar zygapophyseal joint is innervated by the medial branches of two adjacent posterior primary rami. No evidence was found that zygapophyseal joints on one side of the spine receive innervation from the contralateral posterior primary rami.

2. Using transmission electron microscopy and silver and gold chloride impregnation, lower lumbar zygapophyseal joint synovial folds are found to have nerve fibers and/or fasciculi (0.2 μm per fiber to 13 μm per nerve fasciculus) weaving between the fat cells of the subsynovial tissue. Occasionally, nerve fibers (0.5–1.2 μm diameter) were found in the synovial lining membrane. In both the subsynovial tissue and the synovial lining membrane, nerve fibers were found to be paravascular as well as remote from blood vessels. The small-diameter (0.2–1.1 μm) paravascular nerve fibers are considered to have an autonomic vasoregulatory function. Occasionally, encapsulated nerve endings were seen in the fibrous capsule closely related to the attachment of synovial folds.

3. Immunohistochemistry revealed substance P antibody immunofluorescent nerve fibers in the capsule (diameter 3–27 μm, and in the synovial folds 1.5–11 μm). These nerves are considered to have a putative function of nociception.

4. No neural structures could be demonstrated in the ligamentum flavum in the small portions of tissue examined.

5. The synovial folds consist of white adipose tissue i.e., a single droplet of lipid occupies most of the volume of the cell—these fat cells are unilocular, which distinguishes them from brown adipose tissue, which contains multiple small droplets of lipid of varying size and which is therefore multilocular (1). The synovial folds would be expected to contain white adipose tissue, since brown adipose tissue disappears from most sites in humans after the first decade of life.

6. The anatomical arrangement of the lumbosacral zygapophyseal joint differs from that at L4–5 in the following respects:

   a. At the lumbosacral level, there is a much larger synovial fold in the inferior recess which communicates with a very large extracapsular adipose pad. The purpose of this large fat pad is to act as a space filler which could have a cushioning mechanism for the inferior articular process of L5 on the extracapsular fat pad, particularly in order to accommodate extension of L5 on the sacrum during spinal extension.

   b. At the lumbosacral level, an accessory capsule bridges the gap between the ligamentum flavum and the inferior articular process of L5, forming a relatively large opening inferior to the accessory capsule through which the fat, vessels, and nerves in the synovial fold communicate freely with a large extracapsular fat pad.

c. The horizontal joint plane is more coronal at L5–S1 than it is at L4–5.

7. Large lumbosacral intra-articular synovial fold inclusions can project for a distance of up to 9 mm between the hyaline articular cartilage surfaces, although, according to Bogduk and Twomey (2), intra-articular structures of the lumbar zygapophyseal joints project only up to 5 mm into the joint cavity. The intra-articular synovial fold inclusion tip may become pinched between the hyaline articular cartilage surfaces, and this results in fibrous changes of the tip. It is known that chronic inflammation and fibrosis in the synovium and capsule of the zygapophyseal joints may produce persistent severe back pain (3). When large fibrous tips of synovial folds are present (see Fig. 9.4), it is conceivable that these fibrous structures could also cause mechanical dysfunction, with "locking" of a joint at that level.

8. Tinctorial changes may be found in the anteromedial zygapophyseal joint hyaline articular cartilage matrix, with or without fibrillation, indicating degenerative changes within the hyaline articular cartilage of cadavers (mean age = 67 years). Cancellous bone tinctorial changes may also be seen on each side of the anteromedial aspect of the zygapophyseal joint, where the cartilage surfaces press against each other, particularly on spinal flexion.

9. The elastic fibers in the large synovial folds may impart a function of elastic recoil to the synovial fold to protect it during the course of normal joint movements.

10. The ligamentum flavum has small midline intervals with only partial uniting of its left and right halves. This has clinical significance in epidural block injections where the resistance of the ligamentum flavum to the passage of the needle, with a resultant "popping" noise as the needle passes from the ligamentum flavum into the spinal canal, is used to judge the position of the needle for injection of steroid suspension and anesthetic. If the needle should pass through the midline interval, the tip of the needle could be misplaced and thus puncture the dura. This finding supports the recommendation of Pages (4) that the needle puncture should be made 1–1.5 cm from the midline, with the tip of the needle directed medialy. This procedure could prevent some adverse reactions as a result of injecting structures in the wrong region of the spinal canal. However, according to Bromage (5), this oblique approach has the disadvantage that the epidural space is narrower in its lateral parts than medially, and the vertebral veins running in the anterolateral parts of the epidural space are more liable to damage than in the median approach. Nonetheless, it should be noted that the histologic sections described in Chapter 3 (see Fig. 3.8) indicate that Batson's venous plexus is associated mainly with the anterior, and to some extent the anterolateral, parts of the epidural space of the L4–5 and L5–S1 levels.

11. The ligamentum flavum has (a) very small blood vessels irregularly dispersed in its posterolateral regions and (b) one prominent bilateral and symmetrically located vascular channel which passes through it from the spinal canal to each adjacent zygapophyseal joint.

12. As a corollary to the demonstration of probable nociceptive nerves in the synovial folds, two main mechanisms by which pain may arise are proposed:

a. Mechanical pinching of synovial fold tissue, which may result in traction on pain-sensitive tissues and tissue damage with cell rupture and the subsequent release of pain-producing substances, which result in nerve impulses arising from nociceptors; and

b. Traumatic synovitis causing ischemia with the genesis of ischemic pain.

13. The preliminary findings of the histologic study of the effect of leg length

inequality on the lumbar zygapophyseal joints demonstrate that a 1–1.5 cm leg length inequality is associated with a tendency towards asymmetrical changes in the apical and lumbosacral zygapophyseal joints at the center of the facets, where the least biomechanical stresses would be expected to occur between apposing facets in postural scoliosis. These changes are probably due to the asymmetrical load bearing on the convex and concave sides of the curvature. This histologic study, combined with the clinical study, gives support to the view that patients with a leg length inequality of 1 cm or more and a postural scoliosis should wear an appropriate shoe raise to equalize biomechanical stresses between paired left and right lumbar zygapophyseal joints and allow the facet surfaces for a given zygapophyseal joint to function more normally. This may lessen the stresses within a zygapophyseal joint which lead to bumper-fibrocartilage formation due to "thrusting" of the lateral margins of the facets against the pain-sensitive, synovial-lined fibrous capsule. It also may decrease the possibility of intra-articular synovial folds being pinched within a zygapophyseal joint.

Role of the Findings in Low Back Pain with or without Leg Pain

Although pain is the most common presenting complaint for all clinicians, the reasons why a patient hurts can be a subject of endless clinical debate (6), because patients with chronic low back pain often have few objective findings upon which a diagnosis can be made (7). The zygapophyseal joint facet syndrome and some muscle syndromes are common, but because these lesions usually do not demonstrate abnormalities radiographically, they are frequently overlooked (8). According to Frymoyer et al (9), spinal radiographs have minimal value in determining the presence or absence of low back complaints. Also, very little is known about the value of different methods of treatment in patients with back pain (10). However, as long as patients presenting with low back pain are carefully

screened for contraindications to spinal manipulation (11), mobilization is known to be of benefit in patients with nonspecific back pain (12). However, some patients may not respond to mobilization if they have muscular imbalance of the lumbar–pelvis–hip region or lumbosacral transitional anomalies (13). According to Bedbrook (14), manipulation is of use only in recurrent low back pain which is associated with an unstable back, and in these cases relief can be immediate. However, according to Francis (15), 95% of all back pain cases can be relieved by manipulation.

It is important that spinal manipulation should be undertaken only by a practitioner well versed in the art; when this is the case, many patients can be relieved of symptoms arising from the "facet syndrome" (16), even though the pathology is often in doubt (17) and the way in which manipulation works has long been the subject of controversy (18). According to Kuo and Loh (19), lumbar disc protrusions can be effectively treated by spinal manipulation. Their 517 patients underwent routine radiography, followed in the early years of research by myodil myelography, then more recently by water-soluble contrast media; positive findings established the diagnosis of lumbar disc protrusions in the 517 patients manipulated (P. P. Kuo, personal communication, 1987). However, with clinical improvement, there was no need for these patients to undergo repeat myelography to examine the intervertebral disc protrusion, because it was considered that the protrusion may not change much roentgenographically (P. P. Kuo, personal communication, 1987). Therefore, the question arises of whether manipulation gave relief from intervertebral disc protrusion or from the "facet syndrome," to which Kuo and Loh (19) also refer. This is particularly so in view of the findings of Wiesel et al (20) and Heliovaara et al (21) that herniated lumbar intervertebral discs are often asymptomatic when the spinal canal is not narrow. According to Teplick and Haskin (22), spontaneous regression or disappearance of a herniated lumbar intervertebral disc can occur, and apparently occurred in 11 patients who underwent fol low-up computed tomography (CT) studies. However, it must be remembered that CT studies may fail to provide a definitive diagnosis of disc herniation (23), thus raising the question of whether disc herniation regression can be reliably demonstrated by this method.

According to Mennell (24), the difficulty in diagnosing and treating back pain results in part from the failure of physicians to think in mechanical terms when approaching the patient with a back complaint (24). Therefore, in this chapter, a systematic approach to diagnosing low back pain with or without sciatica is given, followed by a hypothesis to show how, when abnormal biomechanical movements occur between adjacent vertebrae and their motion segments, some anatomical structures of the motion segment may cause these symptoms.

Clinical Evaluation

Initially it is imperative to decide whether a particular patient presenting with low back pain with or without sciatica is likely to respond to spine manipulation, with or without shoe-raise therapy to equalize lumbosacral spinal stresses. This can be judged only after a thorough case history; a routine physical examination, including orthopedic and neurologic tests; motion palpation of the spine and sacroiliac joints; erect posture radiographic evaluation for possible biomechanical abnormalities (with or without stress studies being included) and, when indicated, the use of other imaging procedures, such as CT and magnetic resonance imaging; and laboratory investigations as indicated.

The following clinical approach, which has been modified from Sikorski's (25) outline for the evaluation and treatment of low back pain, is suggested (Fig. 14.1).

When considering this treatment outline, caution is suggested if analgesics and/or anti-inflammatory medication are to be prescribed, since many of these types of drugs can have adverse effects on the body—particularly on the gastrointestinal tract. One undesirable adverse effect is constipation. If a patient who has an anular tear or a small nuclear protrusion becomes constipated, he or she may unwittingly bear down excessively to pass a stool, thereby risking an exacerbation of the low back problem. Another example of drugs which could lead to complications is anticoagulants, such as warfarin sodium, which could result in bleeding if blood vessels are damaged during spinal manipulation.

In cases of low back pain with antalgic posture with or without sciatica or neurologic deficits, radiography should be performed in the erect posture when possible. Initially, routine erect posture radiographs should include coned anteroposterior, lateral, and left and right 45° oblique views.

An indication of motion segment dysfunction may be seen on anteroposterior radiographs of patients with antalgic posture (26) and intervertebral disc wedging at one particular spinal level (Fig. 14.2).

The patient in Figure 14.2 was asked to laterally flex (bend) as far as possible to the right side, then to the left side; anteroposterior radiographs were taken in both these positions. The radiographs are shown in Figure 14.3.

The clinical and radiographic findings for this 36-year-old male indicated that further investigations should be performed, and a water-soluble myelogram showed an L4-5 intervertebral disc protrusion which required surgical removal. Following surgery, the patient made a complete recovery.

This case is recorded to show how plain-film erect posture "functional" radiographs may be used as a guide to help in the differential diagnosis of intervertebral disc lesions, as compared with zygapophyseal joint lesions, of the motion segments. This method has also proved to be valuable in defining disc lesions in patients who have been found to have a normal myelogram and yet still suffer from chronic low back pain with or without slight to moderate sciatica. For example, a 42-year-old male with a history of chronic low back pain and a normal myelogram, who periodically experienced acute low back pain with antalgic posture, was found to have abnormal movement at the L4-5 intervertebral level on erect posture anteroposterior lateral flexion radiographs (Fig. 14.4). A follow-up myelogram defined a small intervertebral disc prolapse at the L4-5 level.

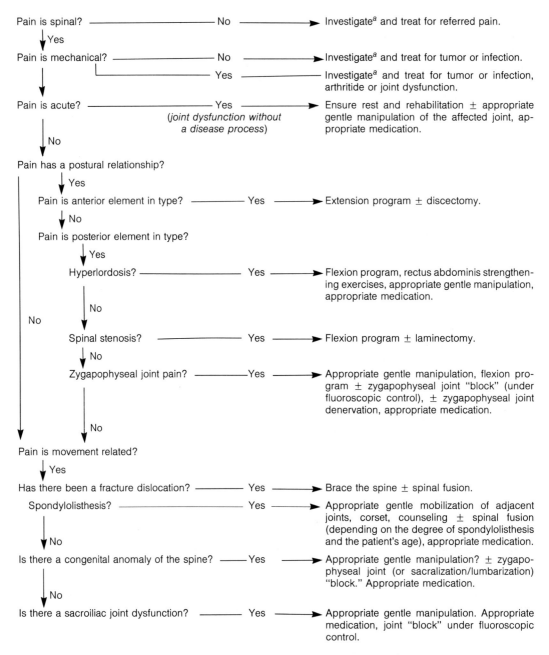

Figure 14.1. Clinical appraoch to evaluation and treatment of low back pain. Presenting symptoms may be secondary to an underlying organic or psychologic disease. Therefore, the possibility of one or more conditions being present simultaneously must never be overlooked. Obviously, treatment should begin with the most conservative method and invasive procedures, such as zygapophyseal joint block, root sleeve injections, zygapophyseal joint denervation, and surgery should be employed only when the least invasive diagnostic and treatment methods fail.

[a]Refers to the use of plain film and/or contrast radiographic procedures and other imaging techniques, such as magnetic resonance imaging, bone scans, and hematology, serology, urinalysis, motion palpation of the spine and sacroiliac joints, sacroiliac joint compression and separation, and any other clinical procedures used in the diagnostic work-up of symptoms. It is expected that the clinician has the necessary clinical judgment to know when tests are indicated. The use of plain film erect posture radiography, as described in Chapter 10, is of paramount importance in investigating low back pain patients to evaluate leg length inequality, pelvic obliquity, and postural scoliosis. Postural stress studies (see Figs. 14.3 and 14.4) can also provide useful diagnostic information. (Modified from Sikorski JM: *Understanding Orthopaedics.* Sydney Butterworths, 1986, p. 68.)

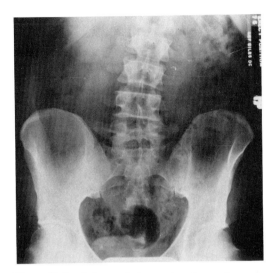

Figure 14.2.   Anteroposterior erect posture radiograph of a 36-year-old male with equal leg lengths and antalgic posture (to the patient's right side), who had lumbosacral pain, slight nonspecific left leg pain, and minor limitation of the left straight leg raising test. Note the wedging of the L4-5 intervertebral disc, which is narrower on the right side.

Erect posture right and left lateral flexion anteroposterior radiographs can also be used when a patient has a leg length inequality and a neurologic deficit indicating the possibility of an intervertebral disc prolapse. Thus, coned and carefully standardized erect posture radiographs not only accurately evaluate leg length, but can be used to show whether the intervertebral discs function ("wedge") normally, that is, whether they conform to the normal pattern of being narrower on the concave side of the spine and wider on the convex side (Fig.14.5).

Correction of postural scoliosis by the use of a shoe raise should result in the vertebral body end-plates becoming approximately parallel on each side of the intervertebral discs at each level, if there is not an associated intervertebral disc prolapse (Fig. 14.6).

In the postural scoliosis shown in Figure 14.5, there will be unequal stresses (*a*) in the postural muscles on each side of the spine and pelvis; (*b*) in the paired zygapophyseal joints at a given spinal level; (*c*) between the left and right halves of each intervertebral

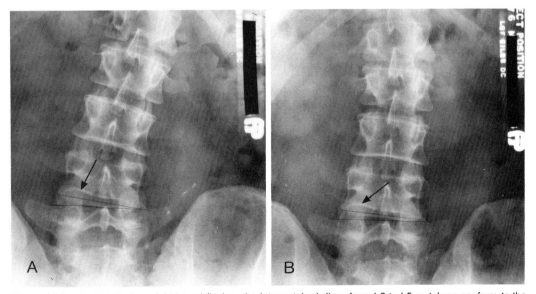

Figure 14.3.   A, Note that on right lateral flexion, the intervertebral discs from L2 to L5 vertebrae conform to the expected pattern of wedging, with the right side being narrower than on the left side, particularly at the L4-5 level. **B**, Note that on left lateral flexion, the wedging of the L4-5 intervertebral disc persists and the intervertebral disc does not become narrower on the left side. The adjacent vertebral bodies do not even become parallel, as they have at the L3-4 level.

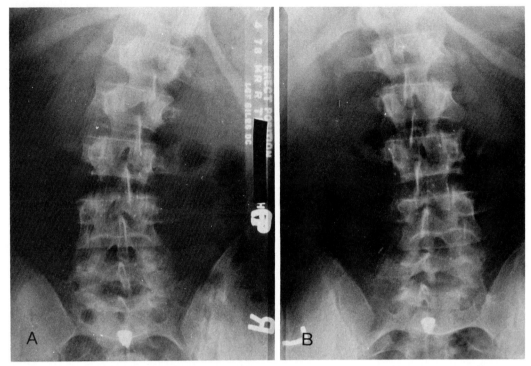

Figure 14.4.   A, Right lateral flexion. **B**, Left lateral flexion. Erect posture anteroposterior right and left lateral flexion studies of a 42-year-old male who complained of chronic low back pain with periodic episodes of acute low back pain with antalgic posture. A myelogram had proved normal. However, on left lateral flexion, the intervertebral discs "wedged" virtually normally; that is, they were narrower on the concave side and wider on the convex side of the spine; the L4–5 intervertebral disc showed exaggeration of the wedging. On right lateral flexion, the L4–5 intervertebral disc did not wedge in conformity with higher spinal levels. These findings indicated a possible motion segment lesion at the L4–5 intervertebral disc level, which was confirmed by myelography.

disc, as a result of wedging of the intervertebral disc, which will cause asymmetrical stresses in the anular fibers between the concave and convex sides of the intervertebral disc as the nucleus pulposus is "squeezed" unilaterally; and (*d*) in the paired sacroiliac joints (which have synovial-lined capsules [27]). There is likely to be some degree of imbrication of the opposing zygapophyseal joint facet surfaces on the concave side of the scoliosis (see Fig. 11.6) because of intervertebral disc wedging, which is narrower on the concave side of the scoliosis. Thinning of the intervertebral disc, as a result of desiccation of nuclear material with increasing age, is known to result in a telescoping or imbrication (subluxation) of the zygapophyseal joint facets (28).

The causes of low back pain in cases of leg length inequality of 1 cm or more and a postural scoliosis are likely to be multifactorial. For example,

1. Myofascial pain due to chronic muscle strain may occur.
2. Postural scoliosis may be the principal etiological factor in osteoarthritis of the spine in patients past middle age (29), because repeated damage to the zygapophyseal joints, especially when associated with subluxation, will lead to osteoarthritis (30).
3. It is conceivable that there would be a greater predisposition to pinching of the large lumbosacral intra-articular synovial folds in postural scoliosis because of asymmetrical stresses at the lum-

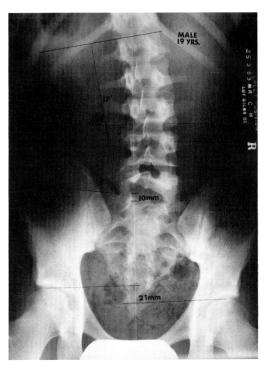

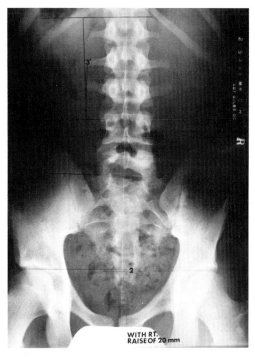

Figure 14.5. Anteroposterior erect posture radiograph of a 19-year-old male complaining of low back pain. There is a right leg length deficiency of 21 mm, a right sacral base obliquity of 10 mm, and a 17° postural scoliosis. Note that all the intervertebral disc spaces conform to the normal pattern of being narrower on the concave side and wider on the convex side of the postural scoliosis.

Figure 14.6. Note that the postural scoliosis has almost completely been eliminated as a result of provision of a right shoe raise of 20 mm. This will lead to a more normal equalization of biomechanical stresses in the zygapophyseal joints, sacroiliac joints, and the postural muscles of the pelvis and lumbar spine.

bosacral zygapophyseal joints and incongruity of the facet surfaces of these joints. Pinching of the synovial folds between articular surfaces (28) could clearly result in traumatic synovitis (31) which may well result in pain due to stimulation of the small-diameter nerve fibers in the zygapophyseal joint synovial folds, which have been ascribed the putative function of nociception (32), or increased pressure within the joint capsule, due to inflammation and hemarthrosis causing tension in the fibrous joint capsule which is innervated by small nociceptors (32).

In the absence of positive neurologic findings and radiologic evidence of intervertebral disc prolapse, traumatic synovitis of the synovial folds (with resulting synovial fold or joint capsule nociceptor stimulation) may be the cause of low back pain, with or without leg pain. Localized reflex muscle spasm is a likely consequence of traumatic synovitis. The components of a simple reflex, resulting in local muscle spasm because of traumatic synovitis or capsular irritation in a zygapophyseal joint, are shown in Figure 14.7.

The sensation of pain would be conveyed to the sensory cortex via the lateral spinothalamic pathway, as shown in Figure 14.8.

In order to lessen the likelihood of low back pain occurring in people with leg length inequality and a postural scoliosis, correction of the postural scoliosis should be considered in a supple spine. Further-

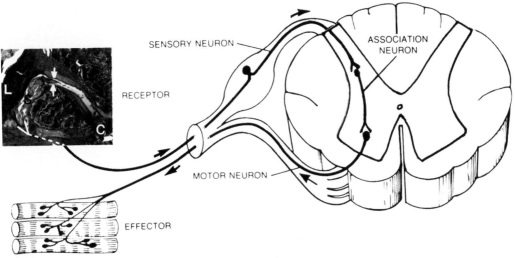

SENSORY NEURON

ASSOCIATION NEURON

RECEPTOR

MOTOR NEURON

EFFECTOR

Components of a generalized reflex arc.

Figure 14.7. Components of a generalized reflex arc. The zygapophyseal joint receptor system includes the synovial fold(s) and the fibrous joint capsule (c). *Arrows* indicate pinching of the synovial fold between the opposing hyaline articular cartilage surfaces. L = ligamentum flavum. (Modified from Tortora GJ, Anagnostakos NP: *Principles of Anatomy and Physiology*, ed 5. New York, Harper and Row, 1987, p. 288. Modified artwork copyright Leonard D. Dank, Medical Illustrations Company, Cutchogue New York.)

more, shoe-raise therapy may be required before lasting relief from low back pain is achieved in low back pain sufferers (34, 35), because a leg length inequality of 1 cm may be biomechanically important (36). The treatment of pelvic obliquity, due solely to leg length inequality, is by equalization of leg lengths by appropriate correction; this may require a shoe-raise or surgical shortening of the long leg or lengthening of the short leg (or both) (37).

In summary, it is suggested that leg length equalization may prevent:

1. Possible recurring synovial fold pinching, with its associated painful traumatic synovitis, as well as the probable tractioning of the synovial fold against the pain-sensitive joint capsule;
2. Mechanical stress against the innervated synovial lining membrane and its associated posterolateral fibrous joint capsule, by preventing the sideways "thrusting" of the lateral margins of the facets of the zygapophyseal joints against this capsule, which results in the formation of

excessive bumper-fibrocartilage (38) (see Fig. 13.9);
3. The formation of osteophytes and traction spurs which are associated with intervertebral disc anulus fibrosus squeezing (on the concave side) and tractioning (on the convex side), as a result of pulling on the periosteum, which is known to be innervated;
4. Unequal biomechanical stresses in the paired sacroiliac joints;
5. Myofascial pain arising from trigger points in the asymmetrically "tensioned" postural muscles on the opposite sides of the spine and pelvis, such as the quadratus lumborum muscles and/or their associated fascia (39).

However, specific rotatory manipulation is usually also required to mobilize the affected joint in order to provide more rapid relief from pain. The therapeutic effects of rotatory spinal manipulation for low back pain may include (*a*) the release of a trapped intra-articular synovial fold, which may explain the dramatic relief from pain and muscle spasm experienced by some

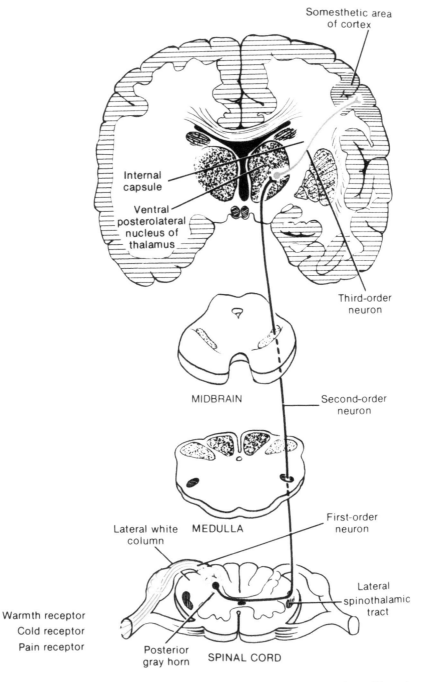

Figure 14.8.   Sensory pathway for pain and temperature—the lateral spinothalamic pathway. (Reproduced with permission from Tortora GJ, Anagnostakos NP: *Principles of Anatomy and Physiology*, ed 5. New York, Harper and Row, 1987.)

patients immediately following manipulation; and (b) stretching of the joint capsule, which may have regions of fibrotic scarring, thus allowing an increased excursion of the joint (40).

Manipulation

According to Sandoz (41), spinal manipulation can be defined as a passive, manual maneuver during which the zygapophyseal joint complex is suddenly carried beyond the normal physiologic range of movement, without exceeding the boundaries of anatomical integrity.

Spinal manipulative therapy is one of the most commonly used treatments for patients with low back pain (42), and the fact that manipulation works is not seriously contested (40). According to Scham (43), rotatory manipulation of the lumbosacral spine has long been known to give symptomatic relief to a large number of patients, with a very low risk of complications, but the

mechanism of the action is ill defined. However, in a group of patients manipulated during operation in the lateral position, the laminae were seen to move apart, stretching the fibers of the ligamentum flavum and the fibrous joint capsule (44). Therefore, it is quite conceivable that as the capsular ligaments are stretched during a rotatory spinal manipulation, the synovial fold could be retracted from between apposing facet surfaces. This concept is supported by Kraft and Levinthal (45), Kirkaldy-Willis (16), and Cui et al (46).

Manipulation Forces

It is necessary to consider what is known about the forces which are thought to take place in axial traction of a metacarpophalangeal joint, as illustrated in Figure 14.9, in order to understand what forces may be involved in manipulation of zygapophyseal joints. The metacarpophalangeal joint axial traction forces are considered to

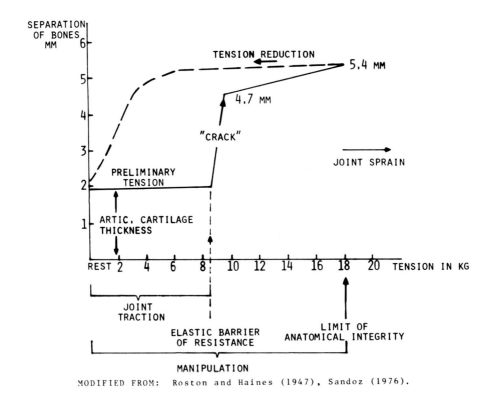

MODIFIED FROM: Roston and Haines (1947), Sandoz (1976).

Figure 14.9. Axial traction of a metacarpophalangeal joint. See text for detailed explanation of this diagram.

be analogous to those of zygapophyseal joints, although it must be remembered that the combined hyaline articular cartilage thickness in zygapophyseal joints is approximately 2–2.4 mm and that the zygapophyseal joints, particularly at the lumbosacral level, have synovial joint anatomy which differs in some respects from that of the matacarpophalangeal joints. However, it is not possible to measure in vivo forces within zygapophyseal joints during manipulation or at any other time, using currently available technology.

According to Roston and Haines (47), who applied axial traction to metacarpophalangeal joints, under radiographic control, in the resting phase, the facet surfaces are separated by hyaline articular cartilage of about 1.8 mm total thickness. They found that when the metacarpophalangeal joint undergoes preliminary tension, up to 8.5 kg, a sudden separation of about 2 mm occurs and a "crack" is heard, and at 9 kg a total separation of facet surfaces of 4.7 mm occurs; a tension of 18.5 kg leads to a total separation of about 5.4 mm. According to Unsworth et al (48), the crack was heard at a load of 10–16 kg and is due to fluid "cavitation": Low pressures are developed in the synovial fluid, and these pressures cause vaporization and gas liberation from the fluid, and at this point, the joint space suddenly springs open. Separation between the joint surfaces does not return to its precracking condition for about 15 minutes (48).

In order to elucidate the significance of the cracking noise often associated with the manipulation of zygapophyseal joints, Meal and Scott (49) used a simultaneous sound and tension recording system to record from axial traction of the metacarpophalangeal joints of eight subjects, and they also made sound recordings from the sounds produced during cervical spine manipulation. They found that the sound wave from a cervical spinal manipulation is the same as that from a metacarpophalangeal joint and therefore concluded that the cracking noise elicited from the spine is from the synovial (zygapophyseal) joints.

From the above, it is obvious that spinal manipulation should be performed within the limit of the elastic barrier of resistance of a synovial joint, and not beyond the limit of anatomical integrity; otherwise a joint sprain will occur (Fig. 14.9). The effect of a carefully performed spinal manipulation which separates the facet surfaces of zygapophyseal joints may well result in the retraction of an entrapped synovial fold and in the stretching of any fibrotic scar tissue which may have formed in the zygapophyseal joint fibrous capsule. Forceful manipulation may well cause an exacerbation of the painful syndrome.

It is suggested that prophylactic care of the low back should be initiated by adolescence in order to determine whether leg length inequality and a postural scoliosis are present. When this is the case, in order to equalize biomechanical stresses and minimize the possible damaging effects of pelvic obliquity on the "motion" segment, a shoe-raise should be provided, unless the leg length inequality is such that orthopedic intervention is necessary. According to Galasko (50), patients whose discrepancy is less than 3 cm should not be considered for surgery. When surgery is considered to be necessary, accurate methods are available for assessing leg length and total hip and knee alignment (51, 52) even when a patient has a contracture of a joint (53). In adults not requiring surgical correction of leg length discrepancy, progression of existing degenerative changes may be arrested or retarded by the use of shoe-raise therapy, coupled with spinal manipulation.

This study presents data which have been collected in an attempt to obtain evidence of the effectiveness of spinal manipulation with or without shoe-raise therapy in the treatment of the costly and debilitating condition of chronic low back pain with or without sciatica.

If the zygapophyseal joints are subjected to sudden and unexpected movements, particularly in the presence of cases of leg length inequality of 1 cm or more and postural scoliosis, or in cases of lumbosacral joint tropism, or if the zygapophyseal joints are held at the extreme of their limit of extension, the strains of everyday living may push the joints past their physiologically permitted limits, thereby producing pain. Eventually the zygapophyseal joint(s) may subluxate (30) and trap the large innervated lumbosacral synovial folds.

In this chapter, the rationale for conservative treatment by spinal manipulation and, when necessary, by shoe-raise therapy, has been considered in the light of recent histologic findings and the radiologic findings associated with leg length inequality. In cases which do not respond rapidly to this conservative approach, the invasive procedure of fluroscopically controlled injections of steroids an anesthetic into zygapophyseal joints may give relief from low back pain with or without sciatica and should be tried, in the absence of contraindications, before surgical procedures are contemplated.

The proposed pain mechanisms probably account for many causes of low back pain with or without leg pain in which no demonstrable lesion is found in spite of a thorough physical examination, imaging procedures (radiography and magnetic resonance imaging), or laboratory investigations.

References

1. Bloom W, Fawcett DW: *A Textbook of Histology*. ed 10. Philadelphia, W.B. Saunders, 1975, pp 197, 199, 202.
2. Bogduk N. Twomey LT: *Clinical Anatomy of the Lumbar Spine*. Melbourne, Churchill Livingstone, 1987, p 31.
3. Pountain GD, Keegan AL, Jayson MIV: Impaired fibrinolytic activity in defined chronic back pain syndromes. *Spine* 12:83-86, 1987.
4. Pages F: Anestesia metamerica. *Rev Sanid Mil Madr* 11:351, 1921.
5. Bromage PR: *Epidural Analgesia*. Philadelphia, W.B. Saunders, 1978, p 177.
6. Buerger AA: *Empirical Approaches to the Validation of Spinal Manipulation*. Springfield, IL, Charles C. Thomas, 1985, pp 193-207.
7. Grubb SA, Hester J, Lipscomb RN, Guilford WB: The relative value of lumbar roentgenograms, metrizamide myelography, and discography in the assessment of patients with chronic low-back syndrome. *Spine* 12:282-286, 1987.
8. Bernard TN, Kirkaldy-Willis WH: Recognizing specific characteristics of nonspecific low back pain. *Clin Orthop* 217:266-280, 1987.
9. Frymoyer JW, Phillips RB, Newberg AH, MacPherson BV: A comparative analysis of the interpretations of lumbar spinal radiographs by chiropractors and medical doctors. *Spine* 11:1021-1023, 1986.
10. Bergquist-Ullman M: Low back pain in industry: a randomized clinical trial. In Buerger AA, Greenman PE (eds): *Empirical Approaches to the Validation of Spinal Manipulation*. Springfield, IL, Charles C. Thomas, 1985, pp 164-173.
11. Kleynhans AM, Terrett AGF: The prevention of complications from spinal manipulative therapy. In Glasgow EF, Twomey LT, Scull ER, Kleynhans AM, Idczak RM (eds): *Aspects of Manipulative Therapy*, ed 2. Melbourne, Churchill Livingstone, 1985, pp 161-175.
12. Young SMS: Controlled trials of mobilization and manipulation for general practitioner and hospital patients. In Buerger AA, Greenman PE (eds): *Empirical Approaches to the Validation of Spinal Manipulation*. Springfield, IL, Charles C. Thomas, 1985, pp 185-192.
13. Schwerdtner HP: Lumbosakrale Ubergangsanomalien als Rezidivursache bei chirotherapeutischen Behandlungstechniken. *Manuelle Medizin* 24:11-15, 1986.
14. Bedbrook GM: Recurrent low back pain. In Twomey LT (ed): *Low Back Pain* (proceedings of a conference on low back pain). Perth, Western Australia Institute of Technology, 1974, pp 137-155.
15. Francis J: Posterior rhizotomy in low back pain. In Twomey LT (ed): *Low Back Pain* (proceedings of a conference on low back pain). Perth, Western Australian Institute of Technology, 1974, pp 156-166.
16. Kirkaldy-Willis WH: Manipulation. In Kirkaldy-Willis (ed): *Managing Low Back Pain*. New York, Churchill Livingstone, 1983, pp 175-183.
17. Winer CER: A survey of controlled clinical trials of spinal manipulation. In Glasgow EF, Twomey LT, Scull ER, Kleynhans AM, Edczak RM (eds): *Aspects of Manipulative Therapy*. ed 2. Melbourne, Churchill Livingstone, 1985, pp 97-108.
18. Kirkaldy-Willis WH: A comprehensive outline of treatment. In Kirkaldy-Willis WH (ed): *Managing Low Back Pain*. New York, Churchill Livingstone, 1983, pp 147-160.
19. Kuo P P-F, Loh Z-C: Treatment of lumbar intervertebral disc protrusions by manipulation. *Clin Orthop* 215:47-55, 1987.
20. Wiesel SW, Tsourmas N, Feffer HL, and associates: A study of computer-assisted tomography: I. The incidence of positive CAT scans in an asymptomatic group of patients. *Spine* 9:549-551, 1984.
21. Heliovaara M, Vanharanta H, Korpi J, Troup JDG: Herniated lumbar disc syndrome and vertebral canals. *Spine* 11:433-435, 1986.
22. Teplick J, Haskin ME: Spontaneous regression of herniated nucleus pulposus. *AJR* 145:371-375, 1985.
23. Mokhtar G, Hodges FJ III, Patel JI: Spine. In Lee JKT, Sagel SS, Stanley RJ (eds): *Computed Body Tomography*. New York, Raven Press, 1983, p 424.
24. Mennell J: McM: *Back Pain Diagnosis and Treatment Using Manipulative Techniques*. Boston, Little, Brown, 1960.
25. Sikorski JM: *Understanding Orthopaedics*. Sydney, Butterworths, 1986, p 68.
26. De Seze S, Rotes Querol J, Djian A: Le diagnostic radiologique de la hernie discale posterieure en station vertecale. *Semaine des Hospitaux de Paris* 26:1297-1307, 1950.
27. Bowen V, Cassidy JD: Macroscopic and microscopic anatomy of the sacroiliac joint from embryonic life until the eight decade. *Spine* 6:620-628, 1981.
28. Hadley LA: *Anatomico-Roentgenographic Studies of the Spine*. Springfield, IL, Charles C. Thomas, 1964, p 174.
29. Cole WV: Disorders of the musculoskeletal system. In Hoag JM, Cole WV, Bradford SG (eds): *Osteopathic Medicine*. New York, McGraw-Hill, 1969, pp 384-426.
30. Macnab I: *Backache*. Baltimore, Williams & Wilkins, 1977, p 86.
31. Giles LGF: Innervation of zygapophyseal joint synovial folds in low-back pain. *Lancet* 2:692, 1987.
32. Giles LGF, Harvey AR: Immunohistochemical demonstration of nociceptors in the capsule and synovial folds of human zygapophyseal joints. *Br J Rheumatol* 26:362-364, 1987.
33. Tortora GJ, Anagnostakos NP: *Principles of Anatomy and Physiology*, ed 5. New York, Harper and Row, 1987, pp 292-294.
34. Giles LGF, Taylor JR: Low-back pain associated with leg length inequality. *Spine* 6:510-521, 1981.

35. Neumann H-D: A concept of manual medicine. In Buerger AA, Greenman PE (eds): *Empirical Approaches to Validation of Spinal Manipulation*. Springfield, IL, Charles C. Thomas, 1985, pp 267-272.

36. Maher RK, Kirby RL, Macleod DA: Simulated leg-length discrepancy. Its effect on mean centre-of-pressure position and postural sway. *Arch Phys Med Rehabil* 66:822-824, 1985.

37. Winter RB, Pinto WC: Pelvic obliquity: its causes and treatment. *Spine* 11:225-234, 1986.

38. Hadley LA: *Anatomico-Roentgenographic Studies of the Spine*. Springfield, IL, Charles C. Thomas, 1976, p 179.

39. Simons DG: Myofascial pain syndromes due to trigger points: (1) Principles, diagnosis, and perpetuating factors. (2) Treatment and single-muscle syndromes. *Manual Medicine* 1:67-77, 1985.

40. Farfan HF: The scientific basis of manipulative procedures. *Clin Rheum Dis* 6:159-178, 1980.

41. Sandoz R: Some physical mechanisms and effects of spinal adjustments. *Annals of the Swiss Chiropractors Association* 6:91-141, 1976.

42. Haldeman S: Spinal manipulative therapy. *Clin Orthop* 179:62-70, 1983.

43. Scham SM: Manipulation of the lumbosacral spine. *Am Orthop* 101:146-150, 1974.

44. Chrisman OD, Mittnacht A, Snook GA: A study of the results following rotatory manipulation in the lumbar intervertebral disc. *J Bone Joint Surg* 46(A):517-524, 1964.

45. Kraft GL, Levinthal DH: Facet synovial impingement: a new concept in the etiology of lumbar vertebral derangement. *Surg Gynecol Obstet* 93:439-443, 1951.

46. Cui G, Li Z, Yang Z, Wang J: Lateral rotary manipulative maneuver in the treatment of subluxation and synovial entrapment of lumbar facet joints. *J Tradit Chin Med* 4(3):211-212, 1984.

47. Roston JB, Haines RW: Cracking in the metacarpophalangeal joint. *J Anat* 81:165-173, 1947.

48. Unsworth A, Dowson D, Wright V: "Cracking joints." A bioengineering study of cavitation in the metacarpophalangeal joint. *Ann Rheum Dis* 31:348-358, 1971.

49. Meal GM, Scott RA: Analysis of the joint crack by simultaneous recording of sound and tension. *J Manipulative Physiol Ther* 9:189-195, 1986.

50. Galasko CSB: Limb length discrepancy. In: *Leg length Inequality: International Orthopedic Symposium on Leg Length Inequality*. Postgraduate Medical Education, Faculty of Medicine, University of Utrecht, the Netherlands, 1984, p 27.

51. Moreland JR, Bassett LW, Hanker GJ: Radiographic analysis of the axial alignment of the lower extremity. *J Bone Joint Surg* 69(A):745-749, 1987.

52. Petersen TD, Rohr W: Improved assessment of lower extremity alignment using new roentgenographic techniques. *Clin Orthop* 219:112-119, 1987.

53. Huurman WW, Jacobsen S, Anderson, JC, Chu W-K: Limb-length discrepancy measured with computerized axial tomographic equipment. *J Bone Joint Surg* 69(A):699-705, 1987.

APPENDIX 1

Definitions and Abbreviations

Antalgic Posture—a posture assumed by patients experiencing acute low back pain, with or without leg pain, in which they lean away from the painful area.

Anteroposterior (A–P)—the position of patients when an x-ray beam is directed to their anterior surface and an x-ray plate is positioned behind them. In this text, the A–P radiographs are viewed from behind the patient; the patient's right side is indicated by a right marker (**R**).

Apical Vertebra—that vertebra which is located at the apex of the postural scoliosis.

Articular Triad—the intervertebral joint and the two zygapophyseal joints at any given level of the spine (1, 2) (below the second cervical vertebra).

Cobb's Method (3)—method for measuring the angle of curvature. The angle of curvature is measured by drawing lines parallel to the superior surface of the uppermost vertebral body of the curvature and to the inferior surface of the lowest vertebra of the curvature.

Intervertebral Load Cell—an instrument consisting of a transducer (inserted into the inferior portion of a cadaveric lumbar vertebral body) which is capable of measuring the intervertebral axial load (4).

Intra-articular Synovial Fold Inclusion—a fibrous or highly vascular fat-filled zygapophyseal joint synovial fold inclusion, which is covered by the sinovial lining membrane, and which projects between the facet surfaces.

Leg Lengths—the types of "leg lengths" (5) (which do not necessarily include the ankle–heel distance) referred to in the

literature are shown diagrammatically in Figure A1.1.

Absolute leg length: distance between the most proximal part of the femoral head and the point of contact of the foot with the ground.

Anatomical leg length: distance between the proximal end of the greater trochanter and the distal end of the lateral malleolus.

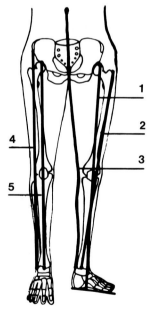

Figure A1.1. Types of leg lengths. *1.* Absolute leg length. *2.* Anatomical leg length. *3.* Apparent leg length. *4.* Clinical leg length. *5.* Relative leg length. (Reproduced with permission from Eichler J: Methodological errors in documenting leg length and leg length discrepancies. In Hungerford DS (ed): *Leg Length Discrepancy: The Injured Knee.* New York, Springer-Verlag, 1977.

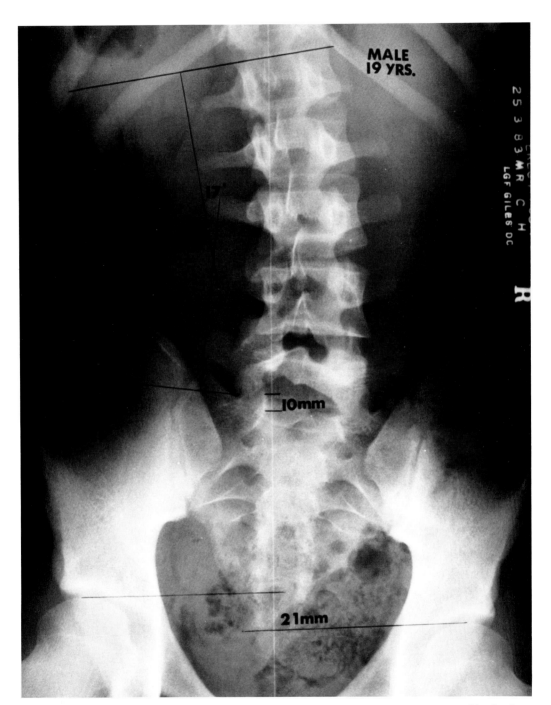

Figure A1.2. An erect posture radiograph of a 19-year-old male showing a right leg length deficiency of 21 mm, sacral base obliquity, and postural scoliosis with a 17° angle of curvature. R = right side of the patient. Note the vertical plumb-line shadow which is used for measuring leg lengths by drawing a horizontal line from the top of each femur head to meet the plumb-line at right angles. Sacral base obliquity is measured by drawing a horizontal line from each superior sacral notch to meet the plumb-line at right angles. The vertical difference between paired horizontal lines gives the difference in leg lengths and the difference in height between the superior sacral notches.

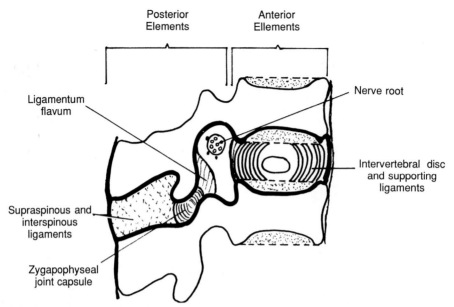

Figure A1.3. The motion (mobile) segment. (Modified from Schmorl G, Junghanns H: *The Human Spine in Health and Disease,* ed 2. New York, Grune and Stratton, 1971, p 37.)

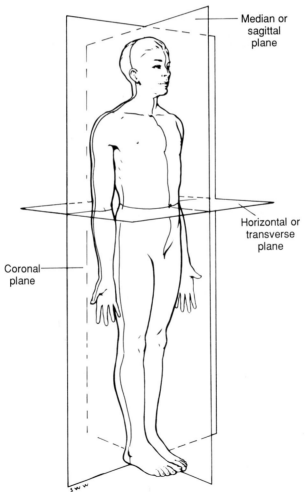

Figure A1.4. The descriptive planes of the body. (Reproduced with permission from Davies DV, Davies F: *Gray's Anatomy. Descriptive and Applied,* ed 33. London, Longmans, Green, 1964, p xix.)

Apparent leg length: distance between the umbilicus and the distal end of the medial malleolus.

Clinical leg length: distance between the anterior superior iliac spine and the distal end of the lateral malleolus.

Relative leg length: distance between the articular surface of the femur head and tibiotalar joint recorded by radiographic measurement.

Leg Length Inequality—the absolute inequality in length of the lower limbs. In this study, the term "leg length deficiency" is used to describe the amount of the absolute inequality. A "significant leg length deficiency" is one where an inequality of 9 mm or more is found, using an accurate method for erect posture radiography (Fig. A1.2).

Low Back Pain—*Chronic* low back pain refers to low back pain of long duration without marked limitation of lumbar spine movements.

Acute low back pain refers to pain of recent onset with marked limitation of lumbar spine movements and antalgic posture.

Lumbosacral Spinal Manipulation—manual manipulation of the lumbosacral joint, performed in this study specifically with each patient lying on his or her side with the short leg side uppermost and both knees partly bent.

Manipulation—the skillful and dextrous mobilization of a synovial joint, within the limit of the joint's elastic barrier of resistance, and *not* beyond its limit of anatomical integrity (see Fig. 14.9).

Motion (Mobile) Segment of Junghanns—all the space between two vertebrae where movement occurs: the intervertebral disc with its cartilaginous plates, the anterior and posterior longitudinal ligaments, the zygapophyseal joints with their fibrous joint capsules and the ligamenta flava, the contents of the spinal canal and the left and right intervertebral canal, and the supraspinous and interspinous ligaments (Fig. A1.3).

Obliquity—*Pelvic obliquity:* a lateral inclination of the pelvis which is tilted downward to the short leg side (Fig. A1.2).

Sacral base obliquity: a lateral inclination of the sacral base (Fig. A1.2).

"Out of Phase" Growth—the unequal dimension of paired bones in a growing individual, e.g., in the lower limbs, due to one bone being more advanced than the corresponding contralateral bone in its maturity.

Pelvic Tilt—tilting of the sacrum in the median (sagittal) plane.

Planes of the Body—the descriptive planes of the body are shown in Figure A1.4.

Scoliosis—*Angle of curvature:* the angle between lines drawn parallel to the superior surface of the upper vertebra of the curvature and to the inferior surface of the lowest vertebra of the curvature (Fig. A1.2).

Postural (compensatory): a lumbar or thoracolumbar scoliosis (lateral curvature) which is an adaptation of the vertebral column to pelvic obliquity and which is convex on the short leg side. The intervertebral discs are wedged from the concave to the convex sides on the A–P radiograph, with the discs being wider on the convex side of the scoliosis (Fig. A1.2). The relationship of the postural scoliosis to sacral base obliquity, and to leg lengths, is schematically summarized in some of the categories shown in Figure A1.5.

Structural idiopathic: a lateral curvature with fixed rotational deformity of the spine, as in idiopathic scoliosis, which is not considered in this text.

Shoe-Raise Therapy—the provision of a shoe raise on the side of the short leg. The raise on the heel is equal to the difference in leg lengths, and the raise on the sole is 5 mm less.

Sphyrion Height—the height of the medial malleolus of the tibia from the sole of the heel.

Spondylosis—osteophytosis secondary to degenerative intervertebral disc disease (9).

Subluxation—the alteration of the normal dynamics or anatomical or physiologic relationships of contiguous articular structures (10). In this text, the term is used when apposing facet surfaces of the

Category 1

Parallel obiquity of
the sacral base
and femur heads
with postural scoliosis.

Category 2

Unequal obliquity of the
sacral base and femoral heads.
The femoral head unleveling is greater.

Category 3

Sacral base obliquity
is greater than the
femoral head unleveling.

Category 4

There is no sacral base
obliquity but femoral head
unleveling is present.

Category 5

Primary sacral base obiquity,
i.e., there is sacral base
obliquity with equal leg
lengths.

Category 6

Contralateral obliquity, i.e., there
is sacral base obliquity opposite
to the unleveling of the
femur heads

Category 7

There is no leg length
inequality or sacral
base obliquity.

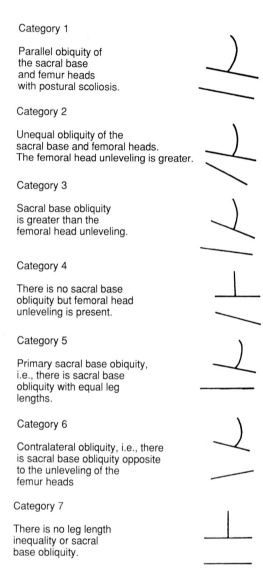

Figure A1.5. Note that the postural scoliosis is compensatory to the sacral base obliquity in each case. In this text, only cases of typical postural scoliosis as defined above, in Category 1, are discussed. A brief comment is made regarding Category 4, in which leg length inequality is present but the sacral base is level due to pelvic osseous anomalies. (Modified from Lloyd PT, Imerbrink JH: Teaching materials. In *Department of Osteopathic Principles and Practice*. Philadelphia, Philadelphia College of Osteopathic Medicine, 1952.)

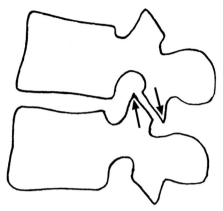

Figure A1.6. Note the subluxation (telescoping, imbrication) of the zygapophyseal joint facet surfaces as indicated by the *arrows.*

zygapophyseal joint are no longer congruous as demonstrated by imbrication (telescoping) of the zygapophyseal joint facet surfaces (11) (Fig. A1.6).

Tropism—asymmetry in the horizontal plane of paired left and right zygapophyseal joints (Fig. A1.7).

Zygapophyseal Joint—the diarthrodial synovial joint between adjacent vertebral arches (apophyseal joint, "facetal" joint, interlaminar joint).

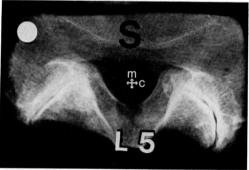

Figure A1.7. Superior-to-inferior radiographic view of paired zygapophyseal joints at the lumbosacral level. The *white dot* shows the left side of the lumbosacral specimen. Note that the left joint is more coronally oriented, while the right is more sagittally oriented. C = coronal plane; M = median (sagittal plane); L5 = lamina junction of the L5 vertebra; S = sacrum. (Reproduced with permission from Giles LGF: Lumbo-sacral zygapophyseal joint tropism and its effect on hyaline cartilage. *Clin Biomech* 2:2-6 1987. Copyright John Wright, Bristol.)

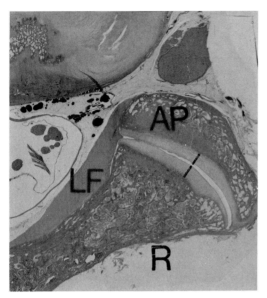

Figure A1.8. The center of the zygapophyseal joint. AP = superior articular process; LF = ligamentum flavum; R = right side.

Zygapophyseal Joint Cartilage—according to Hadley, this is of the hyaline articular cartilage variety and it lines the facet surfaces; extensions of cartilage beyond the facet surface, known as "bumper-fibrocartilage," are not composed of hyaline cartilage (11).

Zygapophyseal Joint Center—the center of each zygapophyseal joint, mid-way between the lateral and medial margins of the joint (see Fig. A1.8).

Zygapophyseal Midjoint Level—the level of the histologic section cut through the middle of the zygapophyseal joint in the horizontal plane.

References

1. Lewin T, Moffet B, Viidik A: The morphology of the lumbar synovial intervertebral joints. *Acta Morphol Neerl Scand* 4:299-319, 1961.
2. Hirsch C, Ingelmark BE, Miller M: The anatomical basis for low back pain. *Acta Orthop Scand* 33:1-17, 1963.
3. Cobb JR: Outline for the study of scoliosis. Instructional course lectures. *Am Acad Orthop Surg* 5:261-275, 1948.
4. Prasad P, King I, Denton RA, Begeman PC: Intervertebral force transducer. In: *Proceedings of the 10th International Conference of Medical Biological Engineers.* Dresden, Medical Biological Engineers, 1973, p 137.
5. Eichler J: Methodological errors in documenting leg length and leg length discrepancies. In Hungerford DS (ed): *Leg Length Discrepancy: The Injured Knee.* New York, Springer-Verlag, 1977, pp 29-39.
6. Schmorl G, Junghanns H: *The Human Spine in Health and Disease,* ed 2. New York, Grune and Stratton, 1971, p 37.
7. Davies DV, Davies F: *Gray's Anatomy. Descriptive and Applied,* ed 33. London, Longmans, Green, 1964, p xix.
8. Lloyd PT, Eimerbrink JH: Teaching materials. In: *Department of Osteopathic Principles and Practice.* Philadelphia, Philadelphia College of Osteopathic Medicine, 1952.
9. Weinstein PR, Ehni G, Wilson CB: Clinical features of lumbar spondylosis and stenosis. In Weinstein PR, Ehni G, Wilson CB (eds): *Lumbar Spondylosis, Diagnosis, Management and Surgical Treatment.* Chicago, Year Book medical Publishers 1977, pp 115-133.
10. Schafer RC: *Chiropractic Physical and Spinal Diagnosis.* Oklahoma City, Oklahoma Associated Chiropractic Academic Press, 1980.
11. Hadley LA: *Anatomico-Roentgenographic Studies of the Spine.* Springfield, IL, Charles C. Thomas, 1964, p 178, 183.
12. Giles LGF: Lumbo-sacral zygapophyseal joint tropism and its effect on hyaline cartilage. *Clin Biomech* 2:2-6, 1987.

APPENDIX 2

Preparation of Cadaveric Spinal Blocks of Tissue for Histology Sections

Method of Processing Spinal Segments

The original celloidin (C) embedding procedure (1, 2) has been largely replaced by a method using low-viscosity nitrocellulose (LVN) (3, 4) because of its relative freedom from shrinkage and fragmentation of tissue (5). The mixture of "LVNC" has been advocated by Disbrey and Rack (5) and Drury and Wallington (6). According to Disbrey and Rack (5), a small proportion of celloidin in the mixture gives flexibility to the LVN, which is otherwise inclined to produce a rather brittle block.

The fixation, decalcification, and embedding of large osseous structures for microtomy is a time-consuming procedure. The preparation of good-quality sections clearly depicting the osseous and adjacent soft tissue structures of large vertebral blocks is possible only by using time-consuming and careful methodology.

A variety of methods using araldite and LVNC and using different periods of time for each procedure were attempted, and finally a method giving good-quality sections was developed as follows:

The spinal blocks were fixed in embalming fluid (glycerine 2.14%, phenol 4.6%, formalin 12.4%, and water 80.72% with a resultant pH of 5) within 24–48 hours of death. The purpose of fixation is to preserve the tissue in as nearly a normal state as possible (7). The blocks were trimmed and then transferred to labeled 50-ml glass jars with secure screw top lids sealed by using Parafilm. They were then subjected to the following 4.8-month histologic processing technique, using an approximate specimen-to-solution volume of 1:5.

Solution A: 2 days
Correction of pH to enhance staining procedures.
Buffered formalin (pH 6.5–6.8) (1 change of solution after 24 hours).

Solution B: 1.5 days
Postfixation, in Heidenhain's (8) Susa fixative, to enhance staining differentiation for histologic purposes.

Solution C: 45 days
Decalcification of osseous structures using the following solutions: 15 parts distilled water, 10 parts formic acid, 4 parts formaldehyde solution. This solution was changed daily until the blocks were totally decalcified, as shown by the decalcification end-point test (9).

Solution D: 14 days
Dehydration in graded concentrations of ethanol and ethanol:diethyl ether as follows to enable the tissues to be embedded with water-immiscible substances:

70% ethanol	1 day
80% ethanol	1 day
95% ethanol (1 change)	2 days
100% ethanol (3 changes)	7 days
Ethanol:diethyl ether (ratio = 1:1)	3 days

Solution E: 81 days
Embedding in a mixture of

178

LVN (fibrous pieces damped with propan-1-ol; Gurr, Hopkin, and Williams, U.K.) and damped celloidin (celloidin wool moistened with butanol; Gurr, Hopkin, and Williams) (5).

Thin LVN and celloidin	9 days
Medium LVN and celloidin	12 days
Thick LVN and celloidin	approx. 60 days

Total	143.5 days

From the time of being immersed in buffered formalin to the end of the medium LVNC stage, the blocks were rotated constantly using electrically driven "Lortone" Gem Sparkle Rock Tumblers (model 33B-NR). These had been slowed down by means of an additional pulley system to 30 revolutions per minute (Fig. A2.1). The specimens were finally embedded, with the superior surface facing down, in flat-bottomed rectangular covered glass staining jars. The specimens were labeled by means of numbered, small, thin cardboard sections simultaneously embedded on the right side of each specimen. The glass staining jars were in turn placed in large closed desiccators. The glass jar lids were gradually opened in stages, over a number of days, to allow the solvents to evaporate *slowly,* so that air bubbles did not appear in the blocks. When the surface of the thick LVNC mixture had hardened enough to prevent sticking to a probe, open glass bottles of chloroform were placed in each desiccator to harden the blocks in the presence of chloroform vapor (10). The blocks were then trimmed to a suitable size and stored in 70% ethanol. As an additional check on orientation, the posterior right-hand corner of each block was cut off in the shape of a triangle (approximately 1 cm equilateral) so that the right-hand side of each section would be easily identifiable after sectioning of the block at the time of mounting.

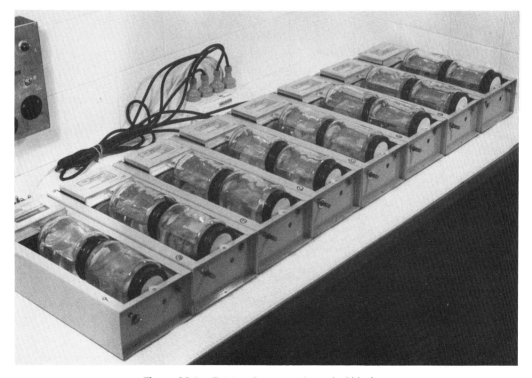

Figure A2.1. Rotators for processing spinal blocks.

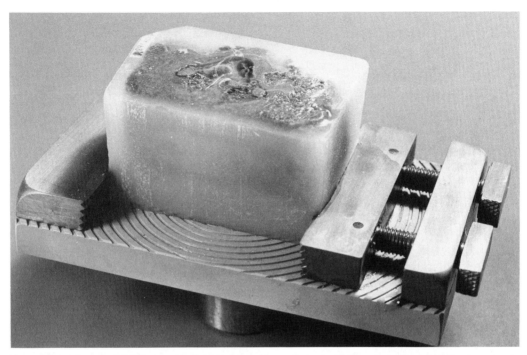

Figure A2.2. A labeled LVNC embedded block clamped in position on a 13.5-cm-long chuck. LVNC refers to a mixture of low-viscosity nitrocellulose and celloidin. (Reproduced with permission from Giles LGF, Taylor JR: Histological preparation of large vertebral specimens. *Stain Technol* 58(1):45-49, 1983. Copyright Williams & Wilkins, Baltimore.)

Sectioning of Embedded Blocks

The large processed blocks were mounted on a block holder (chuck) which was specially designed to hold the large blocks rigid during sectioning (Fig. A2.2).

The blocks were then sectioned horizontally at a thickness of 100 μm and vertically (sagittally) at a thickness of 100 μm, by means of a Jung Tetrander (model K) microtome, using a plano-concave knife (5) set at zero on the knife angle scale. An average number of 137 sections were obtained from each horizontal block, making a total of approximately 4658 sections from the 34 blocks.

The serial sections were numbered using interleaved pieces of paper and then stored in 70% ethanol prior to staining.

Staining and Mounting Procedure for Histologic Sections

The numbered sections were examined under a dissecting microscope for the appearance of the highest part of a joint on either the left or right side. To the first such section was allocated the number *1*, and each successive serial section was numbered in sequence from the superior to inferior dimensions of the joint. The same procedure was adopted for the joint on the opposite side of the spine. This procedure ensured that comparison of the left and right zygapophyseal joints and adjacent structures would relate to corresponding levels of the left and right joints.

The sections were then suspended from a glass rack by means of pieces of half-inch-wide white 3M "Scotch" tape (type 666, double coated) attached to the border of the LVNC mixture surrounding the right-hand side of each section, and each white tape was numbered to identify the section number (Fig. A2.3).

The glass rack was then used to transfer the sections through the following processing stages:

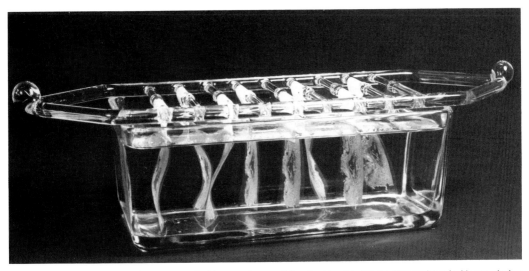

Figure A2.3.   Histologic sections suspended from a glass rack by double-sided tape. (Reproduced with permission from Giles LGF, Taylor JR: Histological preparation of large vertebral specimens. *Stain Technol* 58(1):45-49, 1983. Copyright Williams & Wilkins, Baltimore.)

1. The mercuric chloride crystals (deposited during postfixation in Susa solution) were removed by using 1.0% iodine in 70% alcohol   20 min
2. Distilled water   few dips
3. Removal of iodine color by "Hypo" (2.5% sodium thiosulphate in 50% ethanol)   5 min
4. Running distilled water   5 min
5. Retrogressive staining in Ehrlich's hematoxylin stain   3 min
6. Running distilled water   2 min
7. Differentiation in 0.1% hydrochloric acid in 50% ethanol (to differentiate overstaining with Ehrlich's hematoxylin)   3 min
8. Running distilled water   2 min
9. 0.1% light green stain in 50% ethanol to stain collagen fibers   ½ min
10. Running tap water to "blue" the section   10 min
11. 50% ethanol   overnight if necessary

Each numbered section was then removed from the glass rack and placed on a large horizontal glass slide and transferred by means of a staining "basket" through the following stages:

Dehydration in graded concentrations of ethanol.

75% ethanol	30 sec
95% ethanol (1 change)	½–1 min each
100% ethanol (2 changes)	½–1 min each

Clearing to replace the alcohol used in dehydrating the section by a colorless reagent or mixture of reagents miscible with the mounting medium and with a refractive index of approximately that of glass (7).

Carbolic xylene (6)	15 sec
Xylene (3 changes)	15 sec

Mounting, which consists of applying a colorless "cement" on the tissue to hold the slide, tissue, and cover slip together. The mounting medium provides a refractive index similar to that of glass, so that the specimen appears transparent (7).

Each section was placed on a clean glass slide and then liberally covered with DePex mounting medium before being covered wtih a cover slip. Any air bubbles were removed by carefully applying digital pressure, before using brass weights to maintain some pressure overnight. Care was taken to ensure that the right side of the tissue was on the right-hand side of the slide. Each slide was labeled showing the specimen number and the section number.

Method for Determining Specimen Shrinkage due to Histologic Preparation

A mounted section from the middle of each block was measured across its entire width at the level of the medial aspect of the left and right zygapophyseal joints for comparison with the superior-to-inferior x-ray image of the block.

References

1. Barrett JW: A new method of cutting sections for microscopic examination. *J Anat Physiol* 19:94-96, 1885.
2. Carleton HM, Drury RAB: *Histological Technique,* ed 3. Oxford, Oxford University Press, 1957, pp 47-50.
3. Chesterman W, Leach EH: Low viscosity nitrocellulose for embedding tissues. *Quarterly Journal of Microscopical Science* 90:431-434, 1949.
4. Gurt E: *A Practical Manual of Medical and Biological Staining Techniques.* London, Leonard Hill, 1950, pp 26-29.
5. Disbrey BD, Rack JH: *Histological Laboratory Methods.* Edinburgh, E.&S. Livingstone, 1970.
6. Drury RAB, Wallington EA: *Carleton's Histological Technique,* ed 4. New York, Oxford University Press, 1970.
7. Hopps HC: *Principles of Pathology,* ed 2. New York, Appleton-Century-Crofts, 1964, p 375.
8. Heidenhain M: Über neuere sublimatgemische. *Zeitschrift für Wissenschaftliche Mikroskopie und für Mikroskopische Technik* 33:232-234, 1916.
9. Smith A, Bruton J: *A Colour Atlas of Histological Staining Techniques.* London, Wolfe Medical Publications, 1977.
10. Walter F: *The Microtome: A Guide to Specimen Preparation and Section Cutting.* Wetzlar, Technisch-Paedagogischer Verlag, 1961.
11. Giles LGF, Taylor JR: Histological preparation of large vertebral specimens. *Stain Technol* 58:45-49, 1983.

APPENDIX 3

Preparation of Surgical Material for Histologic Investigations

Glutaraldehyde Fixation with Osmium Tetroxide Postfixation Studies

Fresh surgical specimens were processed as follows (with constant agitation at all stages using an IKA-Vibramax-VXR electronic specimen shaker):

- Immersion fixed in cold Karnovsky's (1) fixative which contained 2 mM calcium chloride in 0.1 M phosphate buffer (pH 7.4) to prevent formation of myelin figures (2–4): 30 min.
- Photographed as a whole mount.
- Sectioned into three parts (ligamentum flavum, posteromedial fibrous capsule, synovial fold).
- Dicing of each part into 2-mm "cubes" (while immersed in fixative). The three groups of "cubes" were kept separate during subsequent processing procedures.
- Stored in fresh fixative at 4° centigrade for 6–8 hours.
- Washed in cold 0.1 M phosphate buffer (pH 7.4), 2 changes: 30 min each.
- Postfixed in 1% osmium tetroxide in 0.1 M phosphate buffer (pH 7.4) at room temperature: 2 hours.
- Washed in 0.1 M phosphate buffer, 4 changes: 10 min each.
- Dehydrated in graded ethanols;
    50%—10 min,
    70%—10 min,
    90%—10 min,
    100%—2 changes: 30 min each.
  1,2-epoxypropane oxide:
    2 changes: 15 min each.
- Embedded in three stages in Epon/Araldite resin (Resin: Epon 812—10 g; Araldite "M"—10 g. Hardener: HY 964—

24 g. Accelerator: DMP 30, 964C DY064—0.4 g):
1. Diluted one part Epon/Araldite to 1 part 1,2-epoxypropane oxide: 4 hours.
2. Diluted 2 parts Epon/Araldite to 1 part 1,2-epoxypropane oxide: 30 min.
3. Undiluted Epon/Araldite: overnight.

The undiluted resin containing the specimen was put into a 60° centigrade vacuum (−102 kPa) for 1 hour before placing it in a labeled plastic mold. Each mold was left for 24 hours in a 60° centigrade oven to polymerize. Sections were cut from each block, at a thickness of 2 μm, on a Nova ultramicrotome, using a glass knife, and were then stained with 0.1% toluidine blue in 1% borax for examination by light microscopy using a Leitz Orthomat microscope. These sections were examined to check the histologic structures and orientation of each tissue block. The araldite block was then further trimmed and ultra-thin sections (silver to pale-yellow interference colors 60–90 nM (5) were cut. These sections were collected on copper grids (150 mesh size) and processed as follows:

- Dried over a hot plate at 60° centigrade.
- Stained in centrifuged 7% uranyl magnesium acetate (6): 15 min.
- Rinsed in double-distilled water: 20 sec.
- Air dried.
- Stained in lead citrate (7): 15 min.
- Washed in double-distilled water: 20 sec.
- Air dried.

Each ultra-thin section was examined by transmission electron microscopy using a

Philips EM 410 microscope, at an accelerating voltage of 60 kV. Areas of interest were photographed using Kodak Electron Image "Plates" and developed according to the method described by Kodak (Pamphlet No. P-116).

The methods of electron microscopy staining and viewing are given in detail since they differ in some respects from methods used for perfusion fixed tissues; e.g., in this study the lead citrate staining time is greater (approximately double) than that usually employed, and the kV for viewing the tissue is lower than usual.

Silver Impregnation Studies: Modified Schofield's Method

Fresh surgical specimens were processed as follows:

- All formalin solutions were made up with tap water.
- Immersion fixed in 10% buffered formalin: 30 min.
- Photographed as a whole mount.
- Sectioned into three parts (ligamentum flavum, posteromedial fibrous capsule, synovial fold).
- Each of the three parts was further subdivided into approximately 5-mm-thick "portions," which were processed separately, so that the tissue type was identifiable at all subsequent stages. The synovial fold, being relatively thin, was usually processed as one "portion."
- Stored in fresh fixative at 4° centigrade: minimum of 4 days.
- Washed in double-distilled water.
- Immersion in pyridine (A. S. Wilson, personal communication, 1986): 3 min.
- Washed in water: 5 min.
- Impregnated with silver (Schofield's method [8] modified by A. S. Wilson [personal communication, 1986][a] to include 2–3 grains of sodium chloride in all formalin solutions to minimize black artifact precipitation.

---

[a] silver nitrate aqueous solution + sodium chloride → silver chloride (white solid) + sodium nitrate

$$AgNO_3 + NaCl \rightarrow AgCl\downarrow + NaNO_3$$

From Holderness and Lambert (29).

1. 10% silver nitrate: 5–10 min.
2. Blotted dry.
3. Dipped in turn into:
   a. 10% formalin; 2 changes: 10 sec.
   b. 2% formalin; 2 changes: 10 sec.
   c. washed in double distilled water: 30 sec.
   d. blotted dry.
   e. 10% aqueous ammoniacal silver nitrate: 10–30 sec.
   f. blotted dry.
   g. 2% formalin until a gold brown color.
- Washed in tap water: 5 min.
- Fixed in 5% sodium thiosulphate solution, with constant agitation: 5 min.
- Washed in tap water.
- Stored in 2% formalin.
- Microscopic examination.

Each "portion" was examined as a whole mount by means of a Wild M400 photomacroscope. These small portions, which, in some cases showed silver-impregnated black structures (neural structures), were photographed and then resected. These included parts of the three separately processed portions: ligamentum flavum, posteromedial fibrous capsule, and adjacent synovial folds. The approximate position of each neural structure within each whole mount (as photographed) was known from the way in which each specimen was divided up into pieces. Where necessary, neural structures were teased in order to separate fibers to show their detailed anatomy. The resected tissue was then dehydrated in 50% aqueous ethyl alcohol (5 min), 70% ethyl alcohol (2 hours) 80% ethyl alcohol (2 hours), 95% oxitol (30 min), 100% oxitol (30 min), and 100% oxitol (1 hour). The tissue was partially cleared in oxitol:methylbenzoate (1:1) (30 min) and methylbenzoate:toluene (1:1) (30 min), then cleared in toluene (1 hour). Those resected parts in which the neural tissue was clearly defined were mounted in DePex and photographed using a Leitz Orthomat microscope for high-power light microscopy. Remaining pieces of tissue containing neural structures which could not be clearly seen in the whole mounts were embedded in Paraplast wax at 60° centigrade (a) for 30 min, (b) for 1 hour, and (c) under a vacuum for 30 min (10)

(−74.5 kPa), then blocked. Serial sections were cut at a thickness of 30 μm, then cleared in toluene (2 changes: 40 min) and mounted in Eukitt mounting medium for further examination and photography. From the 30-μm-thick serial sections of four silver-stained synovial folds, occasional sections were also counterstained with Verhoeff's hematoxylin (11) for general histologic examination of the synovium and subsynovial tissue.

Measurement of Stained Structures

The diameters of neural structures in whole mounts were carefully measured using a Wild M400 photomacroscope with a calibrated scale, in conjunction with a Leitz Mikrometer scale. The diameters of neural structures in the 30-μm-thick serial sections were accurately measured using a Leitz Mikrometer scale in conjunction with a calibrated eye piece graticule in a Leitz Orthomat microscope. Where necessary, a montage was made to show the course of neural structures through the inferior joint recess fibrous capsule and adjacent synovial folds.

Gold Chloride Impregnation Studies

Fresh surgical specimens were processed, as follows, using a modified Zinn and Morin (12) method:

- Immersion fixed in 1 part formic acid to 3 parts 0.001 M citric acid (dark bottle): 30 min.
- Photographed as a whole mount.
- Dark bottle and constant agitation for the following:
  - Washed in distilled water; 3 changes: 10 min.
  - Impregnated with 1% aqueous gold chloride (chloroauric acid/hydrogen tetrachloroaurate/trihydrate) solution: 30–45 min.
  - Washed in distilled water: 10 min.
  - Postfixed in 0.5% formic acid in distilled water: 20 hours.
  - Washed in distilled water; 3 changes: 10 min.
  - Cleared in glycerine: 24 hours.

Each specimen was photographed again as a whole mount, then teased out in a small petri dish containing fresh glycerine, while using the Wild photomacroscope. Small pieces were (a) mounted in glycerine on a glass slide with a cover slip and photographed at a known magnification using a Leitz Orthomat microscope, or (b) immersed in 70% ethanol (2 changes: 24 hours, with constant agitation), then 80% ethyl alcohol (2 hours), 95% oxitol (30 min); 100% oxitol (30 min); and 100% oxitol (1 hour). The tissue was partially cleared in oxitol:methylbenzoate (1:1) (30 min) and methylbenzoate:toluene (1:1) (30 min), then cleared in toluene (1 hour). Specimens from procedure "b" were then embedded in Paraplast wax at 60° centigrade (a) for 30 min, (b) for 1 hour, and (c) under a vacuum for 30 min (21) (−74.5 kPa), then blocked. Serial sections were cut at a thickness of 30 μm, then cleared in toluene (2 changes: 40 min) and mounted in Eukitt mounting medium for further examination and photography.

Measurement of Stained Structures

The diameters of neural structures were accurately measured using a Leitz Mikrometer scale in conjunction with the Leitz Orthomat microscope. Where necessary, a montage was made to show the course of neural structures through the inferior joint recess fibrous capsule and adjacent synovial folds.

Immunohistochemical Studies

Four specimens were processed for immunohistochemistry to substance P antibody to demonstrate any possible reaction sites between specific antigens and antibodies by conjugating antibodies with a fluorescent dye while leaving their capacity of combining with an antigen unchanged (10). The objective was to attempt to demonstrate the presence of substance P-immuno-fluorescent nerves in the zygapophyseal joint inferior recess capsule and its associated synovial folds.

The fresh surgical specimens were processed as follows:

- Immersion fixed in 3.5% ice-cold paraformaldehyde in phosphate-buffered saline (PBS) (13): 30 min.
- Photographed as a whole mount.

- Sectioned into three parts (ligamentum flavum, posteromedial fibrous capsule, synovial fold).
- Each part was subdivided into smaller portions of approximately 3 mm each. The three groups of portions were processed separately so that their "tissue origin" was known.
- Stored in fixative with constant agitation: 12 hours.
- Washed in PBS containing 0.05% thimerosal (methiolate) (PBST); 3 changes: 10 minutes.
- Embedded in optimum cutting temperature medium (OCT) and allowed to set at $-20°$ centigrade in an Ames cryostat: 20 min.

Sections were cut at a thickness of 80 μm, using a Leitz sledge microtome with a cold chuck and a "b" profile knife. Sections were placed in serially numbered compartments in covered Costar culture cluster trays containing PBST, and reacted wtih an ordered series of techniques, the solutions being changed by pipette. The immunohistochemistry was performed by first incubating the specimens in normal sheep serum in PBST (diluted 1:30) at room temperature for 1 hour, to diminish the background fluorescence (24). The specimens were then washed in PBST (10 min × 4 changes) then processed for immunohistochemical detection of substance-P antibody (24) using the primary antibody to substance P (raised in rabbits), and provided by Professor J. Polak, Hammersmith Hospital, London, the specificity of which has previously been confirmed (14). It was applied to the sections in a dilution of 1:400 and they were left in the dark, overnight, at room temperature. The specimens were washed in PBST (10 min × 3 changes), incubated with conjugated sheep anti-rabbit immunoglobulins coupled to fluorescein-isothyocyanate (FITC) (Wellcome Company, United Kingdom) (13), diluted in PBST 1:20, at room temperature for 2 hours, then washed in PBST (10 min × 3 changes).

Immunohistochemical control studies included processing with (*a*) omission of the substance P primary antibody and (*b*) in-cubation with anti-substance P (Sigma Inc., St. Louis, Missouri) (15), 0.014% in PBST.

The specimens were mounted on glass slides in a fluorescent free mounting medium—polyvinyl alcohol (M. Grounds, personal communication, 1986). The specimens were viewed by incident light fluorescence using the Leitz Orthomat microscope with appropriate excitation and barrier filters (the FITC specific barrier filter S525 allows only FITC-specific fluorescence to be observed [16]). Photographs of immunofluorescent structures were taken as soon as they were observed, using fast Agfachrome 1000 ASA 35-mm film, because some fresh FITC specimens can lose up to 75% of their initial fluorescent intensity within the first 10 seconds of excitation (16).

References

1. Karnovsky MJ: A formaldehyde-glutaraldehyde fixative of high osmolality for use in electron microscopy. *J Cell Biol* 27:441, 1965.
2. Baker JR: *Principles of Biological Microtechnique. A Study of Fixation and Dyeing.* London, Methuen, 1958, p 114.
3. Bullock GR, Christian RA, Peters RF, White AM: Rapid mitochondrial enlargement in muscle as a response to triamcinolone acetonide and its relationship to the ribosomal defect. *Biochem Pharmacol* 20:943-953, 1971.
4. Glauert AM: Fixation, dehydration and embedding of biological specimens. In Glauert AM (ed): *Practical Methods in Electron Microscopy.* Amsterdam, North-Holland, 1975, p 47.
5. Peachey LD: Thin sections. I. A study of section thickness and physical distortion produced during microtomy. *Journal of Biophysical and Biochemical Cytology* 4:233, 1958.
6. Gibbons IR, Grimstone AV: On flagellar structure in certain flagellates. *Journal of Biophysical and Biochemical Cytology* 7:697, 1960.
7. Fahmy A: An extemporaneous lead citrate stain for electron microscopy. *Proceedings of the 25th Annual Conference of Electron Microscopy Society of America.* 1967, p 148.
8. Schofield G: The peripheral nervous system. In *Carleton's Histological Technique,* ed 4. Drury RAB, Wallington EA (eds); Oxford, Oxford University Press, 1967, p 384.
9. Holderness A, Lambert J: *School Certificate Chemistry,* ed 4. London, Heinemann, 1954, p. 287.
10. Drury RAB, Wallington EA: *Carleton's Histological Technique,* ed 5. Oxford, Oxford University Press, 1980, p 110.
11. Verhoeff FH: Some new staining methods of wide applicability. Including a rapid differential stain of elastic tissue. *JAMA* 50:876, 1908.
12. Zinn DJ, Morin LP: The use of commercial citric juices in gold chloride staining of nerve endings. *Stain Technol* 37:380-382, 1962.
13. Gronblad M, Korkala O, Liesi P, Karaharju E: Inner-

vation of synovial membrane and meniscus. *Acta Orthop Scand* 56:484-486, 1985.

14. Wharton J, Polak JM, Bloom SR, Will JA, Brown MR, Pearce AGE: Substance P-like immunoreactive nerves in mammalian lung. *Invest Cell Pathol* 2:3, 1979.

15. Korkala O, Gronblad M, Liesi P, Karaharju E: Im-

munohistochemical demonstration of nociceptors in the ligamentous structures of the lumbar spine. *Spine* 10:156-157, 1985.

16. Birk G: *Instrumentation and Techniques for Fluorescence Microscopy.* Sydney, Wild Leitz (Australia), 1984, pp 51, 71.

INDEX

Page numbers in **bold** denote Appendix figures